TRANSDIAGNOSTIC TREATMENTS FOR CHILDREN AND ADOLESCENTS

Transdiagnostic Treatments for Children and Adolescents

PRINCIPLES AND PRACTICE

Edited by

Jill Ehrenreich-May
Brian C. Chu

THE GUILFORD PRESS
New York   London

© 2014 The Guilford Press
A Division of Guilford Publications, Inc.
72 Spring Street, New York, NY 10012
www.guilford.com

Printed in the United States of America

This book is printed on acid-free paper.

Last digit is print number: 9   8   7   6   5   4   3   2   1

The authors have checked with sources believed to be reliable in their efforts to
provide information that is complete and generally in accord with the standards
of practice that are accepted at the time of publication. However, in view of the
possibility of human error or changes in behavioral, mental health, or medical
sciences, neither the authors, nor the editors and publisher, nor any other party
who has been involved in the preparation or publication of this work warrants
that the information contained herein is in every respect accurate or complete,
and they are not responsible for any errors or omissions or the results obtained
from the use of such information. Readers are encouraged to confirm the
information contained in this book with other sources.

Library of Congress Cataloging-in-Publication Data

Transdiagnostic treatments for children and adolescents : principles and
practice / edited by Jill Ehrenreich-May, Brian C. Chu.
    pages cm
Includes bibliographical references and index.
ISBN 978-1-4625-1266-9 (hardcover)
1. Clinical child psychology.   2. Child psychopathology.   3. Adolescent
psychopathology.   I. Ehrenreich-May, Jill, editor of compilation.   II. Chu,
Brian C., editor of compilation.
    RJ503.3C58 2014
    618.92′89—dc23
                                                        2013019532

About the Editors

Jill Ehrenreich-May, PhD, is Director of the Child and Adolescent Mood and Anxiety Treatment Program at the University of Miami, where she is also Associate Professor in the Child Division of the Department of Psychology. She previously was Research Assistant Professor of Psychology and Associate Director of the Child Program in the Center for Anxiety and Related Disorders at Boston University. Dr. Ehrenreich-May's research and clinical work focus on evidence-based treatment of anxiety and depression in youth. She is particularly interested in the transportability and implementation of effective treatments in environments that maximize their impact and benefit for children, including educational, pediatric, and recreational settings. She is author or coauthor of multiple journal articles, book chapters, and other publications.

Brian C. Chu, PhD, is Associate Professor and Assistant Chair of the Department of Clinical Psychology in the Graduate School of Applied and Professional Psychology at Rutgers, The State University of New Jersey. He is a recipient of the Klingenstein Third Generation Foundation Young Investigator Award to support the development of transdiagnostic behavioral activation programs in middle schools. Dr. Chu is Associate Editor of *Cognitive and Behavioral Practice* and serves on the editorial boards of *Behaviour Research and Therapy* and *Journal of Clinical Child and Adolescent Psychology*. His interests include the assessment and treatment of anxiety and depressive disorders in youth, with a special emphasis on the dissemination of evidence-based practices, effectiveness research, and the evaluation of mechanisms of change and within-session therapy processes.

Contributors

Kimberly A. Arditte, MS, Department of Psychology, University of Miami, Coral Gables, Florida

Kelly Banneyer, BA, Department of Educational Psychology, University of Texas at Austin, Austin, Texas

Jessica S. Benas, PhD, Graduate School of Applied and Professional Psychology, Rutgers, The State University of New Jersey, Piscataway, New Jersey

Emily L. Bilek, MS, Department of Psychology, University of Miami, Coral Gables, Florida

Kirstin B. Birtwell, MA, Department of Psychology, Suffolk University, Boston, Massachusetts

Caroline L. Boxmeyer, PhD, Department of Psychiatry and Behavioral Medicine, University of Alabama, Tuscaloosa, Alabama

Brian C. Chu, PhD, Graduate School of Applied and Professional Psychology, Rutgers, The State University of New Jersey, Piscataway, New Jersey

Bruce E. Compas, PhD, Department of Psychology and Human Development, Peabody College, Vanderbilt University, Nashville, Tennessee

Lisa W. Coyne, PhD, Department of Psychology, Suffolk University, Boston, Massachusetts

Thomas J. Dishion, PhD, Child and Family Center, University of Oregon, Eugene, Oregon; Prevention Research Center, Arizona State University, Tempe, Arizona

Jennifer P. Dunbar, MS, Department of Psychology and Human Development, Vanderbilt University, Nashville, Tennessee

Jill Ehrenreich-May, PhD, Department of Psychology, University of Miami, Coral Gables, Florida

B. Heidi Ellis, PhD, Department of Psychiatry, Children's Hospital, Harvard University, Boston, Massachusetts

Haley L. Ford, PhD, Department of Psychology, University of Alabama, Tuscaloosa, Alabama

Maria G Fraire, MS, Department of Psychology, Virginia Polytechnic Institute and State University, Blacksburg, Virginia

Allison G. Harvey, PhD, Department of Psychology, University of California, Berkeley, Berkeley, California

Jutta Joormann, PhD, Department of Psychology, Northwestern University, Evanston, Illinois

Philip C. Kendall, PhD, ABPP, Department of Psychology, Temple University, Philadelphia, Pennsylvania

Annette M. La Greca, PhD, ABPP, Department of Psychology, University of Miami, Coral Gables, Florida

Betty S. Lai, PhD, Departments of Pediatrics and Psychology, University of Miami, Coral Gables, Florida

Daniel Le Grange, PhD, Department of Psychiatry and Behavioral Neuroscience, University of Chicago, Chicago, Illinois

John E. Lochman, PhD, ABPP, Department of Psychology, University of Alabama, Tuscaloosa, Alabama

Katharine L. Loeb, PhD, School of Psychology, Fairleigh Dickinson University, Teaneck, New Jersey

Kristen K. Marciel, PhD, Marcus Autism Center, Atlanta, Georgia

Kristin D. Martinsen, Cand. Psychol., Centre for Child and Adolescent Mental Health, Oslo, Norway

Louise McHugh, PhD, Department of Psychology, School of Human and Health Sciences, Swansea University, Wales, United Kingdom

Alec L. Miller, PsyD, Department of Psychiatry and Behavioral Sciences, Montefiore Medical Center/Albert Einstein College of Medicine, Bronx, New York

Jessica A. Minney, MA, Department of Psychology, University of Alabama, Tuscaloosa, Alabama

Laura Mufson, PhD, Department of Psychiatry, Columbia University College of Physicians and Surgeons and New York State Psychiatric Institute, New York, New York

Thomas H. Ollendick, PhD, Department of Psychology, Virginia Polytechnic Institute and State University, Blacksburg, Virginia

Laura A. Payne, PhD, Pediatric Pain Program, Department of Pediatrics, David Geffen School of Medicine, University of California, Los Angeles, Los Angeles, California

Nicole P. Powell, PhD, Department of Psychology, University of Alabama, Tuscaloosa, Alabama

Alexander H. Queen, MS, Department of Psychology, University of Miami, Coral Gables, Florida

Michelle M. Reising, PhD, Department of Child and Adolescent Psychiatry, Ann & Robert H. Lurie Children's Hospital of Chicago, Chicago, Illinois

Cara S. Remmes, MS, Department of Psychology, University of Miami, Coral Gables, Florida

Lorie A. Ritschel, PhD, Department of Psychiatry and Behavioral Sciences, Emory University School of Medicine, Atlanta, Georgia

Kelly A. O'Neil Rodriguez, PhD, Department of Psychology, Temple University, Philadelphia, Pennsylvania

Glenn N. Saxe, MD, Department of Child and Adolescent Psychiatry, New York University School of Medicine, New York, New York

Sonja K. Schoenwald, PhD, Department of Psychiatry and Behavioral Sciences, Medical University of South Carolina, Charleston, South Carolina

Laura C. Skriner, MA, Department of Psychology, Rutgers, The State University of New Jersey, Piscataway, New Jersey

Justin D. Smith, PhD, Child and Family Center, University of Oregon, Eugene, Oregon; Prevention Research Center, Arizona State University, Tempe, Arizona

Susan H. Spence, PhD, Griffith University, Southport, Queensland, Australia

Alison M. Staples, MS, Department of Psychology, Rutgers, The State University of New Jersey, Piscataway, New Jersey

Kevin D. Stark, PhD, Department of Educational Psychology, University of Texas at Austin, Austin, Texas

Liza M. Suárez, PhD, Institute for Juvenile Research, Department of Psychiatry, University of Illinois at Chicago, Chicago, Illinois

Victoria Taylor, MS, Department of Psychiatry and Behavioral Sciences, Montefiore Medical Center/Albert Einstein College of Medicine, Bronx, New York

Jennie C. I. Tsao, PhD, Pediatric Pain Program, Department of Pediatrics, David Geffen School of Medicine, University of California, Los Angeles, Los Angeles, California

Marianne A. Villabø, PhD, Center for Child and Adolescent Mental Health, Oslo, Norway

Kelly H. Watson, MS, Department of Psychology and Human Development, Vanderbilt University, Nashville, Tennessee

Kelly G. Wilson, PhD, Department of Psychology, University of Mississippi, University, Mississippi

Jami F. Young, PhD, Graduate School of Applied and Professional Psychology, Rutgers, The State University of New Jersey, Piscataway, New Jersey

Lonnie K. Zeltzer, MD, Pediatric Pain Program, Department of Pediatrics, David Geffen School of Medicine, University of California, Los Angeles, Los Angeles, California

Contents

Part III. Transdiagnostic Conceptualizations of Traditional Individual Therapies for Youth

Part IV. Transdiagnostic Treatment Approaches

Part V. Conclusions and Future Directions

TRANSDIAGNOSTIC TREATMENTS
FOR CHILDREN AND ADOLESCENTS

PART I

Introduction

CHAPTER 1

Overview of Transdiagnostic Mechanisms and Treatments for Youth Psychopathology

Jill Ehrenreich-May and Brian C. Chu

Whether in reference to treatment or mechanisms of such, the word *transdiagnostic* seems to evoke a mix of excitement and confusion wherever it is used. Owing to these dueling reactions, we have undertaken this book in an attempt to foster a broader conceptual understanding of potential transdiagnostic mechanisms and treatment approaches for youth and bridge any confusion about what such mechanisms and treatments might look like, why they are relevant at this point in our evolution in clinical child psychology, and what research agenda lies ahead to better understand the long-term implications of transdiagnostic approaches.

Transdiagnostic treatments have certainly been gaining support in the adult literature as efficient and effective approaches to understanding multiple problems within a single conceptual framework (e.g., Barlow, Allen, & Choate, 2004; Fairburn, Cooper, & Shafran, 2003; Harvey, Watkins, Mansell, & Shafran, 2004). A good transdiagnostic approach draws from a unifying theoretical model that explains disparate conditions via common mechanisms. Its treatment strategies are also flexible enough to accommodate diverse problems. Much of the interest in transdiagnostic treatments grows from the vast levels of comorbidity seen in clinical populations, necessitating treatment approaches that reduce redundancies and target the key mechanisms of pathology. In child and adolescent populations, the call for transdiagnostic approaches is even more relevant.

High comorbidity rates, shifting symptom profiles, and complex family contexts all complicate the typical treatment approach.

In many ways, the genesis of the transdiagnostic movement harkens back to the historical argument regarding whether psychopathology should be considered in broader, often dimensional terms or within more discrete, easily definable categories. In other words, decisions about how to classify psychiatric disorders have long been mired in a tension between efforts to either "lump" or "split" clinical problems to best understand them (Mayr, 1982; Taylor & Clark, 2009). As recently reviewed by Taylor and Clark (2009), efforts to lump psychological disorders together call for a small set of broad categories. Such efforts search for universal or common cognitive, emotional, physiological, or interpersonal processes that unify or explain varied clinical phenomena. In many ways, this broader view is also particularly consistent with empirical conceptualizations of youth disorders (e.g., Achenbach, 2005). In contrast, "splitters" prefer a finely sliced taxonomy in which broad concepts such as neurosis are carved into many different disorders. In many ways, endeavors to promote a more transdiagnostic paradigm certainly evolved from a "lumping" mentality, with the fundamental assumption that common processes across disorders imply the possibility of creating broader treatment paradigms.

Such broader treatment paradigms form another primary motivation for the study of transdiagnostic mechanisms and treatments. From the earliest discussions of such an approach, the thought of enhancing the availability of evidence-based treatment principles to the larger community of treatment providers and youth in need of such services has remained a core motivation for this work. Youth treatments have a long tradition of considering broader categories of disorder, although more rarely they cross thresholds between such categories. For instance, in the child anxiety treatment literature, the most common cognitive-behavioral approaches are studied among children with one or any combination of three or four primary anxiety disorders (e.g., separation anxiety disorder, social phobia, generalized anxiety disorder, and sometimes specific phobia), but typically excluded are those with commonly co-occurring conditions such as depressive disorders or pervasive developmental disorders. Admittedly, this is a more advanced state for potential dissemination of evidence-based practices than in the adult treatment literature, in which the norm is to focus more precisely on individual categories of disorder. The dissemination-focused rationale for transdiagnostic approaches in youth suggests that there is yet potential for greater clinician adherence to evidence-based principles should these principles be flexible enough in their application to handle greater variability in caseloads—such as the adolescent with both anxiety and depression, the child with attention-deficit/hyperactivity disorder (ADHD) who has become worried and anxious about her school performance, and so on. Moreover, such approaches may minimize clinician training burden and family treatment time, especially to the degree to which they are focused on straightforward, common mechanisms of change.

Overall, taking a transdiagnostic approach promises benefits to basic science, theory, and clinical practice. Given the decades-long effort to discriminate psychological disorders along observable symptom criteria, a return to basic mechanisms might allow a more refined understanding of the mechanistic commonalities and distinctions among symptom-based syndromes. Psychological treatments that take a transdiagnostic approach have the potential to more efficiently address multiple clinical problems with core techniques and to have more robust, generalizable outcomes by targeting core processes. Together, basic science and treatment will inform theories that focus on the necessary and sufficient components to explain diverse pathologies and their treatments.

In this book, we divide our discussion of youth transdiagnostic theory and research into three broad sections: *basic processes, application of transdiagnostic work to broad theoretical orientations*, and *exemplar treatments*. Before delving further into these varied sections, let's take a step back and consider the terminology used in this book when discussing a transdiagnostic approach.

Transdiagnostic Mechanisms

When considering transdiagnostic mechanisms and treatment, it is critical to consider the level of analysis. In the context of understanding psychopathology, a "transdiagnostic" process can refer to intrapersonal cognitive, behavioral, emotional, and physiological processes. Each of these levels can be divided into smaller levels. Cognitive processes can include attention, memory, and interpretation processes. Emotional processes can include emotional activity, reactivity, and regulation processes. Interpersonally, "transdiagnostic" can refer to peer-to-peer dyad relationships, parent–child relations, and family systems, to name a few. Community processes can involve school climate, neighborhood resources, broader cultural influences, and sociopolitical policies. The unifying theme that underlies each transdiagnostic process is the extent to which any process under investigation can be used to understand a set of related, but distinguishable, phenomena. The target under study can be antisocial behavior, anxiety disorders, academic achievement, or community orientation. If a process can explain some aspect of the onset, development, or maintenance of each target problem, then the process has merit as a transdiagnostic mechanism.

Such discussion raises the question: Can any process be transdiagnostic? Again, the level of analysis is key. If we overgeneralize, we run a risk of being overly inclusive. It might be easy to say that *everything* is caused by multiple factors, and, indeed, many distinguishable problems have at their root several similar if not common factors. For instance, any investigation that leads to the conclusion that "genetics causes everything" would be undesirable. Although true in some general sense, the lack of precision makes such a global statement of little value. This statement provides little information about what type of genetic coding leads to what kind of pathology under what circumstances. And under what circumstances does pathology A differ from pathology B? Under what circumstances are they similar? For this reason, we define a transdiagnostic process as striking the balance between lumping and splitting and seek results that balance explanatory power with parsimony. As a shorthand, to be transdiagnostic, we would expect (1) that any candidate mechanism provide explanatory power in understanding the onset, development, or maintenance of target condition A and target condition B but also (2) that the candidate mechanism provide some kind of unique explanatory power in target conditions A and B that could not be understood through the study of A and B alone.

Naturally, such criteria only provide a conceptual starting point. We recognize the methodological and statistical challenges in achieving such clarity; the methods may not currently exist to satisfy these criteria completely. Still, others have suggested similar approaches. Compas and colleagues (Chapter 3) illustrate three models that are compatible with our recommendation. Model 1 encourages a research agenda that studies how multiple processes relate to the onset or maintenance of a single disorder. Model 2 examines one of the candidate processes in relation to multiple disorders. In Model 3, multiple processes are examined simultaneously in relation to multiple disorders or problem sets. The first two models provide circumstantial evidence for transdiagnostic mechanisms; the third approach permits one to compare the relative strength among candidate mechanisms in their relation to multiple disorders. Mansell, Harvey, Watkins, and Shafran (2009) succinctly refer to this as a *universal, multiple-process* approach that can yield comparative evidence for a single or multiple mechanisms that have universal influence across disorders. Such an approach can be used for diagnostic disorders or symptom-based problem sets, and candidates can be derived from a single therapeutic conceptual model (e.g., cognitive-behavioral therapy) or from multiple theoretical reference points. Nevertheless, the goals of each approach are identical: Transdiagnostic science aims to identify the smallest number of key mechanisms that hold the most explanatory power in understanding psychological disorders.

Transdiagnostic Treatments

Science and theory come together to inform transdiagnostic treatment. The original unifying treatment for anxiety and mood disorders originated in attempts to reconcile the converging evidence linking anxiety and mood disorders (Barlow et al., 2004). The original transdiagnostic treatment for eating disorders (Fairburn et al., 2003) sought to develop a more potent treatment package that addressed "core pathology" across eating disorders. Each treatment approach made use of basic science to inform theory and develop a flexible but robust set of interventions that targeted core mechanisms. In Barlow and colleagues' (2004) unified treatment, poor emotion regulation, behavioral and emotional avoidance, and maladaptive cognitive appraisal processes were targeted for treatment. Over time, Barlow and colleagues (2010) broadened their discussion of unifying core processes to include increasing flexibility in one's thinking and facilitating emotion awareness, particularly awareness of emotions in context. Fairburn and colleagues (2003) identified clinical perfectionism, core low self-esteem, mood intolerance, and interpersonal difficulties as core maintaining mechanisms across bulimia and anorexia nervosa. What should be evident is that, to date, transdiagnostic treatment still focuses on a relatively narrow band of disorders (anxiety/mood and eating disorders), but the focus on core maintaining mechanisms is believed to enhance therapeutic flexibility and effectiveness. At the same time, there are some similarities in the core processes targeted in each (e.g., emotional avoidance, mood intolerance) that have the potential to universally apply across disorders and treatments.

When evaluating transdiagnostic treatments, one should be mindful that multiple levels of analysis exist, too. Transdiagnostic treatment processes can refer to the dysfunctional mechanisms targeted by a treatment, the core therapeutic strategies that are used to intervene, or therapeutic process strategies that underlie the therapeutic endeavor. As discussed earlier, targeted mechanisms can be intra- or interpersonal processes, and therapeutic strategies can be at the level of individual (e.g., cognitive, behavioral), dyad (e.g., communication analysis), family, or community (e.g., multisystemic therapy). The therapeutic process adds an additional level of analysis—therapy-specific interpersonal processes. When a child, adolescent, or family initiates therapy, yet another set of processes is added to consider. These include processes specific to the client: child and family insight, motivation, and expectations for treatment; processes specific to the therapist (background, skill level, education, therapist flexibility and responsiveness); processes specific to the therapy (recommended therapeutic posture, level of structure, goal directedness); and processes specific to client–therapist interactions (therapeutic relationship and alliance). Thus transdiagnostic therapies may be based on the common set of interventions used across disorders (e.g., problem solving, exposure) or to the intratherapy processes that are espoused (e.g., structured goal setting, working alliance). Some examples of universal therapy process are described in Chapter 8 by Kendall and colleagues.

Has DSM-5 Spoiled Everything?

As we write, the American Psychiatric Association (APA) has just completed its decade-long mission of revising and releasing the fifth edition of the *Diagnostic and Statistical Manual of Mental Disorders* (DSM-5; APA, 2013a). Although a number of radical ideas were considered along the way, diagnostic categories remain largely intact and the criteria required for diagnosis remain relatively identical for most disorders (APA, 2013b; Kupfer, Kuhl, & Regier, 2013). There was some reshuffling, such that all autism spectrum disorders were combined under a single diagnosis; posttraumatic stress disorder and other trauma-related disorders received their own chapter instead of falling under the category of anxiety disorders; and obsessive–compulsive disorder has been grouped with other compulsive behaviors instead of with anxiety. However, radical proposals to incorporate a substantial dimensional diagnostic component were not realized (Kraemer, 2007). Instead, each diagnostic category provides indicators or examples of dimensional severity for certain symptoms (Kupfer et al., 2013). These may be common "cross-cutting" features that appear across disorders, such as suicide risk and anxiety, or they may describe dimensional severity of particular symptoms within a disorder, such as the frequency of panic attacks in panic disorder. In so doing, DSM-5 appears to embrace many of the same principles that distinguish transdiagnostic research. It retains a value in conceptualizing distinct disorders while also promoting the research and treatment of symptoms that cross diagnostic boundaries. Likewise, DSM-5 eliminated the DSM-IV-TR (APA, 2000) chapter, "Disorders Usually First Diagnosed in Infancy, Childhood, or Adolescence," and, instead, incorporated aspects of early-onset and developmental factors to each disorder.

The reader of the current volume will notice that many of the dimensional and developmental features championed by transdiagnostic researchers are reflected in, and supported by, the new DSM-5. Still, it is important to note that a transdiagnostic approach to research and treatment transcends individual classification systems. The term *transdiagnosis* implies a grounding in the study of diagnoses, but we cannot emphasize enough the primary focus on the underlying mechanisms and processes. Even without specific diagnoses (certainly as they are currently defined), the study of those underlying processes and mechanisms would still persevere.

Overview of Chapters in This Book

This volume presents current knowledge across the three aforementioned dimensions of transdiagnostic research: transdiagnostic mechanisms, theory, and treatment. Following this overview chapter, Harvey (Chapter 2) provides an overview of the impetus, benefits, and challenges confronting transdiagnostic research and treatment. In particular, she presents the case for the unique challenges and opportunities for transdiagnostic research in child and adolescent populations. Taking a developmental framework, Harvey suggests that a transdiagnostic approach may be uniquely suited to account for developmental differences in typical and atypical development (which may be easier to achieve by considering dimensional constructs), the presence of multiple reporters, and the high rate of comorbidity. She points to a number of general advantages of taking a transdiagnostic approach, including rapid transfer of treatment breakthroughs, an increased attention to basic science in developing our treatments, and an integration of our disciplines.

Part II highlights research on basic intra- and interpersonal processes that influence the development and maintenance of psycho-emotional-behavioral problems across disorder classes. Authors took care to explain how basic mechanisms account for problem development within a transdiagnostic framework. Authors were asked to (1) define their basic process of interest, (2) describe what makes this process transdiagnostic, (3) review the empirical literature describing the relation of the process to multiple diagnostic classes, problem sets, or clinical profiles in youth, and (4) outline future directions for continued research within a transdiagnostic framework.

Compas, Watson, Reising, and Dunbar (Chapter 3) use a developmental framework to explore how stress, coping, and emotion regulations serve as transdiagnostic risk factors to explain diagnostic co-occurrence. They present research on exposure to stressful events and chronic adversity as transdiagnostic sources of risk and the ways that children and adolescents regulate their emotions and cope with stress as transdiagnostic protective factors. Using terms familiar to the developmental psychopathology literature (e.g., *multifinality, equifinality*), they encourage a new way of envisioning transdiagnostic work, including an emphasis on developmental trajectories and multiple causality.

Arditte and Joormann (Chapter 4) review the literature on cognitive processes and the critical roles they play in the experience and regulation of emotion. They distinguish between the multiple levels of cognition (attention, memory, interpretation) and illustrate how each level of cognitive process may universally or distinctively contribute to the onset and maintenance of mood and anxiety disorders.

Chu, Skriner, and Staples (Chapter 5) review evidence for the mechanistic role of behavioral avoidance in promoting and maintaining psychological distress across four major youth diagnostic classes (anxiety, depression, conduct, and impulse disorders). Although research on avoidance predominantly centers on anxiety and mood disorders, the authors make the case that avoidance may play a critical role in maintaining disruptive disorders (e.g., ADHD, oppositional defiant disorder [ODD]), too. Their model proposes that avoidance serves different functions depending on when it manifests itself in the sequence of pathological events.

La Greca and Lai (Chapter 6) provide a comprehensive review of peer relations and interpersonal stressors as transdiagnostic processes. Peer rejection and victimization can serve as universal risk factors for multiple forms of future disorders, and peer acceptance and close friendships can serve as protective factors. This developmental perspective on risk and protective factors creates a road map for examining initial development of problem behavior and also provides direct targets for treatment intervention.

Smith and Dishion (Chapter 7) focus their review on how parent–child interactions might interact with youth problem behavior. The authors make a specific case for mindful parenting as an antidote to the coercive cycle that often builds conflict in the home. They review the evidence for mindful parenting factors, such as positive behavior support, healthy limit setting, and family relationship building, as a universal mechanism for supporting healthy family functioning.

Part III offers a reexamination of traditional therapy models and theories within a transdiagnostic framework. In each chapter, the authors describe how a focus on common processes that underlie disparate diagnostic classes can offer unique insight into client problems and contribute to innovative treatment applications. Authors were asked (1) to describe the "traditional" version of the treatment model, (2) to discuss whether the treatment model was initially designed to be transdiagnostic, and if not, (3) to say what aspects of the treatment merit consideration as a transdiagnostic approach, (4) to review effectiveness data for the treatment model across multiple disorders, and (5) to describe the limits and future directions of the treatment model in transdiagnostic use. Four groups of experts across four major treatment modalities weighed in on this topic.

Kendall, O'Neil, Villabø, Martinsen, Stark, and Banneyer (Chapter 8) review the history and evidence for cognitive-behavioral therapy (CBT) as an integrative treatment model that has broad applicability across numerous disorders. Despite the fact that most evaluations of CBT have been applied to specific identified disorders, the authors make the case that CBT is designed to have broad applicability: the basis of the model is a diathesis–stress model, intervention packages for specific disorders share many common interventions, and aspects of the therapeutic structure are transdiagnostic (therapeutic posture, directiveness, goal orientation).

Young, Mufson, and Benas (Chapter 9) build the case that interpersonal therapy for adolescents (IPT-A) has great promise as a transdiagnostic treatment because the treatment focuses on the universal process of interpersonal relationships. Problems arise and are perpetuated by problematic patterns in interpersonal interactions, whereas quality relations can buffer against problems such as depression and anxiety. The authors review the basic relational mechanisms that explain the onset of mood and anxiety disorders, the critical therapeutic techniques that could be effective across disorder sets, and the outcomes that one would expect to see change.

Dialectical behavior therapy (DBT) was a trendsetter in multiproblem treatments. Ritschel, Miller, and Taylor (Chapter 10) describe how DBT was developed as a principles-based treatment to address the severe and complex presenting problems associated with suicidal behavior and borderline personality disorder. Since its initial development, DBT has been adapted and used for other clinical populations, but because DBT simultaneously drew from multiple theories and implemented diverse therapeutic strategies, it set itself up uniquely as a potential transdiagnostic intervention. In particular, DBT addresses several core mechanisms common to many disorders, including emotion dysregulation, distress tolerance, mindful awareness, social effectiveness, and balanced family interactions.

Coyne, Birtwell, McHugh, and Wilson (Chapter 11) make the case that acceptance and commitment therapy (ACT) is also uniquely suited as a transdiagnostic therapy because it is concerned not with the elimination of syndromes but rather with building broad, flexible behavioral repertoires. Rather than focusing on symptom reduction, ACT promotes acceptance of aversive private experiences in the service of commitment to freely chosen values. Their mechanism of choice is the broader "functional context" of language and behaviors in human experience. To the extent that one can change how one relates to his or her own thoughts, feelings, and actions (i.e., change the relational frame), one can learn to tolerate emotional barriers that interfere with quality living. To the extent that this process is universal to any kind of suffering, this treatment model is inherently transdiagnostic.

Part IV spotlights exemplar treatment protocols that have applied transdiagnostic therapy across diverse clinical settings and client populations. Authors describe the theory underlying their respective approaches, highlight the universal processes that are targeted in the treatment protocol, and report empirical evidence supporting the therapy. Authors were asked to (1) describe the targeted clinical population and treatment intervention, (2) illustrate what makes the treatment explicitly transdiagnostic, (3) discuss distinct developmental considerations in the development or delivery of the treatment, and (4) review the available empirical evidence for the treatment. As this area represents a large domain of future growth, these chapters also highlight future directions in treatment development.

Ehrenreich-May, Queen, Bilek, Remmes, and Marciel (Chapter 12) describe the rationale and subsequent development of two unified protocols, for children and for adolescents, respectively. These protocols follow solidly from the theoretical principles first outlined by Barlow and colleagues (2004; Barlow et al., 2010) in their descriptions of a unified approach to "emotional disorders" but also reflect a lengthy process of iterative treatment development to tailor such work for youth. The protocols are described in detail and, although only open trial and case series results have been published to date, randomized controlled trials (RCTs) of the adolescent (UP-A) and child (UP-C: Emotion Detectives) protocols are nearing completion. These RCT data are viewed as a needed next step to supporting the feasibility and comparative utility of transdiagnostic treatments for anxiety and depressive disorders in youth.

Following this, a fascinating chapter by Lochman, Powell, Boxmeyer, Ford, and Minney (Chapter 13) details the evolution of a treatment, Coping Power, that truly targets a singular mechanism, anger and its regulation, and suggests far-reaching implications for its utility as a transdiagnostic approach. Lochman and colleagues make the case that Coping Power is flexible and comprehensive enough in its structure to accommodate a number of co-occurring problems, beyond the disruptive behavior concerns alone that the intervention was originally designed to influence. Lochman and colleagues illustrate this point throughout their discussion of Coping Power's components, pointedly tying its processes and strategies to their impact on related behavioral and emotional domains.

Much like DBT, multisystemic therapy (MST) is a comprehensive approach somewhat born of the necessity that a highly impaired population, in this case juvenile offenders, requires a variety of flexible and overlapping intervention strategies, guided by an overarching theoretical and systemic view. Helpfully distinguishing the related classes of transdiagnostic, modular, and principle-based interventions for the reader, Schoenwald (Chapter 14) does a masterful job of describing MST as a "principle-based, measurement-based, and flexible" intervention that guides case conceptualization and treatment selection for a variety of target populations. Schoenwald further illustrates how MST provides guidance when a population is sufficiently novel to warrant the inclusion of additional techniques and gives examples of such extensions.

Suárez, Ellis, and Saxe (Chapter 15) provide an example of a treatment, trauma systems therapy for adolescent substance abuse (TST-SA), that started with an existing treatment complexity—youth trauma and its aftermath—then extended its reach to be inclusive of a commonly comorbid problem area, adolescent substance abuse. Rather than simply adding new treatment components to address a related concern, Suárez and colleagues describe how their approach views both youth trauma and substance abuse singularly as "dysregulated emotional and behavioral states that occur in the context of a potentially unstable, and at times threatening, environment" and uses central principles of change to address these challenging problems.

Looking through the lens of eating disorders in youth, Le Grange and Loeb (Chapter 16) then describe how individual eating disorders are fundamentally intertwined with one another, both in terms of current symptom presentations and over the longitudinal course of illness. Although it was originally designed for treatment of anorexia nervosa, Le Grange and Loeb convincingly describe the transdiagnostic applications of family-based treatment (FBT) across eating disorder categories in youth. They support this position through both empirical findings across relevant diagnoses and succinct description of how FBT strategies apply both broadly across dysregulated eating patterns and more specifically within the context of varying clinical presentations.

Chapter 17, by Payne, Tsao, and Zeltzer, discusses a focal application of the unified protocol to a new systemic and intrapersonal context: that of a pediatric population with pain. Payne and colleagues note the high incidence of emotional disorders in pediatric samples, along with the potential common mechanisms of change across emotional disorders and pain management. The authors describe the unified model in further detail, along with the substantive adaptations and revisions they have made to better suit the unique challenges faced by children with chronic pain.

In Part V, following the previous sections' review of contemporary transdiagnostic science and treatment, we were fortunate to have Ollendick, Fraire, and Spence, in Chapter 18, provide commentary on the current state of the research. They critically evaluate the current literature base and acknowledge the promise of current efforts but caution the field to wait until further evidence accumulates.

Returning to the simultaneous excitement and confusion that we sought to address, Chu and Ehrenreich-May (Chapter 19) conclude this book with an endeavor to identify the challenges ahead for the transdiagnotic movement in youth psychopathology. We address the concerns raised by Ollendick and colleagues and look to even further challenges ahead to fully establish the meaning and reach of transdiagnostic research. Although transdiagnostic research and treatment are in their infancy, the current volume demonstrates that they are in a rapid period of development and empirical evaluation. The road ahead is filled with both promise for efficiency in our youth treatments and caution about the need for further research to see this promise fulfilled.

REFERENCES

Achenbach, T. (2005). Advancing assessment of children and adolescents: Commentary on evidence-based assessment of child and adolescent disorders. *Journal of Clinical Child and Adolescent Psychology, 34*, 541–547.

American Psychiatric Association. (2000). *Diagnostic and statistical manual of mental disorders* (4th ed., text rev.). Washington, DC: Author.

American Psychiatric Association. (2013a). *Diagnostic and statistical manual of mental disorders* (5th ed.). Washington, DC: Author.

American Psychiatric Association. (2013b). Highlights of changes from DSM-IV-TR to DSM-5. Retrieved from *www.dsm5.org/documents/changes%20from%20dsm-iv-tr%20to%20dsm-5.pdf.*

Barlow, D. H., Allen, L. B., & Choate, M. L. (2004). Toward a unified treatment for emotional disorders. *Behavior Therapy, 35*, 205–230.

Barlow, D. H., Farchione, T. F., Fairholme, C. P., Ellard, K. K., Boisseau, C. P., Allen, L. B., et al. (2010). *Unified Protocol for the transdiagnostic treatment of emotional disorders: Therapist guide.* New York: Oxford University Press.

Fairburn, C. G., Cooper, Z., & Shafran, R. (2003). Cognitive behaviour therapy for eating disorders: A "transdiagnostic" theory and treatment. *Behaviour Research and Therapy, 41*, 509–528.

Harvey, A., Watkins, E., Mansell, W., & Shafran, R. (2004). *Cognitive behavioural processes across psychological disorders: A transdiagnostic approach to research and treatment.* New York: Oxford University Press.

Kraemer, H. C. (2007). DSM categories and dimensions in clinical and research contexts. *International Journal of Methods in Psychiatric Research, 16*, S8–S15.

Kupfer, D. J., Kuhl, E. A., & Regier, D. A. (2013). DSM-5—The future arrived. *Journal of the American Medical Association, 309*, 1691–1692.

Mansell, W., Harvey, A., Watkins, E., & Shafran, R. (2009). Conceptual foundations of the transdiagnostic approach to CBT. *Journal of Cognitive Psychotherapy, 23*, 6–19.

Mayr, E. (1982). *The growth of biological thought.* Cambridge, MA: Harvard University Press.

Taylor, S., & Clark, D. A. (2009). Transdiagnostic cognitive-behavioral treatments for mood and anxiety disorders: Introduction to the special issue. *Journal of Cognitive Psychotherapy: An International Quarterly, 23*, 3–5.

CHAPTER 2

Transdiagnostic Mechanisms and Treatments for Youth with Psychiatric Disorders

An Opportunity to Catapult Progress?

Allison G. Harvey

Psychopathology in Youth: The Scope of the Challenge

The prevalence of mental illness is staggeringly high, affecting almost 30% of the general population over a 12-month period (Kessler et al., 1994; Regier, Rae, Narrow, Kaelber, & Schatzberg, 1998). The most severe forms (involving psychosis, active suicidality, substance use that threatens jobs and relationships, etc.) have a 12-month prevalence of about 6% (Kessler, Chiu, Demler, Merikangas, & Walters, 2005b), with another 20% or more of the population exhibiting moderate to serious forms, producing substantial impairment. The disability and functional impairments associated with mental illness are serious and wide ranging. Several forms of mental illness are among the "top 10" forms of illness leading to impairment and burden worldwide. Another way of putting this is that among the 20 leading causes of disability worldwide, mental disorders account for 26% of disability (World Health Organization, 2004).

Alarming as this all is, two facts are even more horrifying, and these facts are the reason for this book. First, mental illness begins relatively early in the lifespan, *with half of all lifetime disorders starting by 14 years of age* (Kessler et al., 2008). Second, there are high rates of comorbidity, or the co-occurrence of multiple disorders, with the vast majority of the lifetime disorders showing comorbidity with other disorders (Kessler et al., 1994). Hence, it is quite bizarre that the mechanism and treatment research literature (1) typically focuses on adults (although this has been slowly changing) and (2) takes a "disorder-focused" approach in which researchers and clinicians target one specific disorder, trying to understand its etiology and maintenance and attempting to develop or modify effective treatments for that one disorder (Fairburn, Cooper, & Shafran, 2003; Harvey, Watkins, Mansell, & Shafran, 2004). Indeed, there is minimal knowledge about treating comorbidity, or even why comorbidity is the rule rather than the exception. Accordingly, there is a need for serious consideration of ways to understand *and* derive innovative approaches for effectively treating the co-occurrence of psychiatric disorders in youth. The challenges ahead include carefully examining dimensions that underlie mental illness and gaining insight into mechanisms that underpin the development and maintenance of multiple forms of psychopathology. This pursuit will inevitably require the identification of *underlying transdiagnostic processes that cut across traditional categories of specific single disorders* (Barlow, Allen, & Choate, 2004; Fairburn et al., 2003; Harvey et al., 2004).

What Is a Transdiagnostic Perspective and Could It Catapult Progress?

Research on mental illness is typically dominated by a "disorder focus." That is, researchers have tended to target one specific disorder and tried to understand its etiology and maintenance so as to develop more effective strategies to treat that disorder. There is no doubt that this approach has greatly advanced our understanding of, and ability to treat, several psychiatric disorders (Clark & Fairburn, 1997). Would there be any utility in shifting perspective away from a "disorder focus" toward an "across-disorder," or transdiagnostic, perspective? Three colleagues and I (Harvey et al., 2004), along with several other research groups (e.g., Barlow et al., 2004; Fairburn et al., 2003; Hayes, Wilson, Gifford, Follette, & Strosahl, 1996; Persons, 1989), have been interested in the possibility that studying the processes relevant across disorders may catapult progress in at least three domains.

Classification

The main classification systems for psychiatric disorders are the *Diagnostic and Statistical Manual of Mental Disorders* (DSM-5; American Psychiatric Association, 2013) and the *International Classification of Diseases* (ICD-10; World Health Organization, 1992). Classification systems are attractive because they provide a common language that aids clear communication among clinicians and researchers. Classification systems also facilitate research because studying a reasonably homogeneous group of people with a common set of symptoms assists in developing a picture of what might be contributing to the disorder and how a disorder can best be treated (Adams, Doster, & Calhoun, 1977). However, a categorical conceptualization of psychiatric disorders does not reflect the clinical reality; most of the basic processes and treatments occur on a continuum (Hyman, 2007). This dimensional view assumes that "individuals assigned a [DSM] diagnosis differ from 'normal' persons only in the frequency and/or severity with which they experience the features that form the diagnostic criteria" (Brown, 1996). A dimensional view may also include and/or facilitate the process of identifying, studying, and treating transdiagnostic processes (Harvey et al., 2004). The inclusion of a dimensional approach may well become a reality in the future (Insel et al., 2010; Regier, 2007; Rutter, 2011), a direction that is very much in line with a transdiagnostic perspective.

Importantly for youth, although dimensional approaches are commonly used in child psychiatry and psychology, it is critical to more fully develop and integrate dimensional approaches because the mismatch between the DSM categories and clinical presentation is perhaps greatest for youth (Hyman, 2007). Hudziak, Achenbach, Althoff, and Pine (2007) highlight three additional reasons for the importance of developing dimensional approaches for youth. First, "developmental neurobiology research shows that the connections, anatomy and physiology of the human brain change dramatically across development" (p. S18). There is thus a need to account for differences in typical and atypical development, which is easier to achieve by considering dimensions. Second, there are gender differences in the manifestation and prevalence of various psychiatric disorders in youth. Third, there are nearly always multiple informants (the youth, father, mother, teacher, coach, doctor, etc.) whose reports do not always agree. Whether an average across reports or the most severe problem reported by any informant is ultimately selected as the highest priority for treatment planning and research, the inclusion of a dimensional approach may facilitate both.

Comorbidity

Comorbidity is the coexistence of two or more disorders, either simultaneously or sequentially (de Graaf, Bijl, Smit, Vollebergh, & Spijker, 2002). Comorbidity is the norm, not the exception. A staggering 50% of people who meet diagnostic criteria for a psychiatric disorder in a specific year will meet criteria for more than one disorder (Kessler, Chiu, Demler, Merikangas, & Walters, 2005a). Several accounts of the high rate of comorbidity among the psychiatric disorders have been proposed.

First, comorbidity may reflect poor discriminant validity in that the DSM may distinguish between disorders that would be better combined (Andrews, 1996; Blashfield, 1990; Brown & Barlow, 1992). Another contributor to comorbidity may be the symptom overlap across disorders (Garber & Weersing, 2010).

Second, features of one disorder may act as risk factors for other psychiatric disorders. To give an example, insomnia is a well-established risk factor for the development of first-onset depression (e.g., Ford & Kamerow, 1989), anxiety disorder (Breslau, Roth, Rosenthal, & Andreski, 1996) and substance abuse (Weissman, Greenwald, German, & Dement, 1997), so it is not surprising that insomnia is highly comorbid with these disorders (Harvey, 2001). Anxiety symptoms and disorders in childhood precede the onset of depressive disorders in adolescence and young adulthood, particularly in girls (Garber & Weersing, 2010). Moreover, depression during adolescence is known to predict a fivefold increase in the risk of generalized anxiety disorder in young adulthood (Pine, Cohen, Gurley, Brook, & Ma, 1998).

Third, comorbidity may reflect one or more common vulnerabilities. Examples of factors implicated in the vulnerability to develop *a range of psychiatric disorders* include genetics (Cerdá, Sagdeo, Johnson, & Galea, 2010), anxiety sensitivity (Reiss & McNally, 1985), information-processing biases and negative cognitions (Ernst, Pine, & Hardin, 2005; Pine, 2007), neuroticism (Eysenck, 1973), positive and negative affectivity, as well as somatic tension (Clark & Watson, 1991; Laurent & Ettelson, 2001), high trait anxiety and poor coping skills (Andrews, 1996), trait impulsivity (Beauchaine, Hinshaw, & Pang, 2010), a tendency toward internalizing or externalizing (Kessler et al., 2011), certain parenting behaviors (McLeod, Wood, & Weisz, 2007), and social factors such as childhood adversity and stress, family and peer support, and socioeconomic and academic difficulties (Cerdá et al., 2010).

A final possibility, and the one that is most relevant to the aim of this book, is that perhaps psychiatric disorders co-occur because they share maintaining processes. This possibility is not necessarily inconsistent with the other accounts of comorbidity presented, but it provides an additional explanation.

Garber and Weersing (2010) highlight the critical point that comorbidity varies by age and developmental stage. For example, anxiety is more prevalent in children, rates of depression increase in teens, and comorbid anxiety and depression tend to be more prevalent in older than younger teens. Interestingly, anxiety and depression are not distinguishable in young children (third graders), but they become distinguishable after just a few years more of development (Cole, Truglio, & Peeke, 1997). This change from a unified-construct model to a dual-factor model highlights the challenge and complexity ahead for developmental researchers. To add even more complexity, Pine (2010) points out the importance of context: "behavior changes quite dramatically in the short-term, through the influence of context, and in the long-term, through the influence of development" (p. 533). The youth and their social context dynamically and bidirectionally influence each other, the context surrounding the youth broadens and deepens with age, and the meaning (to the young person) of each social context in which he or she is engaged will determine the potential impact of that context (Boyce et al., 1998). Clearly, a transdiagnostic approach to psychopathology in youth will need to include a crystal-clear focus on age, developmental stage (including pubertal status), and social context.

Rapid Transfer of Treatment Breakthroughs

A third advantage is that a transdiagnostic perspective would encourage greater transfer of theoretical and treatment advances between the disorders. This already happens to some extent. For example, in one of my own fields of research, and as depicted in Figure 2.1, breakthroughs in the treatment of insomnia occurred in the late 1970s. Insomnia is commonly comorbid with a range of other psychiatric disorders, but it took *several decades* for the advances in the treatment of insomnia to be applied to insomnia that is comorbid with other psychiatric disorders (see the dates, in bold, in Figure 2.1). Seeing the success of these treatments in

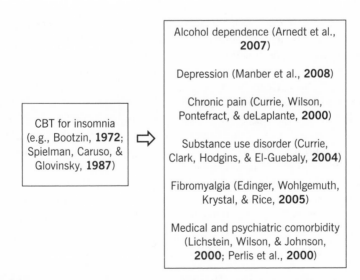

FIGURE 2.1. Transfer of breakthroughs in the treatment of insomnia has been slow (notice the publication dates in **bold**)!

improving not only sleep but also the symptoms associated with the other comorbid disorder, and after considering biological plausibility (Harvey, Murray, Chandler, & Soehner, 2011), we have proposed that sleep disturbance is a plausible transdiagnostic process (Harvey, 2008). We then highlighted the potential of testing a transdiagnostic treatment for sleep disturbance (Harvey, 2009b), including a version that is developmentally adapted for youth (Harvey, 2009a). The main point here is that explicitly taking a transdiagnostic perspective almost ensures more rapid transfer of advances to a broader range of disorders. Moreover, a transdiagnostic approach might lead the field to the ability to specify a single treatment or treatment components that are effective across a wide range of disorders (Harvey et al., 2004). We see examples across several chapters of this book.

What Other Ingredients Are Needed for a Transdiagnostic Perspective to Catapult Progress?

Although progress has been made in developing and disseminating evidence-based treatments for most forms of mental illness across the past few decades, there are gaping holes in our knowledge base. Here, I list a number of issues and facts linked to such barriers.

Lack of Attention to *Childhood* and *Adolescence*

As already mentioned, given the early age of onset of most mental illness, there has been insufficient emphasis on developing and testing interventions that build resilience and prevent the development of mental illness in children and adolescents. Also, treatments for mental illnesses commonly make the mistake of trying to "downsize" adult treatments (Silverman & Hinshaw, 2008). Targeting this early phase of the lifespan is essential for minimizing the adverse effects of psychiatric illness on the expected developmental trajectory. Moreover, there may be specific periods of development that represent unique opportunities for early intervention that change developmental trajectories and prevent a wide range of adverse behavioral and emotional outcomes (Silk et al., 2009). Clearly, the emphasis within this book on developmental psychopathology perspectives is crucial (e.g., Cicchetti & Toth, 2006).

Lack of Knowledge about and Attention to *Basic Processes*

Although evidence-based treatments for most mental illnesses have been developed (Aronson, 2005; Chambless et al., 1996; Silverman & Hinshaw, 2008), there is substantial room for improvement. The effect sizes of most available treatments are small to moderate, gains may not persist, and there are too many patients who derive little or no benefit (Harvey & Tang, 2003; Insel, 2007, 2009; Lambert, 2004; Nathan & Gorman, 2002). Even under optimal conditions, treatment failure is alarmingly common (Lieberman et al., 2005; Thase, 2007; Warden, Rush, Trivedi, Fava, & Wisniewski, 2007).

Traditionally, the development of *psychological treatments* has involved consensus between groups of skilled clinician researchers, and many *medication treatments* have been discovered by serendipity. Hence there have been calls for "increased attention to science" as the optimal path toward developing more highly efficient and effective treatments (Aronson, 2005; Insel, 2009; Salkovskis, 2002). More specifically, whereas knowledge of the basic processes that cause and maintain mental illness has expanded enormously over the past two decades, this knowledge has been minimally leveraged in the service of developing highly efficacious and effective treatments.

As is evident in Part II of this book, transdiagnostic basic processes are identifiable, and the work of defining transdiagnostic processes is leading to novel insights, breakthroughs, and perhaps even transdiagnostic treatments that will reduce the burden on therapists who have to master a wide range of disorder-specific protocols. Furthermore, it is becoming clear that transdiagnostic processes are evident at various levels of explanation. There is already evidence that various cognitive-behavioral processes (Harvey et al., 2004) and emotional processes (Kring & Sloan, 2010) are transdiagnostic. Readers familiar with the neuroscience literature will know that similar brain circuits, structures, neurotransmitters, and genes have been implicated across the disorders (Ellis & Boyce, 2011; Ernst et al., 2006; Shonkoff, Boyce, & McEwen, 2009). The same is true for other levels of explanation, such as personality, temperament, culture, family, and so forth.

I would like to acknowledge that, in many ways, the field of developmental psychopathology has been a guiding light in producing interdisciplinary research on mechanisms that cut across the multiple levels of explanation relevant to youth with psychopathology (Cicchetti & Dawson, 2002; Pellmar & Eisenberg, 2000), including the potential contributing processes of communities, culture, families, schools, and peers. These approaches recognize and embrace the fact that events during development lay the root systems for the development of adult psychiatric conditions (Pine, 2007) and that some problems in childhood predict widespread difficulties in adulthood, whereas others do not (Masten & Cicchetti, 2010). Research groups are even taking on the task of modeling the developmental cascades or the "cumulative consequences for development of the many interactions and transactions occurring in developing systems that result in spreading effects across levels, among domains at the same level and across different systems or generations" (Masten & Cicchetti, 2010). Challenging and exciting!

Lack of Attention to Commonalities across Traditional Therapy Models

Some treatments are explicitly content-focused. For example, some cognitive-behavioral treatments seek to identify and challenge the *content* of negative thoughts and unhelpful assumptions. It seems likely that there will be utility in continuing to incorporate a *process-focused* approach to treatment that seeks to target and reverse the transdiagnostic processes that cause and/or maintain disorders, particularly for patients who do not get better with the current evidence-based treatments and for complex cases in which comorbidity is present (Harvey et al., 2004). These are the patients for whom it may be difficult to determine which disorder is "primary," which disorder to focus on treating, and/or which treatment model to adopt as a guide to treatment. As many randomized controlled trials have excluded patients with comorbid disorders, there may be no evidence base for the particular combination of psychiatric disorders with which the patient presents. Accordingly, targeting transdiagnostic processes as part of a process-based approach may be one way to resolve the tricky question of how to structure therapy in these cases (Harvey et al., 2004). This would contrast with the typical approach of sequentially treating the various comorbid disorders, an approach that invites treatment failure if the disorders are mutually maintaining (e.g., Harvey, 2008).

As is evident across Parts III and IV of this book, even though traditional therapy models such as cognitive-behavioral therapy, interpersonal therapy, dialectical behavior therapy, and acceptance and commitment therapy offer disorder-specific protocols, there is much potential to draw out transdiagnostic versions of these treatments. As these are all multicomponent treatments, let's not forget the problem that we do not know which elements are truly contributing. As highlighted by Clark (1999, 2004), we may be on a path to more efficient and effective psychosocial treatments if we conduct tests of single treatment elements to ensure that each is contributing (e.g., Harvey, Clark, Ehlers, & Rapee, 2000; Tang & Harvey, 2006).

Insularity and *Fragmentation* across Disciplines

It is essential to acknowledge the complex nature of mental health problems. Rather than debating the relative contribution of biological versus psychological risk factors or the relative benefits of biological versus psychosocial treatments (Miller, 2010), we are surely better off focusing on research that provides new insights into how interacting levels of biological, psychosocial, and cultural factors can be targeted in multimodal treatments (Hinshaw et al., 2000) and treatments that reach across individuals, schools, families, and communities. Although this book focuses on psychological processes and treatments, there is much potential for future contributions that crosscut levels of explanations transdiagnostically.

Caveats of a Transdiagnostic Perspective

First, there are ways in which the approach to psychopathology in youth has always been more "transdiagnostic" relative to the adult literature. For example, Coping Cat (Kendall & Hedtke, 2006) is a treatment designed for children ages 8–13 who have generalized anxiety disorder, separation anxiety disorder, or social anxiety disorder. In other words, this treatment cuts *across* anxiety disorders. In adults, there are different protocols for each anxiety disorder.

Second, as we have previously highlighted (Harvey et al., 2004), the proposal to take a transdiagnostic perspective is not new. The importance of cognitive and behavioral processes in psychiatric disorders has long been recognized by clinicians and researchers. For example, research on behavioral processes, such as conditioning and reinforcement contingencies, led to a range of treatments and techniques that were largely transdiagnostic and came to be known collectively as behavior therapy (Pavlov, 1928; Skinner, 1959; Watson & Rayner, 1920; Wolpe, 1958). The recognition of behavior therapy's limitations in treating certain client groups (Rachman, 1997) left the field open and receptive to the novel ideas of clinician researchers such as Beck (1967) and Ellis (1958). Beck and Ellis had a common proposal that they recognized as relevant across the disorders: that cognitive processes, including unhelpful beliefs, illogical thinking, and distorted perception, were crucial to understanding and treating psychiatric disorders. These ideas led to the birth of cognitive therapy and cognitive-behavioral therapy.

Third, my colleagues and I (Harvey et al., 2004) have raised the important limitation of a transdiagnostic perspective: It cannot explain why people with different psychiatric disorders can present so differently. For example, a young person who meets diagnostic criteria for attention-deficit/hyperactivity disorder will, at one level, seem so completely different from a young person diagnosed with obsessive–compulsive disorder (recurrent obsessions experienced as intrusive and inappropriate and compulsions such as hand washing and repeating words silently). Why is this? We have suggested that there are at least three possible explanations.

Current Concerns

One possibility is that the differences between psychiatric disorders may be, at least partly, accounted for by the different concerns inherent to each disorder. The idea of current concerns has been most developed within Eric Klinger's (1996) current concerns theory. Klinger defines a current concern as a nonconscious (latent) processing state initiated when a person commits to pursue a specific goal, which lasts until the goal is either achieved or discarded, and which underpins the goal pursuit by sensitizing emotional responses to and cognitive processing of cues associated with that goal (Klinger, 1996). For example, a teen with anorexia nervosa is concerned about weight and shape, whereas a teen with insomnia is concerned about his or her sleep and a teen with obsessive–compulsive disorder may be concerned with fear of contamination. The follow-up question is: Why do people with different disorders have different current concerns? We have suggested a range of influences on the target of the concern, such as biology (e.g., genes, circuits), personality, learning history, traumatic experiences, and culture (Harvey et al., 2004).

Balance of Common Processes

Perhaps a person with a psychiatric disorder could show any one basic process at any point along a continuum. Accordingly, perhaps the different disorders may be, at least partly, distinguished by their relative balance of the basic transdiagnostic processes. For example, Ernst and colleagues (2006) demonstrate that three systems may contribute to anxiety and depression: the reward system (nucleus accumbens), the harm-avoidance system (amygdala), and the supervisory system (medial/ventral prefrontal cortex). Perhaps the relative strength and efficiency of each system might contribute to explanations of psychiatric disorders that are even broader than anxiety and depression. In other words, perhaps different disorders lie at different points on each continuum. Thus, in principle, differences in the relative balance of these processes may contribute to the differences between the disorders.

Distinct Processes

In our review of the adult literature on cognitive and behavioral processes relevant to Axis 1 disorders, we found some evidence of disorder-specific processes (Harvey et al., 2004). That is, distinct processes appear to be specific to certain disorders or groups of disorders, and the presence of a distinct process may contribute to the differences between disorders. Psychotic disorders were the most prominent example. The empirical evidence we reviewed suggested that psychotic disorders are associated with a data-gathering bias and a bias toward making external attributions for internally generated thoughts and sensations (Harvey et al., 2004). These processing biases have not been found in the other psychiatric disorders. However, it is important to note that comparisons between individuals with psychotic disorders and nonclinical populations may be made along a continuum such that some individuals without psychotic disorders may show the same processing biases under certain conditions. Furthermore, we also found good evidence that psychotic symptoms may be maintained by the processes that we have identified to be *common* across disorders (e.g., internally focused attention, safety behaviors, worry). Nonetheless, this example raises the possible contribution of distinct processes.

Summary

The potential advantages of a transdiagnostic perspective are that it may contribute to progress in classification and comorbidity and that it may encourage rapid transfer of advances made in the context of one disorder to other disorders. However, there have been several barriers to progress, including the lack of attention to research on children and adolescents, the lack of knowledge about basic processes and commonalities across traditional therapy models, and insularity and fragmentation across disciplines. As is evident throughout this book, in many ways developmental psychopathologists have been leading the way in studying basic processes, reaching across disciplines, and developing treatments that cut across disorders. This progress is perhaps necessitated by the complexity of the questions inherent to the study of youth development, which inevitably require a focus on moving targets such as age, pubertal development, and context. Grappling with these and other complexities is the heart and soul of this book, as is the knowledge that *half of all lifetime disorders start by 14 years of age* and have the potential to seriously unravel the health and most basic well-being of individuals and prevent them from thriving in relationships, family life, and career.

ACKNOWLEDGMENT

This research was supported by a National Institute of Mental Health grant (No. R34 MH080958).

REFERENCES

Adams, H. E., Doster, J. A., & Calhoun, K. S. (1977). *A psychologically based system of response classification.* New York: Wiley.

American Psychiatric Association. (2013). *Diagnostic and statistical manual of mental disorders* (5th ed.). Arlington, VA: Author.

Andrews, G. (1996). Comorbidity and the general neurotic syndrome. *British Journal of Psychiatry, 168,* 76–84.

Arnedt, J. T., Conroy, D., Rutt, J., Aloia, M. S., Brower, K. J., & Armitage, R. (2007). An open trial of cognitive-behavioral treatment for insomnia comorbid with alcohol dependence. *Sleep Medicine, 8,* 176–180.

Aronson, J. K. (2005). Drug development: More science, more education. *British Journal of Clinical Pharmacology, 59,* 377–378.

Barlow, D. H., Allen, L. B., & Choate, M. L. (2004). Toward a unified treatment for emotional disorders. *Behavior Therapy, 35,* 205–230.

Beauchaine, T. P., Hinshaw, S. P., & Pang, K. (2010). Comorbidity of attention-deficit/hyperactivity disorder and early-onset conduct disorder: Biological, environmental, and developmental mechanisms. *Clinical Psychology: Science and Practice, 17,* 327–336.

Beck, A. T. (1967). *Depression: Causes and treatment.* Philadelphia: University of Pennsylvania Press.

Blashfield, R. K. (1990). Co-morbidity and classification. In J. Maser & C. R. Cloninger (Eds.), *Comorbidity of mood and anxiety disorders* (pp. 61–82). Washington, DC: American Psychiatric Press.

Bootzin, R. R. (1972). Stimulus control treatment for insomnia. *Proceedings of the American Psychological Association, 7,* 395–396.

Boyce, W. T., Frank, E., Jensen, P. S., Kessler, R. C., Nelson, C. A., & Steinberg, L. (1998). Social context in developmental psychopathology: Recommendations from the MacArthur Network on Psychopathology and Development. *Developmental Psychopathology, 10,* 143–164.

Breslau, N., Roth, T., Rosenthal, L., & Andreski, P. (1996). Sleep disturbance and psychiatric disorders: A longitudinal epidemiological study of young adults. *Biological Psychiatry, 39,* 411–418.

Brown, T. A. (1996). *Validity of the DSM-III-R and DSM-IV classification systems for anxiety disorders.* New York: American Psychological Association.

Brown, T. A., & Barlow, D. H. (1992). Comorbidity among anxiety disorders: Implications for treatment and DSM-IV. *Journal of Consulting and Clinical Psychology, 60,* 835–844.

Cerdá, M., Sagdeo, A., Johnson, J., & Galea, S. (2010). Genetic and environmental influences on psychiatric comorbidity: A systematic review. *Journal of Affective Disorders, 126,* 14–38.

Chambless, D. L., Sanderson, W. C., Shoham, V., Bennett Johnson, S., Pope, K. S., Chrits-Christoph, P., et al. (1996). An update on empirically validated therapies. *Clinical Psychologist, 49,* 5–18.

Cicchetti, D., & Dawson, G. (2002). Editorial: Multiple levels of analysis. *Development and Psychopathology, 14,* 417–420.

Cicchetti, D., & Toth, S. L. (2006). Building bridges and crossing them:

Translational research in developmental psychopathology. *Developmental Psychopathology, 18*, 619–622.

Clark, D. M. (1999). Anxiety disorders: Why they persist and how to treat them. *Behaviour Research and Therapy, 37*(Suppl. 1), S5–S27.

Clark, D. M. (2004). Developing new treatments: On the interplay between theories, experimental science and clinical innovation. *Behaviour Research and Therapy, 42*, 1089–1104.

Clark, D. M., & Fairburn, C. G. (1997). Panic disorder and social phobia. In D. M. Clark & C. G. Fairburn (Eds.), *Science and practice of cognitive behaviour therapy* (pp. 119–154). New York: Oxford University Press.

Clark, L. A., & Watson, D. (1991). Tripartite model of anxiety and depression: Psychometric evidence and taxonomic implications. *Journal of Abnormal Psychology, 100*, 316–336.

Cole, D. A., Truglio, R., & Peeke, L. (1997). Relation between symptoms of anxiety and depression in children: A multitrait-multimethod-multigroup assessment. *Journal of Consulting and Clinical Psychology, 65*, 110–119.

Currie, S. R., Clark, S., Hodgins, D. C., & El-Guebaly, N. (2004). Randomized controlled trial of brief cognitive-behavioural interventions for insomnia in recovering alcoholics. *Addiction, 99*(9), 1121–1132.

Currie, S. R., Wilson, K. G., Pontefract, A. J., & deLaplante, L. (2000). Cognitive-behavioral treatment of insomnia secondary to chronic pain. *Journal of Consulting and Clinical Psychology, 68*, 407–416.

de Graaf, R., Bijl, R. V., Smit, F., Vollebergh, W., & Spijker, J. (2002). Risk factors for 12-month comorbidity of mood, anxiety, and substance use disorders: Findings from the Netherlands Mental Health Survey and Incidence Study. *American Journal of Psychiatry, 159*, 620–629.

Edinger, J. D., Wohlgemuth, W. K., Krystal, A. D., & Rice, J. R. (2005). Behavioral insomnia therapy for fibromyalgia patients: A randomized clinical trial. *Archives of Internal Medicine, 165*, 2527–2535.

Ellis, A. (1958). Rational psychotherapy. *Journal of General Psychology, 59*, 35–49.

Ellis, E. J., & Boyce, W. T. (2011). Differential susceptibility to the environment: Toward an understanding of sensitivity to developmental experiences and context. *Development and Psychopathology, 23*, 1–5.

Ernst, M., Pine, D. S., & Hardin, M. (2006). Triadic model of the neurobiology of motivated behavior in adolescence. *Psychological Medicine, 36*, 299–312.

Eysenck, H. J. (1973). *On extraversion.* New York: Wiley.

Fairburn, C. G., Cooper, Z., & Shafran, R. (2003). Cognitive behaviour therapy for eating disorders: A "transdiagnostic" theory and treatment. *Behaviour Research and Therapy, 41*, 509–528.

Ford, D. E., & Kamerow, D. B. (1989). Epidemiologic study of sleep disturbances and psychiatric disorders: An opportunity for prevention? *Journal of the American Medical Association, 262*, 1479–1484.

Garber, J., & Weersing, V. R. (2010). Comorbidity of anxiety and depression in youth: Implications for treatment and prevention. *Clinical Psychology: Science and Practice, 17*, 293–306.

Harvey, A. G. (2001). Insomnia: Symptom or diagnosis? *Clinical Psychology Review, 21*, 1037–1059.

Harvey, A. G. (2008). Insomnia, psychiatric disorders, and the transdiagnostic perspective. *Current Directions in Psychological Science, 17*, 299–303.

Harvey, A. G. (2009a). The adverse consequences of sleep disturbance in pediatric bipolar disorder: Implications for intervention. *Child and Adolescent Psychiatry Clinics of North America, 18*, 321–338.

Harvey, A. G. (2009b). A transdiagnostic approach to treating sleep disturbance in psychiatric disorders. *Cognitive Behavior Therapy, 38*, 35–42.

Harvey, A. G., Clark, D. M., Ehlers, A., & Rapee, R. M. (2000). Social anxiety and self-impression: Cognitive preparation enhances the beneficial effects of video feedback following a stressful social task. *Behaviour Research and Therapy, 38*, 1183–1192.

Harvey, A. G., Murray, G., Chandler, R. A., & Soehner, A. (2011). Sleep disturbance as transdiagnostic: Consideration of neurobiological mechanisms. *Clinical Psychology Review, 31*, 225–235.

Harvey, A. G., & Tang, N. K. (2003). Cognitive behaviour therapy for primary insomnia: Can we rest yet? *Sleep Medicine Reviews, 7*, 237–262.

Harvey, A. G., Watkins, E., Mansell, W., & Shafran, R. (2004). *Cognitive behavioural processes across psychological disorders: A transdiagnostic approach to research and treatment.* Oxford, UK: Oxford University Press.

Hayes, S. C., Wilson, K. G., Gifford, E. V., Follette, V. M., & Strosahl, K. (1996). Experiential avoidance and behavioral disorders: A functional dimensional approach to diagnosis and treatment. *Journal of Consulting and Clinical Psychology, 64*, 1152–1168.

Helzer, J. E., Kraemer, H. C., Krueger, R. F., Wittchen, H. U., Sirovatka, P. J., & Regier, D. A. (2008). *Dimensional approaches in diagnostic classification: Refining the research agenda for DSM-V.* Arlington, VA: American Psychiatric Association.

Hinshaw, S. P., Owens, E. B., Wells, K. C., Kraemer, H. C., Abikoff, H. B., Arnold, L. E., et al. (2000). Family processes and treatment outcome in the MTA: Negative/ineffective parenting practices in relation to multimodal treatment. *Journal of Abnormal Psychology, 28*, 555–568.

Hudziak, J. J., Achenbach, T. M., Althoff, R. R., & Pine, D. S. (2007). A dimensional approach to developmental psychopathology. *International Journal of Methods in Psychiatric Research, 16*, S16–S23.

Hyman, S. E. (2007). Can neuroscience be integrated into the DSM-V? *Nature Reviews Neuroscience, 8*, 725–732.

Insel, T. R. (2007). Devising prevention and treatment strategies for the nation's diverse populations with mental illness. *Psychiatric Services, 58*, 395.

Insel, T. R. (2009). Translating scientific opportunity into public health impact: A strategic plan for research on mental illness. *Archives of General Psychiatry, 66*(2), 128–133.

Insel, T. R., Cuthbert, B. N., Garvey, M. A., Heinssen, R. K., Pine, D. S., Quinn, K. J., et al. (2010). Research domain criteria (RDoC): Toward a new classification framework for research on mental disorders. *American Journal of Psychiatry, 167*, 748–751.

Kendall, P. C., & Hedtke, K. A. (2006). *Cognitive-behavioral therapy for anxious children: Therapist manual* (3rd ed.). Ardmore, PA: Workbook Publishing.

Kessler, R. C., Chiu, W. T., Demler, O., Merikangas, K. R., & Walters, E. E. (2005a).

Corrections: Errors in byline, author affiliations, and acknowledgment in: Prevalence, severity, and comorbidity of 12-month DSM-IV disorders in the National Comorbidity Survey Replication. *Archives of General Psychiatry, 62,* 709.

Kessler, R. C., Chiu, W. T., Demler, O., Merikangas, K. R., & Walters, E. E. (2005b). Prevalence, severity, and comorbidity of 12-month DSM-IV disorders in the National Comorbidity Survey Replication. *Archives of General Psychiatry, 62,* 617–627.

Kessler, R. C., Heeringa, S., Lakoma, M. D., Petukhova, M., Rupp, A. E., Schoenbaum, M., et al. (2008). Individual and societal effects of mental disorders on earnings in the United States: Results from the National Comorbidity Survey Replication. *American Journal of Psychiatry, 165,* 703–711.

Kessler, R. C., McGonagle, K. A., Zhao, S., Nelson, C. B., Hughes, M., Eshleman, S., et al. (1994). Lifetime and 12-month prevalence of DSM-III-R psychiatric disorders in the United States: Results from the National Comorbidity Study. *Archives of General Psychiatry, 51,* 8–19.

Kessler, R. C., Ormel, J., Petukhova, M., McLaughlin, K. A., Green, J. G., Russo, L. J., et al. (2011). Development of lifetime comorbidity in the World Health Organization World Mental Health Surveys. *Archives of General Psychiatry, 68,* 90–100.

Klinger, E. (1996). Emotional influences on cognitive processing, with implications for theories of both. In P. M. Gollwitzer & J. A. Bargh (Eds.), *The psychology of action: Linking cognition and motivation to behavior* (pp. 168–189). New York: Guilford Press.

Kring, A. M., & Sloan, D. M. (Eds.). (2010). *Emotion regulation and psychopathology: A transdiagnostic approach to etiology and treatment.* New York: Guilford Press.

Lambert, M. J. (Ed.). (2004). *Bergin and Garfield's handbook of psychotherapy and behavior change* (5th ed.). New York: Wiley.

Laurent, J., & Ettelson, R. (2001). An examination of the tripartite model of anxiety and depression and its application to youth. *Clinical Child and Family Psychology Review, 4,* 209–230.

Lichstein, K. L., Wilson, N. M., & Johnson, C. T. (2000). Psychological treatment of secondary insomnia. *Psychology and Aging, 15,* 232–240.

Lieberman, J. A., Stroup, T. S., McEvoy, J. P., Swartz, M. S., Rosenheck, R. A., Perkins, D. O., et al. (2005). Effectiveness of antipsychotic drugs in patients with chronic schizophrenia. *New England Journal of Medicine, 353,* 1209–1223.

Manber, R., Edinger, J. D., Gress, J. L., San Pedro-Salcedo, M. G., Kuo, T. F., & Kalista, T. (2008). Cognitive behavioral therapy for insomnia enhances depression outcome in patients with comorbid major depressive disorder and insomnia. *Sleep, 31,* 489–495.

Masten, A. S., & Cicchetti, D. (2010). Developmental cascades. *Development and Psychopathology, 22,* 491–495.

McLeod, B. D., Wood, J. J., & Weisz, J. R. (2007). Examining the association between parenting and childhood anxiety: A meta-analysis. *Clinical Psychology Review, 27,* 155–172.

Miller, G. A. (2010). Mistreating psychology in the decades of the brain. *Perspectives on Psychological Science, 5,* 716–743.

Nathan, P., & Gorman, J. (Eds.). (2002). *A guide to treatments that work* (2nd ed.). New York: Oxford University Press.

Pavlov, I. (1928). *Lectures on conditioned reflexes.* New York: New York International.

Pellmar, T. C., & Eisenberg, L. (Eds.). (2000). *Bridging disciplines in the brain, behavioral, and clinical sciences.* Washington, DC: National Academy Press.

Perlis, M., Aloia, M., Millikan, A., Boehmler, J., Smith, M., Greenblatt, D., et al. (2000). Behavioral treatment of insomnia: A clinical case series study. *Journal of Behavioral Medicine, 23,* 149–161.

Persons, J. B. (1989). *Cognitive therapy in practice: A case formulation approach.* New York: Norton.

Pine, D. S. (2007). Research review: A neuroscience framework for pediatric anxiety disorders. *Journal of Child Psychology and Psychiatry, 48,* 631–648.

Pine, D. S., Cohen, P., Gurley, D., Brook, J., & Ma, Y. (1998). The risk for early-adulthood anxiety and depressive disorders in adolescents with anxiety and depressive disorders. *Archives of General Psychiatry, 55,* 56–64.

Rachman, S. (1997). The evolution of cognitive behavior therapy. In D. M. Clark (Ed.), *Science and practice of cognitive behavior therapy* (pp. 3–26). New York: Oxford University Press.

Regier, D. A. (2007). Dimensional approaches to psychiatric classification: Refining the research agenda for DSM-V: An introduction. *International Journal of Methods in Psychiatric Research, 16,* S1–S5.

Regier, D. A., Rae, D. S., Narrow, W. E., Kaelber, C. T., & Schatzberg, A. F. (1998). Prevalence of anxiety disorders and their comorbidity with mood and addictive disorders. *British Journal of Psychiatry Supplement, 34,* 24–28.

Reiss, S., & McNally, R. J. (1985). The expectancy model of fear. In S. Reiss & R. Bootzin (Eds.), *Theoretical issues in behavior therapy* (pp. 107–121). New York: Academic Press.

Rutter, M. (2011). Child psychiatric diagnosis and classification: Concepts, findings, challenges, and potential. *Journal of Child Psychology and Psychiatry, 52,* 647–660.

Salkovskis, P. M. (2002). Empirically grounded clinical interventions: Cognitive-behavioural therapy progresses through a multi-dimensional approach to clinical science. *Behavioural and Cognitive Psychotherapy, 30,* 3–9.

Shonkoff, J. P., Boyce, W. T., & McEwen, B. S. (2009). Neuroscience, molecular biology and the childhood roots of health disparities: Building a new framework for health promotion and disease prevention. *Journal of the American Medical Association, 301,* 2252–2259.

Silk, J. S., Siegle, G. J., Whalen, D. J., Ostapenko, L. J., Ladouceur, C. D., & Dahl, R. E. (2009). Pubertal changes in emotional information processing: Pupillary, behavioral, and subjective evidence during emotional word identification. *Development and Psychopathology, 21,* 7–26.

Silverman, W. K., & Hinshaw, S. P. (2008). The second special issue on evidence-based psychosocial treatments for children and adolescents: A 10-year update. *Journal of Clinical Child and Adolescent Psychology, 37,* 1–7.

Skinner, B. F. (1959). *Cumulative record.* New York: Appleton Century.

Spielman, A. J., Caruso, L. S. & Glovinsky, P. B. (1987). A behavioral perspective on insomnia treatment. *Psychiatric Clinics of North America, 10,* 541–553.

Tang, N. K. Y., & Harvey, A. G. (2006). Altering misperception of sleep in insomnia: Behavioral experiment versus verbal feedback. *Journal of Consulting and Clinical Psychology, 74,* 767–776.

Thase, M. E. (2007). STEP-BD and bipolar depression: What have we learned? *Current Psychiatry Reports, 9,* 497–503.

Warden, D., Rush, A. J., Trivedi, M. H., Fava, M., & Wisniewski, S. R. (2007). The STAR*D Project results: A comprehensive review of findings. *Current Psychiatry Reports, 9,* 449–459.

Watson, J. B., & Rayner, R. (1920). Conditioned emotional reactions. *Journal of Experimental Psychology, 3,* 1–14.

Weissman, M. M., Greenwald, S., German, N., & Dement, W. C. (1997). The morbidity of insomnia uncomplicated by psychiatric disorders. *General Hospital Psychiatry, 19,* 245–250.

Wolpe, J. (1958). *Psychotherapy by reciprocal inhibition.* Palo Alto, CA: Stanford University Press.

World Health Organization. (1992). *The ICD-10 classification of mental and behavioral disorders: Clinical descriptions and diagnostic guidelines.* Geneva, Switzerland: Author.

World Health Organization. (2004). *The global burden of disease: 2004 update.* Geneva, Switzerland: Author.

PART II
Transdiagnostic Processes

CHAPTER 3

Stress and Coping
in Child and Adolescent Psychopathology

Bruce E. Compas, Kelly H. Watson, Michelle M. Reising,
and Jennifer P. Dunbar

Psychological symptoms and disorders during childhood and adolescence are characterized by several important features that shape the development of preventive interventions and treatments. First, symptoms and disorders are best characterized *both* on dimensions and as discrete categories. Second, symptom covariation and diagnostic comorbidity are the rule rather than the exception. Third, emerging models of risk and protective factors reflect processes of multifinality in which a wide range of factors are associated with increased or decreased risk for multiple rather than single problems or disorders. And fourth, regulation and dysregulation of emotional, behavioral, cognitive, and physiological processes are important protective and risk factors for most forms of psychopathology. Taken together, these characteristics of psychopathology in young people have contributed to an increasing focus on transdiagnostic models of psychopathology. In this chapter we first briefly consider several aspects of child and adolescent psychopathology that have led to the current interest in transdiagnostic approaches. We then describe evidence for exposure to stress and adversity as a broad, transdiagnostic risk factor and discuss the ways that children and adolescents cope with stress, including the regulation of emotions in response to stress, as a transdiagnostic protective factor. Finally, we present recent evidence from research on children of depressed parents as an example of the translation of research on stress and coping processes into preventive interventions to reduce risk for a wide range of problems and disorders in this high-risk group.

Dimensional and Categorical Approaches to Psychopathology in Childhood and Adolescence

The evolution of models for diagnosing and classifying psychiatric disorders in children and adolescents has followed two rather separate paths. On the one hand, discrete categorical diagnoses, including specific disorders that are hypothesized to emerge in childhood or adolescence, have been represented in the *Diagnostic and Statistical Manual of Mental Disorders* (DSM) from its inception to the current version, DSM-5 (American Psychiatric Association, 2013). In contrast, empirical models that take a dimensional and quantitative approach first identified the two broad dimensions of internalizing and externalizing problems at least 45 years ago (Achenbach, 1966) and have continued to be refined and tested across multiple cultures and age groups (e.g., Achenbach & Rescorla, 2001; Ivanova, Achenbach, Dumenci, et al., 2007; Ivanova, Achenbach, Rescorla, et al., 2007). Until recently, however, categorical and dimensional approaches have developed relatively independently.

A significant shift has occurred with the recognition of substantial problems with the categories and criteria in the DSM-IV (and more recently DSM-5) that has led to pointed calls for the integration of categorical and dimensional approaches. For example, Rutter (2011, p. 647) notes that, "At present, there are far too many diagnoses, and a ridiculously high rate of supposed comorbidity. . . . The overall number of diagnoses should be drastically reduced. Categorical and dimensional approaches to diagnosis should be combined." Similarly, Hyman (2010, p. 167) asserts that "comorbidity is so extensive among DSM-IV diagnoses . . . as to forcefully raise questions about the underlying structure and assumptions of the classification." As part of his call for changes to the DSM, Hyman recommends the use of quantitative scales as alternatives or supplements to current diagnostic criteria and a reclustering of disorders based on findings from research about underlying neural circuitry and genetics.

Along with increasing concerns about DSM categorical approach to diagnoses, continued evidence in support of the broadband factors of internalizing and externalizing psychopathology described by Achenbach (1966) is noteworthy and provides a useful framework for research on transdiagnostic processes (e.g., Krueger & Markon, 2006; Lahey, VanHulle, Singh, Waldman, & Rathouz, 2011; Seeley, Kosty, Farmer, & Lewinsohn, 2011). Diagnostic comorbidity and symptom covariation is most likely to occur within the broad syndromes of internalizing and externalizing problems. For example, anxiety disorders and mood disorders are highly comorbid, both concurrently and sequentially (e.g., Moffitt et al., 2007), and studies based on dimensional models using factor analytic methods have found that symptoms of anxiety and depression load onto a single syndrome (e.g., Ivanova, Achenbach, Dumenci, et al., 2007; Ivanova, Achenbach, Rescorla, et al., 2007). Furthermore, although somewhat less pronounced, there is also considerable comorbidity and covariation across internalizing and externalizing disorders and syndromes. For example, mood disorders and disruptive behavior disorders have high rates of co-occurrence during adolescence (e.g., Costello, Mustillo, Erkanli, Keeler, & Angold, 2003). Moreover, the broadband internalizing and externalizing syndromes are highly correlated (Achenbach & Rescorla, 2001).

If psychopathology is characterized by high levels of symptom covariation and high diagnostic co-occurrence, then a major task for researchers is the identification of transdiagnostic risk factors that can account for this co-occurrence (i.e., individual and environmental factors that predict multiple symptoms and disorders). Similarly, it is important to identify transdiagnostic protective factors that can reduce the risk for multiple problem outcomes. Both of these processes reflect the process of multifinality in which the same etiological processes may lead to multiple disorders (e.g., Cicchetti & Rogosch, 1996).

A useful heuristic for developing transdiagnostic models of psychopathology has been presented by Nolen-Hoeksema and Watkins (2011). They distinguish among distal risk factors, proximal risk factors, and possible mechanisms and moderators of the association between these levels of risk and co-occurring disorders. Distal risk factors are defined as environmental or individual characteristics that do not directly cause symptoms but rather influence symptoms through mediating processes that are more temporally or causally proximal to symptoms. Nolen-Hoeksema and Watkins propose that proximal risk factors directly influence or cause symptoms, follow distal risk factors in time, temporally precede symptoms, and mediate the relations between distal risk factors and symptoms.

Drawing on this heuristic model and perspectives on risk and protective factors in psychopathology, we present research on exposure to stressful events and chronic adversity as transdiagnostic sources of risk and discuss the ways that children and adolescents regulate their emotions and cope with stress as transdiagnostic protective factors. Stressful events and chronic adversity lead to dysregulation of core biological, emotional, cognitive, and behavioral processes (e.g., Cole & Deater-Deckard, 2009; Guerry & Hastings, 2011; Mansell, 2011; Vasilev, Crowell, Beauchaine, Mead, & Gatzke-Kopp, 2009). Conversely, efforts to cope with stress are characterized by conscious and volitional efforts to regulate emotion, cognition, behavior, physiology, and the environment in response to stressful events or circumstances (Compas, Langrock, Keller, Merchant, & Copeland, 2001). We highlight evidence for the role of stress and coping as risk and protective factors, respectively, across multiple types of symptoms and disorders.

Stressful Events and Chronic Adversity as Broad Sources of Risk

In a series of reviews, Grant and colleagues (Grant, Compas, Stuhlmacher, Thurm, & McMahon, 2003; Grant, Compas, Thurm, McMahon, & Gipson, 2004; Grant et al., 2006; McMahon, Grant, Compas, Thurm, & Ey, 2003) identified several overarching findings from research on stress and psychopathology in children and adolescents that are relevant to a transdiagnostic perspective on child and adolescent psychopathology. First, Grant and colleagues (2003) suggest that stress is best conceptualized in terms of the occurrence of acute events or chronic conditions or circumstances (referred to as stressors) that threaten the physical or mental health of the child or adolescent. The nature of events (e.g., parental divorce, family move) and chronic conditions (e.g., poverty, chronic parental conflict and discord) that constitute sources of stress vary as a function of children's development and social context. Second, more than 50 prospective longitudinal studies have provided evidence that exposure to stressful events and chronic adversity predicts increases in both internalizing and externalizing symptoms over time (Grant et al., 2004). Most important, there is substantial evidence that stressful events and adversities at one time point predict increases in both internalizing and externalizing symptoms at a later time point, suggesting that stressors may play a causal role in the development of both types of symptoms. Third, consistent with the heuristic model of Nolen-Hoeksema and Watkins (2011), exposure to stressful life events functions as a distal risk factor whose association with internalizing and externalizing symptoms is mediated by family characteristics, including disrupted parenting and parent–child relationships (Grant et al., 2003, 2006). The evidence is particularly strong for poverty and economic disadvantage as distal risk factors that affect child and adolescent internalizing and externalizing symptoms through their effects on positive and negative parenting (Grant et al., 2003).

Finally, and most germane to understanding transdiagnostic risk factors, McMahon and colleagues (2003) concluded that exposure to stressful events and chronic sources of adversity appears to operate as a nonspecific risk factor that places children and adolescents at risk for the full range of internalizing and externalizing forms of psychopathology. These authors reviewed studies of the effects of a wide range of stressors in childhood and adolescence, including exposure to violence, physical and sexual abuse, divorce or marital conflict, poverty, physical illness, and cumulative life events across multiple domains. Exposure to stressful events and adversity plays a role in virtually all types of psychopathology, including total internalizing and externalizing problems, as well as symptoms of depression, anxiety, eating disorders, aggressive behavior problems, conduct problems, substance use and abuse, and somatization.

One of the central challenges for stress researchers has been to determine whether there are unique relations between some specific types of stressors and specific disorders. McMahon and colleagues (2003) note that across the various stressors examined, the most consistent evidence for specificity was found in the association of sexual abuse with internalizing symptoms, posttraumatic stress disorder (PTSD), and sexual acting-out symptoms across several studies. Subsequent research has shown some evidence for specificity among a wider set of psychosocial risk factors that include but are not limited to stressful events (Shanahan, Copeland, Costello, & Angold, 2008). On the other hand, recent evidence from the National Comorbidity Survey Replication (Green et al., 2010) found that childhood adversities, including interpersonal loss (parental death, parental divorce, and other separation from parents or caregivers), parental maladjustment (mental illness, substance abuse, criminality, and violence), maltreatment (physical abuse, sexual abuse, and neglect), life-threatening childhood physical illness, and extreme childhood family economic adversity, were associated with all types of psychopathology in adulthood.

In summary, stressful events and conditions of chronic adversity exert demands on the regulatory capacities of children and adolescents that contribute to both internalizing and externalizing psychopathology. The comorbidity of disorders and the co-occurrence of symptoms may be the result of dysregulation in processes that are shared by multiple disorders and symptoms; alternatively, stress and adversity may simultaneously trigger the dysregulation of multiple processes that independently lead to separate but co-occurring disorders and symptoms. Based on research to date, there is very little evidence for links between specific types of stress and specific disorders.

Coping as a Broad Protective Factor

Given the importance of exposure to stress and adversity as a major source of risk for psychopathology, it follows that the ways that individuals react to and cope with stress, including but not limited to the regulation of emotions under stress, may play an important role in protecting against the development of psychological symptoms and disorder. In an earlier review of the literature on coping with stress during childhood and adolescence, Compas and colleagues (2001) found evidence that several subtypes of coping were significantly related to both internalizing and externalizing symptoms. For example, the findings generally suggested that engagement forms of coping (i.e., coping efforts directed at the source of stress or one's reactions to the stressor) were related to lower levels of both internalizing and externalizing symptoms, whereas disengagement forms of coping (i.e., coping efforts oriented away from the source of stress or one's reactions to the stressor) were related to higher levels of both types of problems. However, the review by Compas and colleagues was constrained by limitations in the conceptualization and measurement of coping in children and youth up to that time.

A clearer pattern of findings from research on coping in childhood and adolescence can be found in more recent studies guided by a control-based model of coping with stress (Compas, Jaser, Dunn, & Rodriguez, 2012). Within this model, responses to stress are first distinguished along the dimension of automatic versus controlled processes. Coping responses are considered controlled, volitional efforts to regulate cognition, behavior, emotion, and physiological processes, as well as aspects of the environment, in response to stress. Coping responses are further distinguished as primary control engagement (problem solving, emotional modulation, emotional expression), secondary control engagement (acceptance, cognitive reappraisal, positive thinking, distraction), or disengagement (cognitive and behavioral avoidance, denial, wishful thinking). This model has been supported in seven confirmatory factor analytic studies with children, adolescents, and adults coping with a wide range of stressors (e.g., peer stressors, war-related stressors, family stressors, economic stressors, chronic pain, cancer), from diverse socioeconomic and cultural backgrounds and international samples (e.g., European American, Native American Indian, Spanish, Bosnian, Chinese), using multiple informants (Benson et al., 2011; Compas, Beckjord, et al., 2006; Compas, Boyer, et al., 2006; Connor-Smith & Calvete, 2004; Connor-Smith, Compas, Wadsworth, Thomsen, & Saltzman, 2000; Wadsworth, Raviv, Compas, & Connor-Smith, 2005; Yao et al., 2010).

Given the focus on processes of emotion regulation in some current research on transdiagnostic processes (e.g., Nolen-Hoeksema & Watkins, 2011), it is important to note the relation between current conceptualizations of coping and emotion regulation. Coping is at once both *broader* and *more specific* than emotion regulation (Compas, Jaser, & Benson, 2009). Specifically, coping refers to the regulation of emotions *and* other important psychological and biological processes; as such, emotion regulation can be seen as a subset of coping. For example, emotion modulation (e.g., "I keep my feelings under control when I have to, then let them out when they won't make things worse") is part of primary control coping. On the other hand, coping refers to emotion regulation under a *specific* set of circumstances; that is, in response to stress. Because emotion regulation is an ongoing process that occurs under both stressful and nonstressful circumstances, coping is a special case of emotion regulation under stress (e.g., Eisenberg et al., 2001).

Primary control, secondary control, and disengagement coping have been tested in relation to internalizing and externalizing symptoms in three ways (see Figure 3.1). In Model 1 in Figure 3.1, primary control, secondary control, and disengagement coping are examined in relation to a single disorder. Studies using this design cannot address the role of

Model 1:

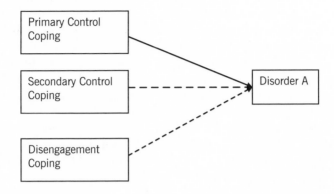

Model 2:

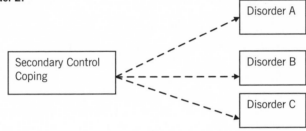

Model 3:

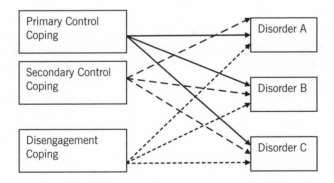

FIGURE 3.1. Models testing the role of coping as a transdiagnostic process in internalizing and externalizing psychopathology.

coping as a transdiagnostic process by virtue of their inclusion of only one type of disorder or problem. Model 2 studies examine one type of coping in relation to multiple disorders or problems. These studies provide potentially important evidence for the role of coping in relation to different disorders and therefore provide transdiagnostic information that is specific to one type of coping. The optimal design for purposes of identifying transdiagnostic processes is represented in Model 3, in which multiple types of coping are examined in relation to multiple types of disorders and problems. This design allows for a complete analysis of the role of each type of coping in relation to multiple problems and disorders and can account for comorbidity among problems and disorders and correlations among the three types of coping. Such an analysis would also permit identifying coping processes that have unique effects for single disorders.

There is considerable evidence that primary control, secondary control, and disengagement coping are all related to a range of internalizing and externalizing symptoms. We have summarized examples of studies with findings bearing on this question in Table 3.1. We have included studies that reflect each of the three models of coping and psychopathology presented in Figure 3.1. For example, a study by Rhoades and colleagues (2007) reflects Model 1, as these investigators examined the association of all three types of coping with a composite measure of internalizing symptoms. Jaser and colleagues (2011) also provides an example of a Model 1 study in their investigation of affective symptoms in children of depressed parents. They found significant associations between primary control, secondary control, and disengagement coping and symptoms of depression. Flynn and Rudolph (2007) found that adolescents' self-reported depressive symptoms were negatively correlated with their use of primary control and secondary control coping but that depressive symptoms were unrelated to disengagement coping strategies. However, none of these studies provides evidence for transdiagnostic processes because only one type of symptom was measured. Although Model 1 studies are useful in understanding relations between coping and specific types of psychopathology, studies using this design may overlook relationships between coping and a wider range of disorders or symptoms because other types of disorders/symptoms are not measured.

An example of Model 2 is found in a study by Jaser and colleagues (2007) in which secondary control coping was examined in relation to affective symptoms and oppositional–defiant problems in children of depressed parents. Children's use of secondary control coping was related to lower levels of both affective symptoms and oppositional–defiant behavior problems. However, neither primary control nor disengagement coping was examined in this study. Thus, although Model 2 studies can provide some evidence about the role of specific subtypes of coping as

TABLE 3.1. Examples of Empirical Studies of Relations between Coping and Psychopathology

Authors	Study design	Sample	Stressor	Symptoms or disorders	Internalizing problems	Externalizing problems
Fear et al. (2009)	Model 3	152 parents with a history of depression and their 204 children (ages 9–15 years, M = 11.5)	Parental depression	Anxiety/depression symptoms (composite YSR and CBCL) Aggression symptoms (composite CBCL and YSR)	Primary control coping: r = -.19 Secondary control coping: r = -.38 Disengagement coping: ns	Primary control coping: r = -.26 Secondary control coping: r = -.36 Disengagement coping: ns
Flynn & Rudolph (2007)	Model 1	510 adolescents (ages 9–15 years, M = 11.7) Calculated correlations based on level of stress reported (low vs. high)	Peer stress	Children's Depression Inventory (CDI)	Primary control coping; r's ranging from -.18 to -.32 Secondary control coping; r's ranging from -.48 to -.60 Disengagement coping; ns	Not tested
Jaser et al. (2005)	Model 3	57 parents with history of depression and their 78 children (ages 10–16 years, M = 12.8)	Parental depression	Anxiety/depression symptoms (composite YSR and CBCL) Aggression symptoms (composite YSR and CBCL)	Primary control coping: ns/ns Secondary control coping: r = -.53/r = -.26 Disengagement coping: ns/ns	Primary control coping: ns/r = -.32 Secondary control coping: r = -.32/ns Disengagement coping: ns/r = .26

(continued)

TABLE 3.1. *(continued)*

Authors	Study design	Sample	Stressor	Symptoms or disorders	Internalizing problems	Externalizing problems
Jaser et al. (2007)	Model 3	50 parents with history of depression and their 73 children (ages 10–16 years, M = 12.7)	Family stress	Anxiety/depression symptoms (composite YSR and CBCL); Aggression symptoms (composite YSR and CBCL)	Primary control coping: ns/ns; Secondary control coping: $r = -.51/ns$; Disengagement coping: ns/ns	Primary control coping: $-.24/ns$; Secondary control coping: $r = -.27/ns$; Disengagement coping: ns/ns
Jaser et al. (2008)	Model 2	34 mothers with history of depression, 38 mothers with no history of depression, and their 72 children (ages 11–14 years, M = 12.2)	Parental depression	Affective symptoms (composite YSR and CBCL); Oppositional–defiant problems (composite YSR and CBCL); Depression symptoms (CDI)	Primary control coping: not tested; Secondary control coping and affective symptoms: $r = -.44$; Secondary control coping and depression symptoms: $r = -.46$; Disengagement coping: not tested	Primary control coping: not tested; Secondary control coping: $r = -.57$; Disengagement coping: not tested
Jaser et al. (2011)	Model 1	34 mothers with history of depression, 38 mothers with no history of depression, and their 72 children (ages 11–14 years, M = 12.2)	Parental depression	Affective problems (composite CBCL and YSR)	Primary control coping: $r = -.53$; Secondary control coping: $r = -.59$; Disengagement coping: $r = .50$	Not tested

44

Study	Model	Sample	Stressor	Outcome		
Langrock et al. (2002)	Model 3	66 depressed parents and their 101 children (ages 7-17 years, M = 11.5)	Parental depression	Anxiety/depression symptoms (CBCL) / Aggression symptoms (CBCL)	Primary control coping: ns Secondary control coping: r = -.45 Disengagement coping: ns	Primary control coping: r = -.20 Secondary control coping: r = -.37 Disengagement coping: ns
Raviv & Wadsworth (2010)	Model 3	24 children (ages 8-12 years, M = 10)	Economic stress	Internalizing symptoms (CBCL) / Externalizing Symptoms (CBCL)	Primary control coping: r = -.74 Secondary control coping: r = -.66 Disengagement coping: (ns)	Primary control coping: r = -.67 Secondary control coping: r = -.57 Disengagement coping: ns
Rhoades, McIntosh, Wadsworth, et al. (2007)	Model 1	154 middle school students (ages 11-14 years, M = 12.2)		Internalizing composite: depression, anxiety, and PTSD	Primary control coping: r = -.20 Secondary control coping: r = -.50 Disengagement coping: ns	Not tested
Wadsworth & Berger (2006)	Model 3	79 adolescents (M = 14.5 years)	Economic strain and family conflict composites (assessed at Time 1)	Anxious/depressed behavior (YSR, Time 2) / Aggressive behavior (YSR, Time 2)	Primary control coping: ns Secondary control coping: ns Disengagement coping: r = .23	Primary control coping: ns Secondary control coping: ns Disengagement coping: ns

(continued)

45

TABLE 3.1. (continued)

Authors	Study design	Sample	Stressor	Symptoms or disorders	Internalizing problems	Externalizing problems
Wadsworth & Berger (2006) (continued)					Primary control coping; anxious/depressed behavior at Time 1 (YSR) and primary control coping at Time 2 (8 months later): $r = -.22$; Secondary control coping; anxious/depressed behavior at Time 1 (YSR) and secondary control coping at Time 2: ns; Disengagement coping; anxious/depressed behavior at Time 1 and disengagement coping at Time 2: ns	Primary control coping; aggressive behavior at Time 1 (YSR) and primary control coping at Time 2 (8 months later): $r = -.25$; Secondary control coping; aggressive behavior at Time 1 and secondary control coping at Time 2: $r = -.27$; Disengagement coping; aggressive behavior at Time 1 and disengagement coping at Time 2: ns
Wadsworth & Compas (2002)	Model 3	364 7th- to 12th-grade students ($M = 14.7$ years)	Economic strain	Anxiety/depression symptoms (YSR); Aggression symptoms (YSR)	Primary control coping: $r = -.18$; Secondary control coping: $r = -.28$; Disengagement coping: $r = .29$	Primary control coping: $r = -.20$; Secondary control coping: $r = -.28$; Disengagement coping: $r = .32$

Study	Predictor	Anxiety/depression symptoms (YSR)	Aggression symptoms (YSR)
Wadsworth & Santiago (2008) Model 3 164 children (n = 82, 6–10 years, n = 82, 11–18 years)	Family conflict	Primary control coping: r = -.27 Secondary control coping: r = -.38 Disengagement coping: r = .27	Primary control coping: r = -.32 Secondary control coping: r = -.41 Disengagement coping: r = .29
	Economic strain	Primary control coping; anxious/depressed (CBCL & YSR composite): r = -.29 Secondary control coping; anxious/depressed: r = -.50 Disengagement coping; anxious/depressed: ns Primary control coping; withdrawn/depressed (CBCL & YSR composite): r = -.30 Secondary control coping; withdrawn/depressed: r = -.36 Disengagement coping; withdrawn/depressed: r = .13	Primary control coping; delinquent problems (CBCL & YSR composite): r = -.18 Secondary control coping; delinquent problems: r = -.36 Disengagement coping; delinquent problems: r = .13 Primary control coping; aggressive behavior (CBCL & YSR composite): r = -.18 Secondary control coping; aggressive behavior: r = -.20 Disengagement coping; aggressive behavior: r = .15-

Note. All correlations statistically significant at $p < .05$. We focused on adolescent self-reports of coping. The *r*'s that appear before the slash represent child self-reports of problems; those that appear after the slash represent parent reports of child problems. CBCL, Child Behavior Checklist; YSR, Youth Self-Report; PTSD, posttraumatic stress disorder.

transdiagnostic factors, these studies also may mistakenly lead to conclusions about the role of a specific type of coping because other coping strategies are not measured.

In several studies, representing Model 3, multiple subtypes of coping were tested in relation to multiple types of internalizing and externalizing symptoms (Fear et al., 2009; Jaser et al., 2005, 2007; Langrock, Compas, Keller, Merchant, & Copeland, 2002; Raviv & Wadsworth, 2010; Rhoades et al., 2007; Wadsworth & Berger, 2006; Wadsworth & Compas, 2002; Wadsworth & Santiago, 2008). These studies are the strongest in testing the role of coping as a general (transdiagnostic) versus disorder-specific process. For example, in two studies of adolescents coping with economic stressors, Wadsworth and Compas (2002) and Wadsworth and Santiago (2008) found significant relationships between primary control and secondary control coping and subtypes of both internalizing (depression, anxiety) and externalizing (aggression, delinquent) symptoms and problems. Specifically, greater use of both types of coping was related to lower levels of all types of symptoms. In contrast, disengagement coping was associated with higher levels of internalizing and externalizing symptoms (Wadsworth & Compas, 2002; Wadsworth & Santiago, 2008).

The significant associations between coping and both internalizing and externalizing disorders and symptoms suggest that coping plays a role in regulating a range of emotions, behaviors, and physiological processes. If coping is involved with the regulation of anxiety, sadness, and anger, this would lead to associations with symptoms of anxiety disorders, mood disorders, and disruptive behavior problems. Furthermore, some types of coping may resolve or reduce sources of stress that drive the development of both internalizing and externalizing symptoms and disorders. It is noteworthy that most of the prior research has examined symptoms of internalizing and externalizing problems and has not examined the relations between coping and categorical diagnoses. However, given the recent emphasis on the importance of dimensional approaches to psychopathology (e.g., Hyman, 2010; Rutter, 2011), this is not inherently a liability of this research.

Children of Depressed Parents: An Example of Transdiagnostic Processes in Risk, Protection, and Intervention

We now turn our attention to a high-risk group, children whose parents suffer from depression, to exemplify the role of stress and coping processes in the development of a wide range of disorders and how these processes can inform the development of preventive interventions to reduce risk and promote resilience. Children of depressed parents are at high risk for *both* internalizing and externalizing psychopathology, including a two- to threefold increased risk of developing depressive disorders (England & Sim, 2009). As much as 50–80% of offspring of depressed parents (i.e., 7.5–12 million children) will likely meet criteria for a psychiatric disorder by young adulthood (England & Sim, 2009). Adolescence marks a particularly important developmental period for increased depression risk, as rates are relatively low during childhood and increase significantly by mid-adolescence (e.g., Hankin et al., 1998). Thus offspring of depressed parents in early to middle adolescence (10–15 years old) are an ideal target for prevention, given their high risk for the development of depression, anxiety, and externalizing behavior problems (England & Sim, 2009). Risk and protective factors for children of depressed parents include biological, psychological, and interpersonal processes (Goodman & Gotlib, 1999). Exposure to chronic stress within the family and the ways in which children and adolescents cope with this stress are two important sources of risk and protection for internalizing and externalizing psychopathology in offspring of depressed parents.

Stress and Parental Depression

Depressive symptoms and episodes of major depression in parents contribute to three types of stressors within the family—parental withdrawal, parental intrusiveness, and marital conflict (e.g., Fear et al., 2009; Jaser et al., 2005; Langrock et al., 2002). Many or most depressed parents vacillate between being emotionally and physically withdrawn from and unavailable to their children and being irritable and overly intrusive in their interactions with their children. These types of parental behaviors most likely lead to low levels of both warmth and structure and create an unpredictable environment for children. Stressors related to both parental withdrawal and parental intrusiveness are related to internalizing and externalizing symptoms in children of depressed parents (e.g., Langrock et al., 2002). Furthermore, exposure to these stressors is associated with heightened levels of stress reactivity, including physiological and emotional arousal (Jaser et al., 2005; Langrock et al., 2002).

Coping with Parental Depression

Several studies have examined children's use of primary control, secondary control, and disengagement coping to manage the stress related to living with a depressed parent (Fear et al., 2009; Jaser et al., 2005, 2007, 2008, 2011; Langrock et al., 2002). There is consistent evidence for relations between secondary control coping and subtypes of both internalizing and externalizing problems, as all of the studies that tested these associations found that secondary control coping was related to subtypes of *both* internalizing problems (r's ranging from –.26 to –.53) and externalizing problems (r's ranging from –.27 to –.57; Fear et al., 2009; Jaser et al. 2005, 2007, 2008; Langrock et al., 2002). In contrast, less consistent evidence has been reported for relations between primary control coping and psychological outcomes in response to this stressor. For example, evidence for associations between externalizing problems and primary control coping was either significant (r's ranging from –.20 to –.32; Fear et al., 2009; Jaser et al. 2005, 2007; Langrock et al., 2002) or the relations were not tested (Jaser et al., 2008, 2011). Evidence for associations between internalizing problems and primary control coping was more limited in that only two of the five studies found a significant relation (r's ranging from –.19 to –.53; Fear et al., 2009; Jaser et al., 2011). Overall, evidence for relations between disengagement coping and subtypes of internalizing and externalizing problems is less consistent. On the one hand, a number of studies found no evidence for associations between disengagement coping and subtypes of internalizing or externalizing problems (Fear et al., 2009; Jaser et al., 2007; Langrock et al., 2002). On the other hand, Jaser and colleagues (2005) found that disengagement coping was related to higher levels of parent-reported aggressive symptoms in their children ($r = .26$), although not significantly related to internalizing problems. Furthermore, Jaser and colleagues (2011) found that disengagement coping was related to higher levels of affective symptoms ($r = .50$) but did not test its relation to subtypes of externalizing problems. Taken as a whole, there is considerable evidence that the ways in which children and adolescents cope in families with a history of depression are related to *both* internalizing and externalizing problems; however, the findings suggest that the associations depend on the specific subtype of coping used and who is reporting psychological symptoms (i.e., parent or child).

Prevention of Internalizing and Externalizing Symptoms and Disorders in Children of Depressed Parents

Drawing on evidence for the importance of stress and coping in families of depressed parents, Compas, Forehand, Keller, and colleagues developed and tested the initial efficacy of a family group cognitive-behavioral (FGCB) preventive intervention for parents with a history of depression and their children (Compas, Keller, & Forehand, 2011; Compas et al., 2001). The preventive intervention is designed to reduce stressful parent–child interactions that are associated with parental withdrawal and irritability or intrusiveness and to enhance children's and parents' use of secondary control engagement coping strategies to reduce the risk for symptoms and disorder in these children.

The FGCB intervention is a manualized 12-session program (8 weekly and 4 monthly follow-up sessions) that is designed to teach coping skills to families with a parent who has a history of a depressive disorder in a small-family-group format. Each family group includes four families and is led by both a mental health professional with extensive training in group facilitation and a doctoral student in clinical psychology. The program is designed for participation by both parents and children. Goals are to educate families about depressive disorders, to increase family awareness of the impact of stress and depression on functioning, to help families recognize and monitor stress, to facilitate the development of children's adaptive coping responses to stress, and to improve parenting skills. Information is presented to group members during 8 weekly sessions, practice and discussion of skills are facilitated during the sessions, and all members are given weekly at-home practice exercises. Four monthly follow-up booster sessions are included to provide additional practice and support in continued development and refinement of the skills learned in the initial weekly sessions.

The intervention is designed to address the hypothesized mediators of the effects of parental depression on children: parental depressive symptoms and negative affect, stressful parent–child interactions, and children's coping with these stressors. The intervention sessions include separate modules targeting parenting skills and children's coping skills. Specifically, the parenting component of the intervention includes building skills to increase parental warmth and involvement with their children, as well as increasing structure and consequences for children's problem behavior. Children are taught skills to cope with their parents' depression, including the use of acceptance, distraction, and cognitive reappraisal.

The coping skills that are taught and practiced as part of the program are designed to enhance the development of secondary control coping strategies (cognitive restructuring, acceptance, distraction) in participants. The research previously summarized has shown that these strategies are effective in coping with stressful parent–child interactions associated with parental depression. One goal of the FGCB intervention is to increase these skills in the children and adolescents coping with depression in their families. Parents are taught to support their children's use of these skills, and they also are encouraged to practice these skills themselves.

The parenting modules of this intervention are drawn from well-established, empirically supported programs for parent training designed to address issues of oppositional behavior in children and adolescents (e.g., Forehand & McMahon, 1981; McMahon & Forehand, 2003) and are similar to modules used in parenting interventions for the treatment of childhood anxiety (e.g., Barrett, Dadds, & Rapee, 1996; Dadds, Spence, Holland, Barrett, & Laurens, 1997; Dadds et al., 1999). The parenting sessions focus on the teaching of basic parenting skills, with an emphasis on areas that are likely to be affected by depression, such as consistency, structure, parental responsiveness, parent–child communication, and involvement in family activities.

The initial efficacy of the intervention has been tested in a clinical trial in which families were randomized to the FGCB intervention or to a written information (WI) comparison condition in which parents and children received information about the nature of depression and its effects on families but did not participate in the group intervention and were not taught coping or parenting skills. Significant effects on children's (ages 9–15 years) mental health favoring the FGCB intervention were found at 2-, 6-, and 12-month follow-ups (Compas, Forehand, et al., 2009), and these effects were generally maintained at 18 months, whereas some effects were found to dissipate at 24 months (Compas, Forehand, et al., 2011). Most pertinent to transdiagnostic processes, the FGCB intervention led to significantly lower levels of Youth Self-Report (YSR) internalizing symptoms at 2, 6, 12, and 18 months and significantly lower externalizing symptoms at 12, 18, and 24 months. There was also an effect for the intervention on a specific YSR measure of depressive symptoms at 12 months and mixed anxiety and depression symptoms at 2, 6, 12, and 18 months. Effects on parents' reports of their children's symptoms were quite limited, with the only significant effect occurring for externalizing symptoms on the Child Behavior Checklist (CBCL) at 12 months. Finally, the FGCB intervention had a significant effect on children's episodes of major depression as measured by diagnostic interviews with the parents and children. Over the 24 months from baseline, fewer children in the FGCB intervention experienced a major depressive episode (14.3%) than children in the WI comparison condition (32.7%); odds ratio = 2.91 (95% CI = 1.12 to 7.58, p = .025).

Mediational analyses examined whether changes in children's coping and changes in parenting behaviors accounted for the effects of the FGCB on children's mental health outcomes. Specifically, changes in coping from baseline to the 6-month follow-up were examined as mediators of the effects of the intervention on children's internalizing and externalizing symptoms at 12 months (Compas et al., 2010). This design allowed for a test of the temporal precedence of changes in coping and parenting in relation to children's mental health. Significant effects were found for changes in children's coping as a mediator of the intervention, as changes in secondary control coping from baseline to 6 months mediated intervention effects on changes in children's depression, mixed anxiety and depression, internalizing, and externalizing symptoms from baseline to 12-month follow-up. Anecdotally, we also tested for possible effects of the intervention on children's primary control coping, and there were no significant effects; that is, the intervention was specific in its effects on secondary control coping. Thus strong evidence was found for secondary control coping as a transdiagnostic protective factor for both internalizing and externalizing symptoms.

Summary and Future Directions

There is now considerable support for the role of stress and coping as important transdiagnostic processes in internalizing and externalizing psychopathology in children and adolescents. Several areas are of high priority for future research.

Stress as a Transdiagnostic Risk Factor

At a broad level, exposure to stressful events and circumstances that are characterized by chronic levels of adversity (e.g., poverty) are associated with all subtypes of internalizing and externalizing psychopathology during childhood and adolescence. The strongest evidence for these associations comes from prospective studies in which stressful events and adversity predict increases in symptoms over a period of months or years (Grant et al., 2004). Furthermore, chronic adversities in childhood are associated with all types of psychopathology in adulthood, suggesting lasting, long-term nonspecific effects of exposure to stress early in development (Green et al., 2010).

Coping as a Transdiagnostic Protective Factor

Support has been found for the association between three subtypes of coping (primary control, secondary control, disengagement) within a control-based model of coping and symptoms of internalizing and externalizing psychopathology. The evidence is strongest for the role of primary control and secondary control coping as protective factors in coping with several different types of stressors and chronic conditions. The evidence is less clear with regard to disengagement coping, but some studies have shown that this subtype of coping is associated with increased risk for both internalizing and externalizing symptoms. Furthermore, there is now evidence that interventions to enhance at least secondary control coping can lead to reductions in both internalizing and externalizing symptoms.

Directions for Future Research

First, research is needed that provides a closer examination of specificity in relations between types of stressor and types of psychopathology. Second, further delineation of the mechanisms linking stress to psychopathology is a high priority. For example, research is needed on the links between distal risk factors (e.g., chronic adversity due to poverty), proximal risk mediators and moderators (e.g., parenting), and types of psychopathology. Third, although there is considerable evidence for the association between coping and internalizing and externalizing symptoms in cross-sectional studies, prospective studies of coping and psychopathology are needed. Moreover, the vast majority of stress and coping research has used dimensional measures of psychopathology; future research using categorical diagnostic measures is needed. We anticipate that similar effects will be found with categorical measures, but this needs to be tested. Fourth, similar to the need for studies of the mechanisms of stress, further research is needed to understand how coping affects diverse disorders and symptoms. And finally, continued development and testing of interventions to reduce exposure to stress and enhance coping skills on a wide range of types of psychopathology are needed.

REFERENCES

Achenbach, T. (1966). The classification of children's psychiatric symptoms: A factor-analytic study. *Psychological Monographs: General and Applied, 80*, 1–37.

Achenbach, T. M., & Rescorla, L. A. (2001). *Manual for ASEBA School-Age Forms and Profiles.* Burlington: University of Vermont, Research Center for Children, Youth, and Families.

American Psychiatric Association. (2013). *Diagnostic and statistical manual of mental disorders* (5th ed.). Arlington, VA: Author.

Barrett, P. M., Dadds, M. R., & Rapee, R. M. (1996). Family treatment of childhood anxiety: A controlled trial. *Journal of Consulting and Clinical Psychology, 64*, 333–342.

Benson, M. A., Compas, B. E., Layne, C. M., Vandergrift, N., Pasalic, H., Katalinski, R., et al. (2011). Measurement of post-war coping and stress responses: A study of Bosnian adolescents. *Journal of Applied Developmental Psychology 32,* 323–335.

Cicchetti, D., & Rogosch, F. A. (1996). Equifinality and multifinality in developmental psychopathology. *Development and Psychopathology, 8*, 597–600.

Cole, P. M., & Deater-Deckard, K. (2009). Emotion regulation, risk and psychopathology. *Journal of Child Psychology and Psychiatry, 50*, 1327–1330.

Compas, B. E., Beckjord, E., Agocha, B., Sherman, M. L., Langrock, A., Grossman, C., et al. (2006). Measurement of coping and stress responses in women with breast cancer. *Psycho-Oncology, 15*, 1038–1054.

Compas, B. E., Boyer, M. C., Stanger, C., Colletti, R. B., Thomsen, A. H., Dufton, L. M., et al. (2006). Latent variable analysis of coping, anxiety/depression, and somatic symptoms in adolescents with chronic pain. *Journal of Consulting and Clinical Psychology, 74*, 1132–1142.

Compas, B. E., Champion, J. E., Forehand, R., Cole, D. A., Reeslund, K. L., Fear, J., et al. (2010). Coping and parenting: Mediators of 12-month outcomes of a family group cognitive-behavioral preventive intervention with families of depressed parents. *Journal of Consulting and Clinical Psychology, 78,* 623–634.

Compas, B. E., Forehand, R., Keller, G., Champion, A., Reeslund, K. L., McKee, L., et al. (2009). Randomized controlled trial of a family cognitive-behavioral preventive intervention for children of depressed parents. *Journal of Consulting and Clinical Psychology, 77,* 1009–1020.

Compas, B. E., Forehand, R., Thigpen, J. C., Keller, G., Hardcastle, E. J., Cole, D. A., et al. (2011). Family group cognitive-behavioral preventive intervention for families of depressed parents: 18- and 24-month outcomes. *Journal of Consulting and Clinical Psychology, 79,* 488–499.

Compas, B. E., Jaser, S. S., & Benson, M. (2009). Coping and emotion regulation: Implications for understanding depression during adolescence. In S. Nolen-Hoeksema & L. Hilt (Eds.), *Handbook of depression in adolescents* (pp. 419–440). New York: Routledge/Taylor & Francis.

Compas, B. E., Jaser, S., Dunn, M. J., & Rodriguez, E. M. (2012). Coping with chronic illness in childhood and adolescence. *Annual Review of Clinical Psychology, 8,* 455–480.

Compas, B. E., Keller, G., & Forehand, R. (2011). Preventive intervention in families of depressed parents: A family cognitive-behavioral intervention. In T. J. Strauman, P. R. Costanzo, & J. Garber (Eds.), *Depression in adolescent girls: Science and prevention* (pp. 318–340). New York: Guilford Press.

Compas, B. E., Langrock, A. M., Keller, G., Merchant, M. J., & Copeland, M. E. (2001). Children coping with parental depression: Processes of adaptation to family stress. In S. H. Goodman & I. H. Gotlib (Eds.), *Children of depressed parents: Mechanisms of risk and implications for treatment* (pp. 227–252). Washington, DC: American Psychological Association.

Connor-Smith, J. K., & Calvete, E. (2004). Cross-cultural equivalence of coping and involuntary responses to stress in Spain and the United States. *Anxiety, Stress, and Coping, 17,* 163–185.

Connor-Smith, J. K., Compas, B. E., Wadsworth, M. E., Thomsen, A. H., & Saltzman, H. (2000). Responses to stress in adolescence: Measurement of coping and involuntary stress responses. *Journal of Consulting and Clinical Psychology, 68,* 976–992.

Costello, E. J., Mustillo, S., Erkanli, A., Keeler, G., & Angold, A. (2003). Prevalence and development of psychiatric disorders in childhood and adolescence. *Archives of General Psychiatry, 60,* 837–844.

Dadds, M. R., Holland, D. E., Laurens, K. R., Mullins, M., Barrett, P. M., & Spence, S. (1999). Early intervention and prevention of anxiety disorders in children: Results at 2-year follow-up. *Journal of Consulting and Clinical Psychology, 67,* 145–150.

Dadds, M. R., Spence, S. H., Holland, D., Barrett, P. H., & Laurens, K. (1997). Early intervention and prevention of anxiety disorders: A controlled trial. *Journal of Consulting and Clinical Psychology, 65,* 627–635.

Eisenberg, N., Cumberland, A., Spinrad, T. L., Fabes, R. A., Shepard, S. A., Reiser, M., et al. (2001). The relations of regulation and emotionality to children's externalizing and internalizing problem behavior. *Child Development, 72,* 1112–1134.

England, M. J., & Sim, L. J. (Eds.). (2009). *Depression in parents, parenting, and children: Opportunities to improve identification, treatment, and prevention.* Washington, DC: National Academies Press.

Fear, J. M., Champion, J. E., Reeslund, K. L., Forehand, R., Colletti, C., Roberts, L., et al. (2009). Parental depression and interparental conflict: Adolescents' self-blame and coping responses. *Journal of Family Psychology, 23,* 762–766.

Flynn, M., & Rudolph, K. D. (2007). Perceptual asymmetry and youths' responses to stress: Understanding vulnerability to depression. *Cognition and Emotion, 21,* 773–788.

Forehand, R. L., & McMahon, R. J. (1981). *Helping the noncompliant child: A clinician's guide to parent training.* New York: Guilford Press.

Goodman, S. H., & Gotlib, I. H. (1999). Risk for psychopathology in the children of depressed mothers: A developmental model for understanding mechanisms of transmission. *Psychological Review, 106,* 458–490.

Grant, K. E., Compas, B. E., Stuhlmacher, A. F., Thurm, A. E., & McMahon, S. D. (2003). Stress and child/adolescent psychopathology: Moving from markers to mechanisms of risk. *Psychological Bulletin, 129,* 447–466.

Grant, K. E., Compas, B. E., Thurm, A. E., McMahon, S. D., & Gipson, P. Y. (2004). Stressors and child/adolescent psychopathology: Measurement issues and prospective effects. *Journal of Clinical Child and Adolescent Psychology, 33,* 412–425.

Grant, K. E., Compas, B. E., Thurm, A. E., McMahon, S. D., Gipson, P. Y., Campbell, A. J., et al. (2006). Stressors and child and adolescent psychopathology: Evidence of moderating and mediating effects. *Clinical Psychology Review, 26,* 257–283.

Green, J. G., McLaughlin, K. A., Berglund, P. A., Gruber, M. J., Sampson, N. A., Zaslavsky, A. M., et al.(2010). Childhood adversities and adult psychiatric disorders in the National Comorbidity Survey Replication I: Associations with first onset of DSM-IV disorders. *Archives of General Psychiatry, 67,* 113–123.

Guerry, J. D., & Hastings, P. D. (2011). In search of HPA axis dysregulation in child and adolescent depression. *Clinical Child and Family Psychology Review, 14,* 135–160.

Hankin, B. L., Abramson, L. Y., Moffitt, T. E., Silva, P. A., McGee, R., & Angell, K. E. (1998). Development of depression from preadolescence to young adulthood: Emerging gender differences in a 10-year longitudinal study. *Journal of Abnormal Psychology, 107,* 128–140.

Hyman, S. E. (2010). The diagnosis of mental disorders: The problem of reification. *Annual Review of Clinical Psychology, 6,* 155–179.

Ivanova, M. Y., Achenbach, T. M., Dumenci, L., Rescorla, L. A., Almqvist, F., Weintraub, S., et al. (2007). Testing the 8-syndrome structure of the Child Behavior Checklist in 30 societies. *Journal of Clinical Child and Adolescent Psychology, 36,* 405–417.

Ivanova, M. Y., Achenbach, T. M., Rescorla, L. A., Dumenci, L., Almqvist, F., Bilenberg, N., et al. (2007). The generalizability of the Youth Self-Report syndrome structure in 23 societies. *Journal of Consulting and Clinical Psychology, 75,* 729–738.

Jaser, S. S., Champion, J. E., Dharamsi, K. R., Reising, M. M., & Compas, B. E. (2011). Coping and positive affect in adolescents of mothers with and without a history of depression. *Journal of Child and Family Studies, 20,* 353–360.

Jaser, S. S., Champion, J. E., Reeslund, K., Keller, G., Merchant, M. J., Benson, M., et al. (2007). Cross-situational coping with peer and family stressors in adolescent offspring of depressed parents. *Journal of Adolescence, 30*, 917–932.

Jaser, S. S., Fear, J. M., Reeslund, K. L., Champion, J. E., Reising, M. M., & Compas, B. E. (2008). Maternal sadness and adolescents' responses to stress in offspring of mothers with and without a history of depression. *Journal of Clinical Child and Adolescent Psychology, 37*, 736–746.

Jaser, S. S., Langrock, A. M., Keller, G., Merchant, M. J., Benson, M., Reeslund, K., et al. (2005). Coping with the stress of parental depression: II. Adolescent and parent reports of coping and adjustment. *Journal of Clinical Child and Adolescent Psychology, 34*, 193–205.

Krueger, R. F., & Markon, K. E. (2006). Reinterpreting comorbidity: A model-based approach to understanding and classifying psychopathology. *Annual Review of Clinical Psychology, 2*, 111–133.

Lahey, B. B., Van Hulle, C. A., Singh, A. L., Waldman, I. D., & Rathouz, P. J. (2011). Higher-order genetic and environmental structure of prevalent forms of child and adolescent psychopathology. *Archives of General Psychiatry, 68*, 181–189.

Langrock, A. M., Compas, B. E., Keller, G., Merchant, M. J., & Copeland, M. E. (2002). Coping with the stress of parental depression: Parents' reports of children's coping and emotional/behavioral problems. *Journal of Clinical Child and Adolescent Psychology, 31*, 312–324.

Mansell, W. (2011). Core processes of psychopathology and recovery: "Does the Dodo bird effect have wings?". *Clinical Psychology Review, 31*, 189–192.

McMahon, R. J., & Forehand, R. L. (2003). *Helping the noncompliant child: Family-based treatment for oppositional behavior* (2nd ed.). New York: Guilford Press.

McMahon, S. D., Grant, K. E., Compas, B. E., Thurm, A. E., & Ey, S. (2003). Stress and psychopathology in children and adolescents: Is there evidence of specificity? *Journal of Child Psychology and Psychiatry, 44*, 1–27.

Moffitt, T. E., Harrington, H., Caspi, A., Kim-Cohen, J., Goldberg, D., Gregory, A. M., et al. (2007). Depression and generalized anxiety disorder: Cumulative and sequential comorbidity in a birth cohort followed prospectively to 32 years. *Archives of General Psychiatry, 64*, 651–660.

Nolen-Hoeksema, S., & Watkins, E. R. (2011). A heuristic for developing transdiagnostic models of psychopathology: Explaining multifinality and divergent trajectories. *Perspectives on Psychological Science, 6*, 589–609.

Raviv, T., & Wadsworth, M. E. (2010). The efficacy of a pilot prevention program for children and caregivers coping with economic strain. *Cognitive Therapy and Research, 34*, 216–228.

Rhoades, G. K., McIntosh, D. N., Wadsworth, M. E., Ahlkvist, J. A., Burwell, R. A., Gudmundsen, G. R., et al. (2007). Forgiving the perpetrators of September 11th: Associations with religiosity, responses to stress, and psychological distress. *Anxiety, Stress, and Coping, 20*, 109–128.

Rutter, M. (2011). Research review: Child psychiatric diagnosis and classification: Concepts, findings, challenges, and potential. *Journal of Child Psychology and Psychiatry, 52*, 647–660.

Seeley, J. R., Kosty, D. B., Farmer, R. F., & Lewinsohn, P. M. (2011). The modeling of internalizing disorders on the basis of patterns of lifetime comorbidity:

Associations with psychosocial functioning and psychiatric disorders among first-degree relatives. *Journal of Abnormal Psychology, 120,* 308–321.

Shanahan, L., Copeland, W., Costello, E. J., & Angold, A. (2008). Specificity of putative psychosocial risk factors for psychiatric disorders in children and adolescents. *Journal of Child Psychiatry and Psychology, 49,* 34–42.

Vasilev, C. A., Crowell, S. E., Beauchaine, T. P., Mead, H. K., & Gatzke-Kopp, L. M. (2009). Correspondence between physiological and self-report measures of emotion dysregulation: A longitudinal investigation of youth with and without psychopathology. *Journal of Child Psychology and Psychiatry, 50,* 1357–1364.

Wadsworth, M. E., & Berger, L. (2006). Adolescents coping with poverty-related family stress: Prospective predictors of coping and psychological symptoms. *Journal of Youth and Adolescence, 35,* 57–70.

Wadsworth, M. E., & Compas, B. E. (2002). Coping with family conflict and economic strain: The adolescent perspective. *Journal of Research on Adolescence, 12,* 243–274.

Wadsworth, M. E., Raviv, T., Compas, B. E., & Connor-Smith, J. K. (2005). Parent and adolescent responses to poverty-related stress: Tests of mediated and moderated coping models. *Journal of Child and Family Studies, 14,* 283–298.

Wadsworth, M. E., & Santiago, C. D. (2008). Risk and resiliency processes in ethnically diverse families in poverty. *Journal of Family Psychology, 23,* 399–410.

Yao, S., Xiao, J., Zhu, X., Zhang, C., Auerbach, R. P., McWhinnie, C. M., et al. (2010). Coping and involuntary responses to stress in Chinese university students: Psychometric properties of the Responses to Stress Questionnaire. *Journal of Personality Assessment, 92,* 356–361.

CHAPTER 4

Cognitive Biases in Child Psychopathology

Kimberly A. Arditte and Jutta Joormann

Individual differences in cognitive processes, such as attention, memory, and interpretation, are known to play a critical role in the experience and regulation of emotion (Gross, 2007; Lazarus, 1994). Indeed, cognitive theories of emotion propose that one's cognitive appraisal, or interpretation, of a situation determines one's emotional response (Lazarus & Folkman, 1984). Consequently, modifying cognition is a primary route through which emotion is regulated. Imagine a child standing alone at the playground, watching a game of pickup basketball, and hoping to join in with his peers. What this child attends to (*Is he watching the bully on the court or his three other friends who are playing?*), how he remembers similar past experiences (*Is he thinking of that time he successfully joined in last week?*), and the way he interprets ambiguous environmental cues (*"What did that kid mean when he asked if I was good at basketball?"*) may directly relate to this child's emotional response to the situation.

Transdiagnostic theory looks to explain disparate psychological conditions via common mechanisms (Taylor & Clark, 2009). Biases in cognitive processing have been documented within a number of clinical disorders, including anxiety, mood, substance use, and eating disorders (Benas & Gibb, 2011; Bowler, Bowler, & James, 2011; Mathews & MacLeod, 2005). Also central to these disorders is an inability to effectively regulate emotions and mood states (Kring & Sloan, 2010). Recent accounts of emotional disorders have proposed that the presence of cognitive biases contributes to difficulties in emotion regulation, which then leads to the onset, maintenance, and/or recurrence of psychological disorders (Joormann & D'Avanzato, 2010). Experimental research has supported this hypothesis, demonstrating, for example, that the induction of a bias in attention toward negative material leads to increased emotional reactivity in response to an acute stressor (e.g., MacLeod, Rutherford, Campbell, Ebsworthy, & Holker, 2002).

The goal of this chapter is to examine the evidence for the existence of cognitive biases among children and adolescents across a range of psychological disorders. Relative to the adult literature, little attention has been paid to this area of research. Yet understanding the role of cognitive biases within these younger populations may have important implications for both theory and treatment. For example, elucidating the developmental trajectory of cognitive biases, particularly in conjunction with the onset of other symptoms, may allow us to better understand the causal mechanisms underlying the development of psychological disorders. In addition, the identification of biased cognitive processes across disorders may allow a point of entry for transdiagnostic treatments for children and adolescents.

Unfortunately, given the confines of this chapter, it would be impossible to adequately cover the existing theory and research on every cognitive bias for every psychological disorder. Given this, we do not intend this chapter to be an exhaustive review. Rather, we have chosen to focus on three of the most commonly studied cognitive processes (attention, memory, and the interpretation of ambiguous stimuli) as they relate to mood and anxiety disorders. These processes have all been previously identified as transdiagnostic (Harvey, Watkins, Mansell, & Shafran, 2004) and may be particularly so among mood and anxiety disorders, which have been shown to be highly comorbid and to share a number of vulnerability factors (Dozois, Seeds, & Collins, 2009). According to cognitive accounts, maladaptive schemata, or core beliefs about oneself, the world, or the future, underlie anxiety and mood disorders (e.g., Beck & Clark, 1997; Beck, Rush, Shaw, & Emery, 1979). Individuals experiencing depression or anxiety are more likely to attend to, remember, or interpret ambiguous stimuli or situations in a manner that is congruent with these schemata. For example, individuals with anxiety disorders may maintain a hyperoperative danger schema (Beck, Emery, & Greenberg, 1985). Filtering information through such a schema is thought to lead individuals with anxiety to interpret ambiguous information in a threatening manner, even in cases in which threat is not present. However, the interpretation of ambiguous situations as threatening will likely exacerbate symptoms of anxiety and may maintain them by eliciting avoidance behavior, thereby reinforcing threat-related cognitions (Creswell, Schniering, & Rapee, 2005). Similarly, people may attend to, encode, or recall information in a manner congruent with negative schemata, feeding into a cycle of exacerbated psychological symptoms, further activated schemata, and increasingly biased cognitive processes. In this way, biases in attention, memory, and interpretation are each proposed to play an important role in the onset, maintenance, and recurrence of emotional disorders.

In the following sections, we provide summaries of the extant child and adolescent literature for each of the three above-mentioned cognitive biases. Within these summaries, we have used the labels *child* and *adolescent* as authors of specific studies have used them. Generally, research examining cognitive biases has focused on children ranging from 8 to 12 years of age and adolescents ranging from 13 to 18 years of age.

Attentional Biases

Conceptually, biased attention involves a preference to visually attend to emotion-relevant stimuli in one's environment. Theory suggests that individuals with emotional disorders will display attentional biases congruent with their moods and/or activated schemata, and research on attention within clinical samples of adults has largely confirmed this. Anxiety disorders are often found to be associated with an initial orienting toward threat-related stimuli (e.g., Mogg, Bradley, Miles, & Dixon, 2004). Yet studies examining attention to stimuli presented for longer durations has produced mixed results, with some evidence for maintained attention toward threat (Weierich, Treat, & Hollingworth, 2008) and other evidence suggesting avoidance of threat over time (Mogg et al., 2004). Finally, rather than demonstrating an initial orientation to negative stimuli, adults with depression appear to demonstrate an inability to disengage from dysphoric content presented for an extended period of time (Caseras, Garner, Bradley, & Mogg, 2007; Kellough, Beevers, Ellis, & Wells, 2008).

Research on attentional biases has relied primarily on versions of the Stroop (Stroop, 1935) and dot-probe tasks (MacLeod, Mathews, & Tata, 1986). In the Stroop task, individuals are presented with a series of words printed in inks of various colors. They are then instructed to identify the color of the ink the word is printed in as quickly as possible while ignoring the content of the word. Attentional orienting toward word content will lead to increased color-naming latencies on the task, and biased attention is identified when individuals take longer to respond to words associated with a particular theme. For example, Taghavi, Dalgleish, Moradi, Neshat-Doost, and Yule (2003) demonstrated that, in contrast to healthy controls, children and adolescents diagnosed with generalized anxiety disorder (GAD) took significantly longer to respond to threat-relevant (i.e., *worried*) than neutral words.

In the dot-probe task, participants are simultaneously presented with two stimuli (e.g., words or images). One stimulus is neutral in content, whereas the other is emotionally valenced. Once the stimuli disappear from the screen, a probe appears in the same spatial location as one of the two stimuli. The participants are instructed to respond to the probe by indicating whether it appeared on the left or the right side of the screen. Congruent trials occur when the probe appears in the spatial location of the previously displayed emotionally valenced stimulus, and incongruent trials occur when the probe appears in the spatial location of the previously displayed neutral stimulus. If participants maintain an attentional bias for emotional content, it is expected that they will demonstrate decreased latencies on congruent trials, as their attention will already be oriented to that side of the screen. Using this task, children and adolescents diagnosed with anxiety disorders (i.e., separation anxiety disorder [SAD], social phobia [SP], or GAD), have been found to demonstrate an attentional bias for angry facial expressions (Roy et al., 2008).

As seen in Table 4.1, research on attentional biases among children and adolescents with emotional disorders has produced variable findings. In keeping with the adult literature, results from a number of studies have confirmed the existence of biased attention toward negative stimuli using the modified Stroop (Moradi, Taghavi, Neshat-Doost, Yule, & Dalgleish, 1999; Taghavi et al., 2003) and dot-probe tasks (Brotman et al., 2007; Dalgleish, Moradi, Taghavi, Neshat-Doost, & Yule, 2001; Dalgleish et al., 2003; Roy et al., 2008; Taghavi, Neshat-Doost, Moradi, Yule, & Dalgleish, 1999; Waters, Mogg, Bradley, & Pine, 2008). For example, using the Stroop task, Moradi and colleagues (1999) examined attentional biases for trauma-related words (e.g., *terrified*) among children and adolescents with a primary diagnosis of posttraumatic stress disorder (PTSD) and nonpsychiatric controls matched on age, sex, verbal IQ, and reading ability. A significant group-by-word-type interaction was reported such that children and adolescents with PTSD had longer color-naming latencies for trauma-related as compared with neutral words. Similarly, using the dot-probe task, children and adolescents diagnosed with either PTSD or GAD, as compared with their nonpsychiatric peers, have demonstrated an attentional preference for threat-related words (Dalgleish et al., 2003).

However, other studies have found little to no evidence for attentional biases among children and adolescents with anxiety (Benoit, McNally, Rapee, Gamble, & Wiseman, 2007; Vervoort et al., 2011; Waters, Lipp, & Cobham, 2000; Waters, Lipp, & Spence, 2004), and, indeed, some have even reported evidence of orienting attention away from threatening stimuli (Benoit et al., 2007; Gamble & Rapee, 2009; Monk et al., 2006; Pine et al., 2005). Using the Stroop task with images of children and adults displaying angry, disgusted, happy, or neutral expressions, Benoit and colleagues (2007) found that children with anxiety, like control participants, did not display an attentional preference for emotional faces. Furthermore, adolescents with anxiety demonstrated longer color-naming latencies for neutral rather than angry or disgusted faces. This latter result was interpreted as an attentional avoidance of negative emotional

TABLE 4.1. Studies on Attentional Biases and Their Corresponding Characteristics, Including Sample, Methodology Used, and Summary of Primary Results

Authors	Sample	Assessment of attentional biases	Summary of results
Benoit et al. (2007)	n = 52 children/adolescents with diagnosis of at least one anxiety disorder; n = 46 child/adolescent nonpsychiatric controls	Modified Stroop task utilizing child and adult faces displaying one of four expressions: anger, disgust, happiness, or neutral	No evidence for attentional biases was found among children with anxiety. However, adolescents with anxiety demonstrated a bias for neutral rather than angry or happy faces.
Brotman et al. (2007)	n = 20 children/adolescents with BD and a comorbid anxiety disorder (BD + ANX); n = 11 children/adolescents with BD and no anxiety disorder (BD – ANX); n = 14 nonpsychiatric controls	Attentional dot-probe paradigm with 500-millisecond display of angry, happy, or neutral faces	Only the BD + ANX group demonstrated biased attention toward threat. The BD – ANX and control groups did not differ from each other and showed no preference for angry over neutral faces.
Dalgleish et al. (2001)	n = 24 children/adolescents with PTSD; n = 24 children/adolescent healthy controls	Attentional dot-probe paradigm with 1,500-millisecond display of physical threat, social threat, depression, and neutral words	Compared with healthy controls, children/adolescents with PTSD demonstrated bias toward social threat words and away from depression-related words.
Dalgleish et al. (2003)	n = 19 adolescents with MDD; n = 24 adolescents with PTSD; n = 24 adolescents with GAD; n = 26 nonpsychiatric controls	Attentional dot-probe paradigm with 1,500-millisecond display of threat-related, depression-related, and neutral words; modified Stroop task utilizing threat-related, depression-related, and neutral words	On the attentional dot-probe task, adolescents with anxiety (i.e., the PTSD and GAD groups) demonstrated an attentional bias toward threat-related words not seen among adolescents with depression or controls. The Stroop task did not yield significant results.

(continued)

TABLE 4.1. (continued)

Authors	Sample	Assessment of attentional biases	Summary of results
Gamble & Rapee (2009)	$n = 43$ children/adolescents with an anxiety disorder (i.e., GAD, SP, specific phobia, SAD, OCD); $n = 49$ matched, child/adolescent healthy controls	Eye-tracking paradigm in which images of negative (anger, disgust, fear, sadness), positive (happy), or neutral facial expressions were presented for 500 or 3,000 milliseconds	Adolescents with anxiety demonstrated an initial attentional preference for angry faces, whereas children with anxiety demonstrated an initial attentional avoidance of happy faces. No late-stage biases were seen for either group.
Monk et al. (2006)	$n = 18$ adolescents with GAD; $n = 15$ adolescent healthy controls	Attentional dot-probe paradigm with 500-millisecond display of angry, happy, or neutral faces.	Adolescents with GAD demonstrated greater attentional biases away from angry faces.
Moradi et al. (1999)	$n = 23$ children/adolescents with PTSD; $n = 23$ matched child/adolescent healthy controls	Modified Stroop task utilizing happy, neutral, dysphoric, threat-relevant, and trauma-related words	Participants with PTSD demonstrated greater color-naming latencies for trauma-related words than for neutral words as compared with healthy controls.
Neshat-Doost et al. (2000)	$n = 19$ children/adolescents with MDD; $n = 26$ children/adolescents with no history of emotional disorders	Attentional dot-probe paradigm with 1,500-millisecond display of depression, threat, and neutral words	No evidence of depression-related attentional bias.
Pine et al. (2005)	$n = 29$ children with PTSD; $n = 21$ children with no history of trauma	Attentional dot-probe paradigm with 500-millisecond display of angry, happy, or neutral faces	Compared with children without a trauma history, children with PTSD demonstrated greater attentional avoidance of angry faces.
Roy et al. (2008)	$n = 101$ children/adolescents with primary anxiety disorder (i.e., SP, GAD, or SAD); $n = 51$ child/adolescent healthy controls	Attentional dot-probe paradigm with 500-millisecond display of angry, happy, or neutral faces.	Children with anxiety demonstrated attentional bias toward angry, but not happy, faces as compared with children without anxiety. No biases were found for specific anxiety disorders.
Taghavi et al. (1999)	$n = 24$ children/adolescents with GAD; $n = 19$ children/adolescents	Attentional dot-probe paradigm with 1,500-millisecond display of physical	The GAD group demonstrated an attentional bias toward threat but not depression

Study	Sample	Method	Results
	with mixed anxiety-depressive disorder; $n = 24$ children/adolescent nonpsychiatric controls	threat, social threat, depression, and neutral words	related words. The mixed anxiety-depression and control groups did not demonstrate attentional biases.
Taghavi et al. (2003)	$n = 19$ children and adolescents with GAD; $n = 19$ children and adolescent healthy controls	Modified Stroop task utilizing happy, neutral, dysphoric, threat-relevant, and trauma-related words	A Stroop interference effect was found for negatively valenced words among children and adolescents with GAD.
Vervoort et al. (2011)	$n = 39$ adolescents with an anxiety disorder (i.e., SAD, SP, specific phobia, panic disorder, or GAD); $n = 35$ adolescent healthy controls	Attentional dot-probe paradigm with 500-millisecond and 1,250-millisecond conditions displaying neutral or threat-related IAPS images	No evidence for anxiety-related attentional biases.
Waters et al. (2000)	$n = 16$ children diagnosed with an anxiety disorder (i.e., SAD, GAD, specific phobia, SP, or OCD)	Startle eyeblink modification (SEM) paradigm utilizing threat and neutral words	With regard to startle magnitude, no differences were found for threat and neutral words. However, startle latency supported bias toward threat in early stages of information processing.
Waters et al. (2004)	$n = 23$ clinically anxious children with diagnosis of GAD, SAD, SP, or specific phobia; $n = 23$ unselected children	Attentional dot-probe paradigm with 500-millisecond display utilizing fear-related, neutral, or pleasant images from the International Affective Picture System (IAPS)	Children both with and without anxiety demonstrated initial attentional biases for fear-related images. However, no differences in attentional biases were found between children with and without anxiety.
Waters, Mogg, et al. (2008)	$n = 23$ children with GAD; $n = 25$ control children without anxiety	Attentional dot-probe paradigm with 500-millisecond display of angry, happy, or neutral faces	Attentional biases toward both angry and happy faces were seen in children with high levels of anxiety. Those with low levels of anxiety and healthy controls did not demonstrate attentional biases.

Note. BD, bipolar disorder; MDD, major depressive disorder; PTSD, posttraumatic stress disorder; GAD, generalized anxiety disorder; SP, social phobia; SAD, separation anxiety disorder; OCD, obsessive–compulsive disorder.

expressions. Likewise, children with PTSD and adolescents with GAD have demonstrated attentional avoidance of angry facial expressions on the dot-probe task (Monk et al., 2006; Pine et al., 2005).

Studies examining attentional biases among samples of children and adolescents with depression or mixed anxiety and depression have found no evidence of attentional biases (Dalgleish et al., 2003; Neshat-Doost, Moradi, Taghavi, Yule, & Dalgleish, 2000; Taghavi et al., 1999). These results may indicate that children and adolescents with depressive symptoms differ from adults in their attentional preference for mood-congruent stimuli. Alternatively, as studies have failed to directly examine attentional disengagement among depressed youth, further research is needed to confidently draw conclusions about the presence of attentional biases within these populations.

Moreover, though research has relied heavily on the Stroop and dot-probe paradigms, neither is without its methodological weaknesses. Some researchers have been critical of the emotional Stroop task, arguing that it is unclear whether color-naming latencies are reflective of interference due to attention allocation (e.g., MacLeod et al., 2002; Roy et al., 2008). Likewise, critics of the dot-probe task argue that this paradigm provides only cross-sectional data on attention allocation, missing potentially important information on how attention to emotional stimuli changes over time (e.g., Caseras et al., 2007). To further elucidate the time course of attentional biases, emerging research has turned to the tracking of natural gaze patterns. Eye-tracking provides a richer and more ecologically valid understanding of biased attention because it allows for the continuous evaluation of focal attention. However, to date, only one known study has examined attentional biases among children and adolescents using eye-tracking technology (Gamble & Rapee, 2009).

In their study, Gamble and Rapee (2009) found evidence for an early-stage attentional bias among adolescents with a primary diagnosis of anxiety (i.e., GAD, SP, specific phobia, SAD, or obsessive–compulsive disorder [OCD]). Specifically, they found that adolescents with anxiety were more likely to initially orient toward angry faces than their counterparts without anxiety. However, when the negative emotional expressions were presented for longer durations (i.e., 3000 ms), the tracking of eye movements yielded no significant evidence for attentional biases toward threat. Results from this study highlight the fact that eye-tracking provides a more comprehensive assessment of attentional biases as compared with the Stroop and dot-probe paradigms, and employing eye-tracking in future research may elucidate inconsistent findings.

Selective attention to external stimuli has been previously identified as a transdiagnostic cognitive process (Harvey et al., 2004). Review of the child and adolescent literature provides some support for the presence of a negative attentional bias common across a range of anxiety disorders.

However, evidence of such biases in children and adolescents with depression has yet to be found, indicating that attention is, perhaps, more critical to the onset or maintenance of the anxiety disorders than it is to major depression. Continued examination of attention as a transdiagnostic mechanism should focus on issues yet to be addressed in the child and adolescent literature. Research should look to investigate attentional biases as a function of the stimuli used. Documentation of attentional biases within specific disorders may require the use of disorder-specific stimuli. In addition, employing emotionally valenced words, rather than images, may yield different results, particularly when examining biases from a developmental perspective.

Memory Biases

As with attentional biases, it has been theorized that individuals with activated depression- or anxiety-related schemata will demonstrate enhanced encoding and recall of material congruent with such schemata (Beck et al., 1979). Furthermore, certain thought processes, including an overly narrow or analytical self-focus common to many of the emotional disorders, may lead to deficits in the recall of autobiographical memories (Mathews & MacLeod, 2005).

Within the adult literature, there is strong evidence for the existence of depression-related memory biases (for a review, see Mathews & MacLeod, 2005). Research also suggests that depressed individuals will tend to remember autobiographical memories in an overgeneralized fashion. It has been hypothesized that these biases relate to separate memory processes; overgeneral memory is thought to relate to poorly employed retrieval tactics, whereas mood-congruent memory biases may relate to the selective processing or ruminative elaboration of schema-congruent material.

Less consistent support has been found for anxiety-related memory biases. Researchers have often failed to find evidence for enhanced memory for threat-relevant stimuli (see Coles & Heimberg, 2002) and have proposed that anxiety disorders may be characterized by avoidance of semantic processing or the perceptual encoding of threat information (e.g., Brewin, 2001a). However, some studies report enhanced recall of threat-related words among individuals with panic disorder, particularly when words have been deeply encoded (e.g., Cloitre, Shear, Cancienne, & Zeitlin, 1994). Similarly, adults diagnosed with PTSD exhibit enhanced recall of details central to trauma-related autobiographical memories (Brewin, 2001b) and in some studies have demonstrated better recall of trauma-related, as compared with neutral, words (e.g., Vrana, Roodman, & Beckham, 1995).

Memory biases have been most commonly assessed in one of two ways: via the free recall or recognition of emotionally valenced words or by using the Autobiographical Memory Test (AMT; Williams & Broadbent, 1986). In the free-recall task, participants are instructed to remember a series of positive, negative, and neutral words and are later asked to recall as many words as possible. Free recall is sometimes followed up with a recognition test in which participants are instructed to respond "yes" or "no" to whether a word had been previously included in the learning phase.

In the AMT, participants are given a series of positive and negative emotional cue words. For each cue, participants are given a short period of time (e.g., 30–60 seconds) to recall a detailed autobiographical memory. Specifically, they are instructed to think of a *time* and *place* when something happened to them occurring on *one* day. Latency to the first word of the recalled memory is recorded. If no memory is recalled within the allotted time, the cue is coded as an omission. Researchers have varied in how they have opted to code memories, with some choosing to dichotomously code variables as "specific" versus "overgeneral" (e.g., Kuyken, Howell, & Dalgleish, 2006) and others opting for a more complex coding system assessing multiple facets of the recalled memory (e.g., Park, Goodyer, & Teasdale, 2002). Other paradigms, including self-referent encoding tasks and tests of implicit memory, have also been used to examine emotional memory biases, but rarely within the child and adolescent literature. Because of this, detailed descriptions of these paradigms are beyond the scope of this chapter.

Given the pattern of findings within the adult literature, it is unsurprising that research on memory biases among children and adolescents has primarily focused on depressed and trauma-exposed populations. However, unlike the adult literature, evidence for emotional memory biases among children and adolescents has been equivocal (Table 4.2). Some studies using free recall/recognition paradigms have found evidence for a negative memory bias, but only on the free-recall task. For example, Neshat-Doost, Taghavi, Moradi, Yule, and Dalgleish (1998) found that the proportion of negative to positive or neutral words recalled by children and adolescents with diagnoses of major depressive disorder (MDD) was significantly higher than that recalled by child and adolescent controls. The same pattern was revealed when examining children and adolescents with and without a diagnosis of PTSD (Moradi, Taghavi, Neshat-Doost, Yule, & Dalgleish, 2000). In contrast, Dalgleish and colleagues (2003) did not find evidence for a negative memory bias, though their analyses compared children and adolescents with depression with those with anxiety and mixed anxiety and depression and did not include positive word recall. Similarly, when comparing children and adolescents who formerly had depression with their peers who currently have or never had depression on the proportion of negative to neutral words, no significant evidence of a negative memory bias emerged (Timbremont, Braet, Bosmans, & Vlierberghe, 2008).

Research employing the AMT has produced strong evidence for an overgeneral memory bias within clinical samples (Arie, Apter, Orbach, Yefet, & Zalzman, 2008; de Decker, Hermans, Raes, & Eelen, 2003; Kuyken et al., 2006; Park et al., 2002; Swales, Williams, & Wood, 2001; Vrielynck, Deplus, & Philippot, 2007). Children and adolescents with emotional disorders have repeatedly exhibited difficulty detailing specific autobiographical memories, instead recalling memories in a categorical (i.e., memory is a general class of events), extended (i.e., memory extends over the period of multiple days), or repeated (i.e., the same memory is recalled for multiple cues) fashion. At the time of publication, only one study has failed to find evidence for this general memory deficit using the AMT (Kuyken & Howell, 2000). However, when the authors of this study employed the Self-Defining Memory Test (SDMT; Singer & Moffitt, 1991-1992), a task in which participants are asked to recall any memory they believe to be self-defining in some way, they found that adolescents with depression were more likely than nonpsychiatric controls to recall recent memories from an observer's perspective, perhaps indicating some sort of specificity deficit.

Still, it remains unclear whether this overgeneral memory bias applies to autobiographical memories associated with a particular valence. Whereas de Decker and colleagues (2003) found that teenage psychiatric inpatients with severe trauma history were more likely to recall positive memories overgenerally, Park and colleagues (2002) found that adolescents with depression were more likely to recall negative autobiographical memories in an overgeneralized manner. Most studies have found that, across disorders, positive and negative memories are equally as likely to be remembered in an overgeneral way (Arie et al., 2008; Kuyken et al., 2006; Swales et al., 2001; Vrielynck et al., 2007). Importantly, the AMT does not include neutral cues, and, as such, it remains unknown whether this lack of memory specificity relates to all or only emotionally valenced memories.

Finally, one study has examined emotional memory biases among children and adolescents with a history of MDD using emotionally valenced and neutral facial expressions (Pine et al., 2004). The memory task used in this study consisted of both an encoding and a recognition phase. In the encoding phase, participants were presented with images of 24 actors portraying one of three emotional expressions (angry, happy, or fearful). Thirty minutes later, participants completed a recognition phase in which they were presented with 48 actors, all portraying a neutral face. Participants were asked whether or not they recognized the actor from the encoding portion of the task. Results indicated that participants with

TABLE 4.2. Studies on Memory Biases and Their Corresponding Characteristics, Including Sample, Methodology Used, and Summary of Primary Results

Authors	Sample	Assessment of memory biases	Summary of results
Arie et al. (2008)	n = 25 adolescent, psychiatric inpatient, suicide attempters; n = 25 adolescent, psychiatric inpatient, suicide nonattempters; n = 25 healthy community participants	Modified version of the Autobiographical Memory Test	Suicide attempters demonstrated the least specific autobiographical memories. Suicide nonattempters demonstrated less specific memory recall than the control group. No within-group differences on specificity as a function of valence were reported.
Dalgleish et al. (2003)	n = 19 adolescents with MDD; n = 24 adolescents with PTSD; n = 24 adolescents with GAD; n = 26 nonpsychiatric controls	Free-recall and recognition procedure composed of depression-related, threat-related, trauma-related, positive, and neutral words	No group differences in the proportion of negative to neutral words recalled.
de Decker et al. (2003)	n = 28 adolescent, psychiatric inpatients (diagnoses unspecified)	Modified version of the Autobiographical Memory Test	More severe trauma history was associated with less specific memory recall. This relation was most pronounced in the recall of positive memories.
Kuyken & Howell (2000)	n = 34 adolescents with MDD; n = 31 adolescent controls who never had depression	Autobiographical Memory Test and the Self-Defining Memory Test	Compared with controls, adolescents with depression had memories that were more recent, from the observer perspective, marginally less pleasant, and rated as more personally important.
Kuyken et al. (2006)	n = 12 adolescents with MDD but no trauma; n = 22 adolescents with MDD plus trauma; n = 28 never depressed controls	Autobiographical Memory Test	Adolescents with MDD but no trauma remembered more overgeneral memories than those with MDD plus trauma or never-depressed controls. No evidence for a Group × Cue Valence interaction was found.
Moradi et al. (2000)	n = 24 children/adolescents with PTSD; n = 25 child/adolescent nonpsychiatric controls, with no history of trauma	Free-recall and recognition procedure composed of depression-related, threat-related, trauma-related, positive, and neutral words	Participants with PTSD recalled a higher proportion of negative relative to neutral/positive words than control participants.

Study	Sample	Measure	Findings
Neshat-Doost et al. (1998)	$n = 19$ children/adolescents with MDD; $n = 19$ child/adolescent healthy control participants	Free-recall and recognition procedure composed of positive and negative trait adjectives and semantically related neutral words	In contrast to the control group, the MDD group recalled significantly more negative than positive or neutral words.
Park et al. (2002)	$n = 40$ adolescents with MDD; $n = 26$ adolescents with clinical diagnoses other than depression (psychiatric group); $n = 33$ community controls	Autobiographical Memory Test	Categoric, overgeneral memory recall was more common among MDD and psychiatric groups than among controls. In addition, within the MDD group, overgeneral memory was more common for negative than positive cues.
Pine et al. (2004)	$n = 19$ children/adolescents with MDD; $n = 133$ children/adolescents without MDD	Face-memory task utilizing images of happy, angry, fearful, and neutral facial expressions	Face memory for actors depicting fearful expressions was significantly reduced in children/adolescents with MDD as compared with those without MDD. No differences were found in memory for happy or angry faces.
Swales et al. (2001)	$n = 26$ diagnostically mixed, adolescent psychiatric inpatients; $n = 24$ adolescent, nonpsychiatric controls	Autobiographical Memory Test	Compared with controls, the psychiatric group recalled less specific memories for both positive and negative cues.
Timbremont et al. (2007)	$n = 18$ currently depressed children or adolescents; $n = 16$ formerly depressed children or adolescents; $n = 39$ never depressed children or adolescents with another DSM-IV diagnosis	Self-referent encoding task followed by word recall	No significant within-group differences were found on the recall of positive versus negative self-referent words.
Vrielynck et al. (2007)	$n = 15$ children with clinical depression; $n = 25$ children with clinical disorder other than depression; $n = 23$ child control participants	Autobiographical Memory Test	The depressed clinical group recalled less specific, more generic, and more extended memories than the control group. The nondepressed clinical group recalled less specific and more general memories than the control group. No evidence for a Group $\times$ Cue Valence interaction was found.

Note. MDD, major depressive disorder; PTSD, posttraumatic stress disorder; GAD, generalized anxiety disorder.

a history of MDD were less able to recognize actors who had portrayed fearful expressions during the encoding phase. Findings appear to be in contrast with the majority of the adult literature but are consistent with Park and colleagues' (2002) finding that children and adolescents vulnerable to depression display deficits in negative memory recall. Because this is the first and only study of its kind, future research on biased emotional memory for facial expressions is necessary to replicate findings.

As with attention, explicit selective memory has been identified as a transdiagnostic cognitive mechanism (Harvey et al., 2004). Indeed, findings suggest that across the emotional disorders, children and adolescents display overgeneral recall of both positive and negative autobiographical memories. Evidence for enhanced recall of mood-congruent memory among children and adolescents is less robust than in adult populations and appears to be most pronounced in individuals with depression. One possible explanation for this is that memory biases are disorder-specific. Emotion regulation strategies frequently used in depression (e.g., rumination) may lead to increased elaboration and encoding of negative material, whereas strategies associated with anxiety (e.g., distraction or avoidance) may lead to reduced encoding of threat material. In addition, differences in the use of emotion regulation strategies among children, adolescents, and adults may account for discrepancies in memory biases across age groups. However, little work has been done to explore reliance on emotion regulation strategies from a developmental perspective, and such hypotheses require empirical examination.

Interpretation Biases

In their review of the adult literature, Mathews and MacLeod (2005) state that interpretation biases have been documented in most, if not all, of the emotional disorders. Consistent with theoretical models, findings from experimental research with adults have shown that individuals with anxiety are more likely to interpret ambiguous information in a negative manner (e.g., Richards, Austin, & Alvarenga, 2001). This bias may be particularly pronounced when possible interpretations of ambiguous stimuli correspond to the threats relevant to a particular disorder. For example, Stopa and Clark (2000) found that adults with social phobia were most likely to predict negative outcomes for ambiguous social situations. Using self-report measures, adults with depression also demonstrate negative interpretation biases (e.g., Carver, Ganellen, & Behar-Mitrani, 1985), though experimental research has rarely been able to replicate these results. It has been argued, however, that the lack of experimental findings to support a depression-related bias may be a function of the stimuli employed (as they often do not correspond with depression-based schemata; Wisco, 2009).

As with other cognitive biases, multiple methods have been used to assess biased interpretation. Within the child and adolescent literature, research has primarily relied on two experimental paradigms, which involve making interpretations of ambiguous scenarios or determining the meaning of a homophone or homograph. In paradigms using ambiguous situations, participants are presented with a series of situations, each of which could be interpreted in either a neutral or a threatening manner. Situations are typically designed to elicit possible feelings of separation anxiety, social anxiety, general worry, or physical threat. For example, a scenario that may elicit general worry could be "You are busy doing your school work in class when your teacher walks up beside your desk and says that he wants to talk to you after class today" (Waters, Craske, Bergman, & Treanor, 2008). Outcome measures for studies using ambiguous scenarios have been variable and have included open-ended questions (e.g., "How would you feel if you were in this situation?"; Bögels & Zigterman, 2000), multiple-choice responses (e.g., "Which of these interpretations [two neutral and two threat-related] do you think is most likely?"; Barrett, Rapee, Dadds, & Ryan, 1996), and judgment ratings using Likert scales (e.g., "Do you think this situation is dangerous?"; Waters, Craske, Bergman, & Treanor, 2008).

Homophone and homograph tasks rely on children and adolescents to derive a meaning from an ambiguous word. Homophones are words that sound alike but may have multiple spellings (e.g., *bury* vs. *berry*). Within these tasks, one variant of the presented homophone has a threat-relevant meaning, and the other has a neutral meaning. Homographs are words that have multiple meanings, even though they are spelled the same way (e.g., *sink* as in a kitchen vs. *sink* as a boat might). Again, when homographs have been used within interpretation bias tasks, one variant of the word has a threat-relevant interpretation, and the other is neutral. Homophones and homographs have been presented aurally and/or visually. For example, Gifford, Reynolds, Bell, and Wilson (2008) opted to present homophones aurally while displaying images of both threat and neutral interpretations of the words. Children were then asked to select which image was representative of the word. In contrast, Taghavi, Moradi, Neshat-Doost, Yule, and Dalgleish (2000) visually presented a homograph to children and adolescents and asked them to construct a sentence with it.

Research indicates that children and adolescents with anxiety disorders consistently demonstrate biases in favor of threat-related interpretations (Table 4.3). When asked open-ended questions, children with anxiety report more negative cognitions in response to the ambiguous scenarios than children without anxiety do (Bögels & Zigterman, 2000; Chorpita, Albano, & Barlow, 1996). In addition, children with a primary diagnosis of an anxiety disorder (e.g., SP, SAD, GAD, or overanxious disorder) are more likely than their peers without anxiety to choose a

TABLE 4.3. Studies on Interpretation Biases and Their Corresponding Characteristics, Including Sample, Methodology Used, and Summary of Primary Results

Authors	Sample	Assessment of interpretation bias	Summary of results
Barrett et al. (1996)	n = 152 children with a primary diagnosis of an anxiety disorder (i.e., SAD, overanxious disorder, simple phobia, SP); n = 27 children with ODD; n = 26 nonclinical children	12 ambiguous scenarios related to physical or social threat	All groups differed significantly in their interpretation of the ambiguous scenarios. Children with ODD were most likely to interpret the situations as threatening, and the nonclinical children were least likely.
Bögels & Zigterman (2000)	n = 15 children with a primary diagnosis of anxiety (i.e., SAD, SP, GAD); n = 15 children with an externalizing disorder (i.e., ODD, ADHD, or conduct disorder); n = 15 nonclinical controls	9 ambiguous stories about social, separation, and general worry areas	Children with anxiety had significantly more negative cognitions than the externalizing group. In addition, when given closed response options, children with anxiety perceived the most danger and had less perceived ability to influence the situation.
Chorpita et al. (1996)	n = 4 clinically anxious children; n = 8 child controls	Ambiguous Situations Questionnaire	Significant correlation found between anxiety symptoms and threatening interpretations of ambiguous situations.
Creswell et al. (2005)	n = 27 children with unspecified anxiety disorders; n = 33 nonclinical children	12 ambiguous scenarios related to physical or social threat	Children with anxiety demonstrated more threat interpretations than children without anxiety. Anxiety symptoms were positively correlated with threat biases.
Gifford et al. (2008)	n = 18 children with anxiety; n = 15 children with externalizing disorder; n = 23 nonclinical children	Homophone task	Children with anxiety made significantly more biased interpretations than children without anxiety. Children with externalizing disorders did not differ from either of the other groups.
Taghavi et al. (2000)	n = 17 children and adolescents with GAD; n = 40 non-psychiatric child and adolescent controls	Modified homograph test	Participants with anxiety chose the threatening meaning of homographs more often than the neutral meaning, as compared with controls.
Waters, Craske, et al. (2008)	n = 15 children with principal diagnosis of an anxiety disorder; n = 16 children at-risk for developing an anxiety disorder; n = 14 child controls	12 ambiguous stories about social, separation, and general worry areas	Children with anxiety expected to feel significantly more negative emotion and had less perceived ability to influence the situation than either of the other groups.

Note. SAD, separation anxiety disorder; SP, social phobia; ODD, oppositional defiant disorder; GAD, generalized anxiety disorder; ADHD, attention-deficit/hyperactivity disorder.

threatening interpretation of an ambiguous situation (Barrett et al., 1996; Creswell et al., 2005). Interestingly, when Barrett and colleagues (1996) examined biases as a function of anxiety diagnosis, no differences in threat interpretations were found. Finally, evidence suggests that children with anxiety make more anxiety-related judgments of ambiguous situations. For example, Bögels and Zigterman (2000) found that children with anxiety were more likely to rate ambiguous situations as dangerous and to perceive themselves as having less influence over the situation than their counterparts without anxiety. Similarly, Waters, Craske, and colleagues (2008) found that anxious and nonanxious groups differed with respect to their perceived influence over the situations, as well as their predicted emotional reactions to them (i.e., children with anxiety were more likely to respond that they would experience "a lot" of negative emotion in response to the situation).

Findings from homophone and homograph tasks have confirmed the existence of anxiety-related interpretation biases in children and adolescents. In one study, children and adolescents meeting criteria for a primary diagnosis of GAD were more likely than healthy controls to make threat-related interpretations of a series of visually presented homographs (Taghavi et al., 2000). In a second study, children with anxiety disorders were significantly more likely to select the threatening interpretations of ambiguous homophones or homographs than were children with no history of psychological disorders (Gifford et al., 2008).

Overall, studies examining interpretation biases in children and adolescents have found strong evidence for the existence of negative biases, similar to those found among adults. Threat interpretations are present across anxiety disorders, including GAD, SAD, and SP. Moreover, research suggests that similarities across disorders may outweigh differences between them, as Barrett and colleagues (1996) found no significant differences as a function of diagnosis. These results suggest that interpretation biases are one of the most robust transdiagnostic cognitive processes. Given this, research has begun to examine the nature of interpretation biases in children with externalizing disorders but has produced mixed results (Barrett et al., 1996, but also see Bögels & Zigterman, 2000; Gifford et al., 2008). Further research is needed to elucidate the nature of interpretation biases in externalizing populations and to extend research to children and adolescents with MDD.

Conclusion

In this chapter, we examined the role of cognitive biases across a range of diagnoses, reviewing the extant research on attention, memory, and interpretation biases as they relate to anxiety and depression. Though a great deal of work has been done to document the existence of such biases among adults, relatively little work has been done to investigate the presence of biases among children and adolescents. Cognitive theory implicates these biases in the etiology and maintenance of emotional disorders, and therefore identifying biases in child and adolescent populations may provide insight into common mechanisms underlying these disorders and could provide a target for transdiagnostic interventions for these age groups.

However, to date, results from research on attentional and memory biases in children and adolescents have been mixed at best. Though a number of studies have found support for biased attention similar to what has been documented in the adult literature, others have not found evidence for such biases and have sometimes found evidence for a preference to avoid emotional stimuli. Similarly, though children and adolescents with disorders such as MDD or PTSD appear to demonstrate overgeneral recall of autobiographical material, the evidence for enhanced memory for schema-related content remains equivocal.

In contrast, the literature on interpretation biases has consistently demonstrated that children and adolescents with clinical levels of anxiety are more likely to interpret ambiguous information in a threatening manner. Interestingly, most of the studies examining interpretation biases have not differentiated among anxiety disorders. In fact, when Barrett and her colleagues (1996) examined biases as a function of specific disorders, no significant differences were found. Threat interpretations appear to be common to multiple childhood anxiety disorders and, as a result, may be especially important to consider from a transdiagnostic framework.

Given that research on cognitive biases among children and adolescents is still in its nascency, we believe that there are a number of limitations to the existing body of literature and, subsequently, areas of future inquiry that are worth noting. For one thing, there has been a large amount of heterogeneity with regard to the methodology and stimuli used to assess cognitive biases. This may have important implications, particularly from a developmental perspective. For example, within the literature on attentional bias, many studies have relied on word stimuli (e.g., Dalgleish et al., 2001; Moradi et al., 2000; Taghavi et al., 2003). However, it is likely that children's ability to understand and/or process such semantic information may change over time. Instead, studies may want to examine attentional biases using such stimuli as emotional images or facial expressions. However, even here researchers are urged to be aware of methodological issues. Would we expect children to respond in the same manner to an emotion expressed by a same-age peer as to one by an adolescent or adult? Little research has been devoted to addressing such methodological questions, yet adequately adapting tasks for children and adolescents will be essential to understanding biased processes with these populations. Moreover, some researchers have questioned whether children and adolescents demonstrate more marked variability in the presentation of attentional biases due to developmental changes that occur over time, such as the ability to react quickly to stimuli (Van Damme & Crombez, 2009). Eye-tracking technology should be used in future studies on attentional biases, as this methodology relies on the monitoring of natural gaze patterns rather than on such factors as executive functioning or fine motor coordination that may affect a child's reaction times.

Research has been similarly inconsistent with regard to how clinical samples are selected or how comorbid diagnoses are accounted for. For example, a number of studies examining memory biases relied on samples of psychiatric inpatients with unspecified diagnoses (Arie et al., 2008; de Decker et al., 2003; Swales et al., 2001). Rarely do studies report whether participants were diagnosed with more than one disorder. In addition, given the proposition that cognitive biases underlie a range of disorders, more studies are needed that extend research on these biases to disorders other than depression and anxiety, including disorders primarily diagnosed in childhood and that may predispose for the onset of adult psychopathology, such as attention-deficit/hyperactivity disorder (ADHD). Although some studies have begun to examine interpretation biases in children with externalizing disorders (Barrett et al., 1996; Bögels & Zigterman, 2000; Gifford et al., 2008), this research remains absent from the attention and memory literature.

Additionally, more work is needed to identify how specific biases operate in different psychological disorders. The adult literature has demonstrated, for example, that attentional biases characterize both anxiety and depression. Yet, whereas participants with anxiety quickly orient to threat-relevant material, those with depression demonstrate difficultly disengaging from depression-relevant stimuli (Caseras et al., 2007). Conducting studies that differentiate early- and late-stage attentional processing in children with anxiety and depression could lend further support for attention as an important transdiagnostic process. In this way, it will also be important to identify how transdiagnostic cognitive processes causally relate to the development of specific disorders. For example, it has been proposed that biases in attention, memory, and interpretation may differentially relate to the etiology or maintenance of disorders in three ways (Mansell, Harvey, Watkins, & Shafran, 2009). First, if biases are mood- or schema-congruent, then the content of an individual's concerns will affect his or her manifest symptoms. Children and adolescents demonstrating a preference for dysphoric content will be more likely to experience depressive symptoms, whereas those exhibiting attentional vigilance for threat may be more likely to experience symptoms of anxiety. Additionally, specific biases may be more or less pronounced among certain disorders. Extant research suggests that, among children and adolescents, attentional biases may be more closely related to the development of anxiety disorders, whereas emotional memory biases may be more strongly associated with depression. Finally, it remains possible that certain processes are disorder-specific and should not be considered from a transdiagnostic perspective. Given the relatively small literature that exists on cognitive processes in children and adolescents, more research is needed to determine whether, and in what capacity, attention, memory, and interpretation should be considered transdiagnostic mechanisms within these populations.

Beyond documenting the existence of cognitive biases in psychological disorders, it will be important to examine how cognitive processes and disorders causally relate to each other. It remains unclear, for example, whether cognitive biases among children and adolescents are simply correlates of their depression or anxiety symptoms or whether such biases contribute to the onset or maintenance of emotional disorders. One method of examining this question will be to identify the point of onset for cognitive biases, both clinically and developmentally, as implications of such research may be far reaching. Studies examining cognitive biases in high-risk samples, such as the biological offspring of mothers with depression, will greatly help to elucidate the temporal presentation of cognitive biases and psychological symptoms (Joormann, Talbot, & Gotlib, 2007).

In addition, emerging research on cognitive bias modification (CBM) in adults has looked to uncover the causal relations between these variables by modifying biases and examining the subsequent change in psychological symptoms (see Koster, Fox, & MacLeod, 2009). For example, Amir, Beard, Burns and Bomyea (2009) conducted an eight-session attention training with a sample of adults diagnosed with GAD. Findings of this study revealed that participants trained to deploy attention away from threat-related words reported fewer symptoms of anxiety and depression and were significantly less likely to meet diagnostic criteria for GAD (50%) as compared with participants in a no-training control group (13%). These results also indicate that biases may be effective targets of intervention. Though studies have begun to investigate the effects of these trainings in child and adolescent samples (e.g., Bar-Haim, Morag, & Glickman, 2011), much more research in this area is needed.

Finally, studies examining the proposition that cognitive biases in children and adolescents impair emotion regulation, thereby setting the stage for the onset and maintenance of psychological disorders, are still missing. Studies on CBM in adults have found that modifying attention or interpretation bias alters their ability to regulate negative affect and respond to stress (Schartau, Dalgleish, & Dunn, 2009; Tran, Siemer, & Joormann, 2011). As the relation between cognitive processes and emotion regulation seems a particularly important area of study from a transdiagnostic perspective, and given the promising nature of these results in the adult literature, it is essential that research continue to explore the relation between cognitive biases, emotion regulation, and psychological disorders within children and adolescents.

REFERENCES

Amir, N., Beard, C., Burns, M., & Bomyea, J. (2009). Attention modification program in individuals with generalized anxiety disorder. *Journal of Abnormal Psychology, 118*, 28–33.

Arie, M., Apter, A., Orbach, I., Yefet, Y., & Zalzman, G. (2008). Autobiographical memory, interpersonal problem solving, and suicidal behavior in adolescent inpatients. *Comprehensive Psychiatry, 49*, 22–29.

Bar-Haim, Y., Morag, I., & Glickman, S. (2011). Training anxious children to disengage attention from threat: A randomized controlled trial. *Journal of Child Psychology and Psychiatry, 52*, 861–869.

Barrett, P. M., Rapee, R. M., Dadds, M. M., & Ryan, S. M. (1996). Family enhancement of cognitive style in anxious and aggressive children. *Journal of Abnormal Child Psychology, 24*, 187–203.

Beck, A. T., & Clark, D. A. (1997). An information processing model of anxiety: Automatic and strategic processes. *Behaviour Research and Therapy, 35*, 49–58.

Beck, A. T., Emery, G., & Greenberg, R. L. (1985). *Anxiety disorders and phobias: A cognitive perspective.* New York: Basic Books.

Beck, A. T., Rush, A. J., Shaw, B. F., & Emery, G. (1979). *Cognitive therapy of depression.* New York: Guilford Press.

Benas, J. S., & Gibb, B. E. (2011). Cognitive biases in depression and eating disorders. *Cognitive Therapy and Research, 35*, 68–78.

Benoit, K. E., McNally, R. J., Rapee, R. M., Gamble, A. L., & Wiseman, A. L. (2007). Processing of emotional faces in children and adolescents with anxiety disorders. *Behaviour Change, 24*, 183–194.

Bögels, S. M., & Zigterman, D. (2000). Dysfunctional cognitions in children with social phobia, separation anxiety disorder, and generalized anxiety disorder. *Journal of Abnormal Child Psychology, 28*, 205–211.

Bowler, J. L., Bowler, M. C., & James, L. R. (2011). The cognitive underpinnings of addiction. *Substance Use and Misuse, 46*, 1060–1071.

Brewin, C. R. (2001a). A cognitive neuroscience account of posttraumatic stress disorder and its treatment. *Behaviour Research and Therapy, 39*, 373–393.

Brewin, C. R. (2001b). Memory processes in post-traumatic stress disorder. *International Review of Psychiatry, 13*, 159–163.

Brotman, M. A., Rich, B. A., Schmajuk, M., Reising, M., Monk, C. S., Dickstein, D. P., et al. (2007). Attention bias to threat faces in children with bipolar disorder and comorbid lifetime anxiety disorders. *Biological Psychiatry, 61*, 819–821.

Carver, C. S., Ganellen, R. J., & Behar-Mitrani, V. (1985). Depression and cognitive style: Comparisons between measures. *Journal of Personality and Social Psychology, 49,* 722–728.

Caseras, X., Garner, M., Bradley, B. P., & Mogg, K. (2007). Biases in visual orienting to negative and positive scenes in dysphoria: An eye movement study. *Journal of Abnormal Psychology, 116,* 491–497.

Chorpita, B. F., Albano, A. M., & Barlow, D. H. (1996). Cognitive processing in children: Relation to anxiety and family influences. *Journal of Clinical Child Psychology, 25,* 170–176.

Cloitre, M., Shear, M. K., Cancienne, J., & Zeitlin, S. B. (1994). Implicit and explicit memory for catastrophic associations to bodily sensation words in panic disorder. *Cognitive Therapy and Research, 18,* 225–240.

Coles, M. E., ,& Heimberg, R. G. (2002). Memory biases in the anxiety disorders: Current status. *Clinical Psychology Review, 22,* 587–627.

Creswell, C., Schniering, C. A., & Rapee, R. M. (2005). Threat interpretation in anxious children and their mothers: Comparison with nonclinical children and the effects of treatment. *Behaviour Research and Therapy, 43,* 1375–1381.

Dalgleish, T., Moradi, A. R., Taghavi, M. R., Neshat-Doost, H. T., & Yule, W. (2001). An experimental investigation of hypervigilance for threat in children and adolescents with post-traumatic stress disorder. *Psychological Medicine, 31,* 541–547.

Dalgleish, T., Taghavi, M. R., Neshat-Doost, H. T., Moradi, A., Canterbury, R. & Yule, W. (2003). Patterns of processing bias for emotional information across clinical disorders: A comparison of attention, memory, and prospective cognition in children and adolescents with depression, generalized anxiety, and posttraumatic stress disorder. *Journal of Clinical Child and Adolescent Psychology, 32,* 10–21.

de Decker, A., Hermans, D., Raes, F., & Eelen, P. (2003). Autobiographical memory specificity and trauma in inpatient adolescents. *Journal of Clinical Child and Adolescent Psychology, 32,* 22–31.

Dozois, D. J. A., Seeds, P. M., & Collins, K. A. (2009). Transdiagnostic approaches to the prevention of depression and anxiety. *Journal of Cognitive Psychotherapy, 23,* 44–59.

Gamble, A. L., & Rapee, R. M. (2009). The time-course of attentional bias in anxious children and adolescents. *Journal of Anxiety Disorders, 23,* 841–847.

Gifford, S., Reynolds, S., Bell, S., & Wilson, C. (2008). Threat interpretation bias in anxious children and their mothers. *Cognition and Emotion, 22,* 497–508.

Gross, J. J. (Ed.). (2007). *Handbook of emotion regulation.* New York: Guilford Press.

Harvey, A. G., Watkins, E. R., Mansell, W., & Shafran, R. (2004). *Cognitive behavioural processes across psychological disorders: A transdiagnostic approach to research and treatment.* Oxford, UK: Oxford University Press.

Joormann, J., & D'Avanzato, C. (2010). Emotion regulation in depression: Examining the role of cognitive processes. *Cognition and Emotion, 24,* 913–939.

Joormann, J., Talbot, L., & Gotlib, I. H. (2007). Biased processing of emotional information in girls at risk for depression. *Journal of Abnormal Psychology, 116,* 135–143.

Kellough, J. L., Beevers, C. G., Ellis, A. J., & Wells, T. T. (2008). Time course of selective attention in clinically depressed young adults: An eye tracking study. *Behaviour Research and Therapy, 46,* 1238–1243.

Cognitive Biases 81

Koster, E. H. W., Fox, E., & MacLeod, C. (2009). Introduction to the special section on cognitive bias modification in emotional disorders. *Journal of Abnormal Psychology, 118*, 1-4.

Kring, A. M., & Sloan, D. M. (2010). *Emotion regulation and psychopathology: A
transdiagnostic approach to etiology and treatment.* New York: Guilford Press.

Kuyken, W., & Howell, R. (2000). Facets of autobiographical memory in adolescents with major depressive disorder and never-depressed controls. *Cognition and Emotion, 20*, 466-487.

Kuyken, W., Howell, R., & Dalgleish, T. (2006). Overgeneral autobiographical
memory in depressed adolescents with, versus without, a reported history of
trauma. *Journal of Abnormal Psychology, 115*, 387-396.

Lazarus, R. S. (1994). *Emotion and adaptation.* Oxford, UK: Oxford University
Press.

Lazarus, R. S., & Folkman, S. (1984). *Stress, appraisal, and coping.* New York:
Springer.

MacLeod, C., Mathews, A., & Tata, P. (1986). Attentional bias in emotional disorders. *Journal of Abnormal Psychology, 95*, 15-20.

MacLeod, C., Rutherford, E., Campbell, L., Ebsworthy, G., & Holker, L. (2002).
Selective attention and emotional vulnerability: Assessing the causal basis
of their association through the experimental manipulation of attentional
bias. *Journal of Abnormal Psychology, 111*, 107-123.

Mansell, W., Harvey, A., Watkins, E., & Shafran, R. (2009). Conceptual foundations of the transdiagnostic approach to CBT. *Journal of Cognitive Psychotherapy: An International Quarterly, 23*, 6-19.

Mathews, A., & MacLeod, C. (2005). Cognitive vulnerability to emotional disorders. *Annual Review of Clinical Psychology, 1*, 167-195.

Mogg, K., Bradley, B. P., Miles, F., & Dixon, R. (2004). Time course of attentional
bias for threat scenes: Testing the vigilance–avoidance hypothesis. *Cognition
and Emotion, 18*, 689-700.

Monk, C. S., Nelson, E. E., McClure, E. B., Mogg, K., Bradley, B. P., Leibenluft, E.,
et al. (2006). Ventrolateral prefrontal cortex activation and attentional bias
in response to angry faces in adolescents with generalized anxiety disorder.
American Journal of Psychiatry, 163, 1091-1097.

Moradi, A. R., Taghavi, M. R., Neshat-Doost, H. T., Yule, W., & Dalgleish, T.
(1999). Performance of children and adolescents with PTSD on the Stroop
colour-naming task. *Psychological Medicine, 29*, 415-419.

Moradi, A. R., Taghavi, R., Neshat-Doost, H. T., Yule, W., & Dalgleish, T. (2000).
Memory bias for emotional information in children and adolescents with
posttraumatic stress disorder: A preliminary study. *Journal of Anxiety Disorders, 14*, 521-534.

Neshat-Doost, H. T., Moradi, A. R., Taghavi, M. R., Yule, W., & Dalgleish, T.
(2000). Lack of attentional bias for emotional information in clinically
depressed children and adolescents on the dot probe task. *Journal of Child
Psychology and Psychiatry, 41*, 363-368.

Neshat-Doost, H. T., Taghavi, M. R., Moradi, A. R., Yule, W., & Dalgleish, T.
(1998). Memory for emotional trait adjectives in clinically depressed youth.
Journal of Abnormal Psychology, 107, 642-650.

Park, R. J., Goodyer, I. M., & Teasdale, J. D. (2002). Categoric overgeneral autobiographical memory in adolescents with major depressive disorder. *Psychological Medicine, 32,* 267–276.

Pine, D. S., Lissek, S., Klein, R. G., Mannuzza, S., Moulton, J. L. III, Guardino, M., et al. (2004). Face-memory and emotion: Associations with major depression in children and adolescents. *Journal of Child Psychology and Psychiatry, 45,* 1199–1208.

Pine, D. S., Mogg, K., Bradley, B. P., Montgomery, L., Monk, C. S., McClure, E., et al. (2005). Attention bias to threat in maltreated children: Implications for vulnerability to stress-related psychopathology. *American Journal of Psychiatry, 162,* 291–296.

Richards, J. C., Austin, D. W., & Alvarenga, M. E. (2001). Interpretation of ambiguous interoceptive stimuli in panic disorder and nonclinical panic. *Cognitive Therapy and Research, 25,* 235–246.

Roy, A. K., Vasa, R. A., Bruck, M., Mogg, K., Bradley, B. P., Sweeney, M., et al. (2008). Attention bias toward threat in pediatric anxiety disorders. *Journal of the American Academy of Child and Adolescent Psychiatry, 47,* 1189–1196.

Schartau, P. E. S., Dalgleish, T., & Dunn, B. D. (2009). Seeing the bigger picture: Training in perspective broadening reduces self-reported affect and psychophysiological response to distressing films and autobiographical memories. *Journal of Abnormal Psychology, 118,* 15–27.

Singer, J. A., & Moffitt, K. H. (1991–1992). An experimental investigation of specificity and generality in memory narratives. *Imagination, Cognition, and Personality, 11,* 233–257.

Stopa, L., & Clark, D. M. (2000). Social phobia and interpretation of social events. *Behaviour Research and Therapy, 38,* 273–283.

Stroop, J. R. (1935). Studies of interference in serial verbal reactions. *Journal of Experimental Psychology, 18,* 643–662.

Swales, M. A., Williams, J. M. G., & Wood, P. (2001). Specificity of autobiographical memory and mood disturbance in adolescents. *Cognition and Emotion, 15,* 321–331.

Taghavi, M. R., Dalgleish, T., Moradi, A. R., Neshat-Doost, H. T., & Yule, W. (2003). Selective processing of negative emotional information in children and adolescents with generalized anxiety disorder. *British Journal of Clinical Psychology, 42,* 221–230.

Taghavi, M. R., Moradi, A. R., Neshat-Doost, H. T., Yule, W., & Dalgleish, T. (2000). Interpretation of ambiguous emotional information in clinically anxious children and adolescents. *Cognition and Emotion, 14,* 809–822.

Taghavi, M. R., Neshat-Doost, H. T., Moradi, A. R., Yule, W., & Dalgleish, T. (1999). Biases in visual attention in children and adolescents with clinical anxiety and mixed anxiety-depression. *Journal of Abnormal Child Psychology, 27,* 215–223.

Taylor, S., & Clark, D. A. (2009). Transdiagnostic cognitive-behavioral treatments for mood and anxiety disorders: Introduction to the special issue. *Journal of Cognitive Psychotherapy: An International Quarterly, 23,* 3–5.

Timbremont, B., Braet, C., Bosmans, G., & Van Vlierberghe, L. (2008). Cognitive biases in depressed and non-depressed referred youth. *Clinical Psychology and Psychotherapy, 15,* 329–339.

Tran, T. B., Siemer, M., & Joormann, J. (2011). Implicit interpretation biases affect emotional vulnerability: A training study. *Cognition and Emotion, 25,* 546–558.

Van Damme, S., & Crombez, G. (2009). Measuring attentional bias to threat in children and adolescents: A matter of speed? *Journal of Behavior Therapy and Experimental Psychiatry, 40,* 344–351.

Vervoort, L., Wolters, L. H., Hogendoorn, S. M., Prins, P. J., de Haan, E., Boer, F., et al. (2011). Temperament, attentional processes, and anxiety: Diverging links between adolescents with and without anxiety disorders? *Journal of Clinical Child and Adolescent Psychology, 40,* 144–155.

Vrana, S. R., Roodman, A., & Beckham, J. C. (1995). Selective processing of trauma-relevant words in posttraumatic stress disorder. *Journal of Anxiety Disorders, 9,* 515–530.

Vrielynck, N., Deplus, S., & Philippot, P. (2007). Overgeneral autobiographical memory and depressive disorder in children. *Journal of Clinical Child and Adolescent Psychology, 36,* 95–105.

Waters, A. M., Craske, M. G., Bergman, R. L., & Treanor, M. (2008). Threat interpretation bias as a vulnerability factor in childhood anxiety disorders. *Behaviour Research and Therapy, 46,* 39–47.

Waters, A. M., Lipp, O. V., & Cobham, V. E. (2000). Investigation of threat-related attentional bias in anxious children using the startle eyeblink modification paradigm. *Journal of Psychophysiology, 14,* 142–150.

Waters, A. M., Lipp, O. V., & Spence, S. H. (2004). Attentional bias toward fear-related stimuli: An investigation with nonselected children and adults and children with anxiety disorders. *Journal of Experimental Child Psychology, 89,* 320–337.

Waters, A. M., Mogg, K., Bradley, B. P., & Pine, D. S. (2008). Attentional bias for emotional faces in children with generalized anxiety disorder. *Journal of the American Academy of Child and Adolescent Psychiatry, 47,* 435–442.

Weierich, M. R., Treat, T. A., & Hollingworth, A. (2008). Theories and measurement of visual attentional processing in anxiety. *Cognition and Emotion, 22,* 985–1018.

Williams, J. M., & Broadbent, K. (1986). Autobiographical memory in suicide attempters. *Journal of Abnormal Psychology, 95,* 144–149.

Wisco, B. E. (2009). Depressive cognition: Self-reference and depth of processing. *Clinical Psychology Review, 29,* 382–392.

CHAPTER 5

Behavioral Avoidance across Child and Adolescent Psychopathology

Brian C. Chu, Laura C. Skriner, and Alison M. Staples

Avoidance and escape are well-documented etiological behavioral processes in the development and maintenance of anxiety. But what roles do they play in other childhood disorders? In this chapter, we define avoidance/escape and its related constructs. We then review evidence for the mechanistic role of avoidance in promoting and maintaining psychological distress across four major youth diagnostic classes (anxiety, depression, conduct, and impulse disorders) to identify its potential as a transdiagnostic mechanism. Various study designs are reviewed, including longitudinal, observational, experimental, and clinical trial research, to understand how different methodologies contribute to our understanding of avoidance. The chapter concludes by proposing a model that pinpoints the different functions of avoidance along a continuum of time. That is, dysfunctional avoidance in various psychological disorders may be differentiated depending on when it manifests itself in the sequence of pathological events. This model will provide direction for future study of avoidance in youth, including recommendations for common terminology and assessment methods across disorders.

Defining Avoidance and Related Constructs

The terms *behavioral escape* and *avoidance* refer to situations in which an individual does not enter, or prematurely leaves, a fear-evoking or distressing situation (henceforth shortened to *avoidance* unless otherwise specified). Cognitive and emotional processes can be invoked during avoidance (e.g., distraction, experiential avoidance); however, this chapter primarily focuses on behavioral forms. We touch on cognitive and emotional avoidance, which are important areas for research growth, but the majority of existing research focuses on behaviors.

Why is avoidance bad? Several theories try to explain how avoidance maintains psychological distress. As summarized by Harvey, Watkins, Mansell, and Shafran (2004), most suggest that avoidance interferes with proper emotional processing and learning. According to the habituation model of anxiety, prolonged exposure is required to decrease physiological aspects of anxiety (brief exposure periods may "sensitize" patients to feared stimuli). According to the emotion processing model of anxiety (Foa, Huppert, & Cahill, 2006), pathological fear structures contain associations among a stimulus, a response, and meaning representations that distort reality. Repeated avoidance prevents sufficient activation of the fear network, precluding new, anti-anxiety information from being learned. In both the habituation and emotion processing models, avoidance prevents prolonged exposure. Learning theory assigns a number of impairing functions to avoidance. First, avoidance behavior is often negatively reinforced because it provides immediate relief through escape. Second, avoidance denies the person opportunities for positive reinforcement and contributes to a deprived environment (Ferster, 1973; Jacobson, Martell, & Dimidjian, 2001). Third, it may exacerbate self-focused attention and ruminative thinking because avoidance narrows the person's interests and reduces his or her exposure to external stimuli. From a cognitive perspective, avoidance removes the opportunity to disconfirm negative beliefs (Salkovskis, 1991). Finally, avoidance behavior is intrinsically problematic because sheer absence from school, play, or social environments interferes with socio-occupational functioning. By contrast, preventing avoidance can increase a sense of self-control and self-efficacy that promotes approach behavior. No matter the theory, behavioral, emotional, and cognitive processes are affected when avoidance is used as a solution to a stressful trigger.

But doesn't avoidance work sometimes? Research in adult depression suggests that avoidance strategies such as distraction can attenuate dysphoric mood (e.g., Morrow & Nolen-Hoeksema, 1990; Nolen-Hoeksema, Morrow, & Fredrickson, 1993). However, in these circumstances, distraction is defined as an active response that prevents cognitive rumination and encourages pursuit of pleasurable activities. Thus "avoidance" of a pathological process may be desirable to the extent that it encourages approach behavior in other domains of life (cf., "pragmatic truth criterion"; Jacobson et al., 2001). A second line of research presents the possible beneficial effect of thought suppression. When individuals use thought suppression techniques to distract from intrusive thoughts and worry, distressing thoughts do tend to abate—but only in the short term. Distraction and suppression of intrusive thoughts and worry are subject to "rebound effects" wherein suppressed thoughts often return with greater frequency and intensity after the suppression ceases (Abramowitz, Tolin, & Street, 2001; Wegner, Schneider, Carter, & White, 1987).

Figure 5.1 illustrates the short- and long-term impact of avoidance in the case of a school-refusing youth. Following the habituation model, psychological distress should naturally spike in anticipation of, or following exposure to, a fearful stimulus. Claims of sickness, dread, and physical resistance increase as the youth's parents prompt the youth to prepare for school. Complaints and resistance increase during bathroom time, breakfast, the car ride to school, and finally school and classroom entry. At any point in time, the youth could choose to escape as his distress increases. He could resist rising from bed, refuse to get in the car, or refuse to enter school. Choosing to avoid/escape has two effects. First, distress immediately drops. Resisting a parent's prompts to rise from bed until the parent stops leads to almost instantaneous relief ("I get to stay home!"). Over time, the youth draws the eminently logical conclusion that, "Escaping a distressing situation makes me feel better." Although this conclusion makes logical sense, a second consequence results. The youth never learns that distress would naturally lessen or abate with sufficient perseverance. With time, natural habituation would decrease distress, prompting the

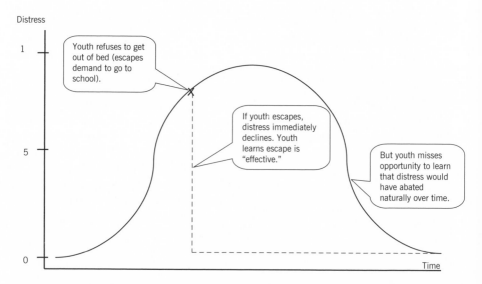

FIGURE 5.1. Effect of escape on learning in the case of a school-refusing youth. Escape is negatively reinforced by its immediate impact on distress reduction.

conclusion, "Things get better with time." Escape prevents the second lesson from occurring but reinforces the first. This illustration highlights the interactive roles that behavioral avoidance, emotional habituation, and cognitive beliefs play in reinforcing future avoidance behavior.

Figure 5.1 provides a straightforward example. Some notes: First, the habituation curve is rarely "smooth." Distress levels often follow smaller peaks and valleys as parent and child negotiate and bargain and alternate between resistance and concession. For example, a child might refuse to dress, leading the parent to relent momentarily to attend to other children. This momentary success alleviates distress until the parent returns to resume the fight, reescalating distress. Any habituation curve could reflect this "scalloped" form of mini-peaks and valleys. Second, avoidance can be complete or partial. Ineffective safety behaviors (e.g., relying on presence of parent, medication, food, drink, or talisman) are ways the youth can "remove" oneself from a situation behaviorally, cognitively, or emotionally to reduce distress. Such behaviors prevent full exposure to the stimulus and prevent access to contradictory information. Finally, extinction bursts should be expected. A dutiful parent may execute "planned ignoring" to help the child habituate, but one should expect a sharp peak of distress (and outwardly expressed opposition!) as the parent ignores the oppositional behavior without positive reinforcement.

Avoidance in Youth Anxiety Disorders

The remainder of the chapter reviews the research on the various processes described in Figure 5.1, including escape, avoidance, safety behaviors, and ineffective coping strategies. We start with reviewing anxiety disorders, as substantial research has established the etiological and maintaining role of avoidance.

Experimental Studies of Avoidance in Anxiety

Experimental studies have explored both the causal role of avoidance in triggering anxiety and avoidance as a consequence of teaching fear-valenced information. For example, Huijding and colleagues (2009) completed an experiment with 95 nonclinical youth (ages 9–13 years) to show that behavioral training of approach–avoidance behaviors without any additional information could lead to changes in evaluations of novel stimuli, differences in fear beliefs, and further behavioral avoidance. Using a computer approach–avoidance task, youth participants were instructed to repeatedly push away (avoid) or pull closer (approach) pictures of novel animals using a joystick. Trait anxiety and fear ratings of the novel animal were measured with self-report questionnaires and global evaluations with a visual analogue scale (e.g., "Do you think this [animal] is positive?"). Implicit attitudes were assessed with an Implicit Association Test (IAT). Avoidance tendencies (posttraining) were measured using a "nature reserve task," in which the child was asked to place himself or herself at varying distances from the approached or avoided animal in a series of pictorial scenarios. The computer approach–avoidance training produced greater positive evaluations toward the pulled animals and more negative evaluations to the pushed animals for all children. Both fear and avoidance tendencies (nature reserve task) toward avoided animals increased for girls, but not for boys. Implicit attitudes were not affected by the experiment. Stronger prior trait anxiety was related to stronger changes in self-reported attitudes and, in boys, also produced stronger fear beliefs, suggesting that trait vulnerability may be required to produce avoidance effects in boys. The results suggest that behavioral avoidance can have emotional and attitudinal consequences, as well as produce further avoidance, even when the child is presented with minimal verbal information.

Likewise, ample evidence has demonstrated that negative verbal and visual information about a novel animal can prospectively drive avoidance behaviors. In a series of experiments, Field and colleagues recruited nonclinical youth (ages 6–9) to demonstrate how information about novel animals would produce emotional, attitudinal, and behavioral avoidance. Field and Lawson (2003) reported that 59 children received negative and positive information (short stories) about novel animals. The children were evaluated for self-reported fear beliefs, behavioral avoidance (latency to approach three touch boxes that contained an animal), and implicit attitudes (response latencies on an IAT). Fear beliefs grew more intense after negative information and less intense after positive information (no change after no information). Data from the IAT demonstrated that fear beliefs could be trained at the implicit semantic level. On the behavioral avoidance task, children took a longer than average time to approach the box if negative information had been given and a significantly shorter than average time to approach the box if positive information had been given. These results are several steps away from linking fear beliefs to diagnosable disorders, but findings demonstrate that fear information can produce behavioral avoidance in youth without dispositional anxiety.

Follow-up studies using this paradigm have demonstrated several additional facts about the learning process. Elevated fear beliefs and behavioral avoidance can be taught using nonverbal pairings of fearful faces with an animal (compared with happy and unpaired), and these fear beliefs can last over a 3-month period (Askew & Field, 2007). Furthermore, when threat information (e.g., "an animal might bite you") is paired with a compatible experience (e.g., a mechanical animal "leaps out" and surprises the child when they reach into a touch box), fear beliefs and avoidance tendencies are greater than when either receiving threat information or experiencing a surprise alone (Field & Storksen-Coulson, 2007). Also, fear beliefs held by children prior to the negative experience exacerbated the effect of the negative experience, suggesting that prior cognitive conditions make some youth more vulnerable to fear experiences. Together, this series of studies confirms the reciprocal relations among behavioral, cognitive, and emotional learning, demonstrating that learned avoidance can promote attitudinal and emotional deficits and that behavioral avoidance can be a consequence of learned fear.

Experimental and Observational Family Studies of Youth Anxiety

A complementary experimental literature illustrates how parent messages and modeling of avoidance can foster anxiety. An early experimental study coined a phenomenon, the "FEAR effect" (Family Enhancement of Avoidant Responses; Barrett, Rapee, Dadds, & Ryan, 1996), to describe how parents foster children's selection of avoidant choices when managing ambiguous situations. Youth (ages 7–14) read ambiguous situations with potential social or physical threat and then provided responses coded for threat interpretations and avoidant solutions. Youth with anxiety, compared with oppositional and nonclinical youth, offered a greater number of threat interpretations than nonclinical youth (though less than oppositional youth) and more avoidant plans than either group. After a subsequent 5-minute conversation with their parents, twice as many anxious youth chose an avoidant solution than had done so before the family discussion. Follow-up analysis indicated that parents were more likely to discourage nonavoidant responses and reciprocate their child's avoidant communication during discussions (Dadds, Barrett, Rapee, & Ryan, 1996). A later replication found that maternal distress also predicted increases in anxious–avoidant responding after family discussion (Shortt, Barrett, Dadds, & Fox, 2001).

Since the FEAR effect was identified, a number of observational and semiexperimental studies have illustrated how parents communicate fear and avoidance through modeling fears and threat information (Fisak & Grills-Taquechel, 2007). Questionnaire studies show that youth notice a parent's anxious parenting and avoidant behavior, and that this has been associated with higher internalizing symptoms. Observational studies show that mothers with anxiety tend to model more catastrophizing than mothers without anxiety (Moore, Whaley, & Sigman, 2004; Whaley, Pinto, & Sigman, 1999). Experimental data show that mothers of youth with anxiety exhibit greater anxious parenting (focus on negatives/dangers, expression of doubt that child could succeed) than parents without anxiety for children both with and without anxiety (Barrett, Fox, & Farrell, 2005) and that communication of fears and negative information is influential in shaping child fear beliefs and subsequent avoidant behavior (Field & Lawson, 2003). Other studies carefully demonstrate that the arrow can point in both directions, such that there can be an interaction between mother's and child's anxiety in predicting maternal catastrophizing (Moore et al., 2004; Schrock & Woodruff-Borden, 2010); in some cases, it is the child's anxiety status that predicts parenting style, regardless of parent anxiety (Hudson, Doyle, & Gar, 2009). In sum, youth with anxiety transmit messages of distress and desires to avoid, and parents often respond by permitting avoidance or escalating fear and catastrophizing. In this way, not only is avoidance reinforced by its natural reinforcing properties but it also may become a fixed pattern through modeling and social learning.

Youth Self-Report of Avoidant Coping Strategies

In cross-sectional studies, youth-reported avoidant strategies have been linked to internalizing and externalizing symptoms. In a series of community and clinical studies, Compas, Connor-Smith, and colleagues identified three broad stress-response styles: engagement coping, disengagement coping, and involuntary responding (Compas, Connor-Smith, Saltzman, Thomsen, & Wadsworth, 2001; Connor-Smith, Compas, Wadsworth, Thomsen, & Saltzman, 2000). *Engagement coping* is conscious effort directed toward a stressor (e.g., problem solving, emotional regulation, cognitive restructuring) that is consistent with approach behavior. *Disengagement* (or *avoidant*) *coping* includes most mental and behavioral conscious efforts to avoid stressors (e.g., denial, wishful thinking, behavioral avoidance). *Involuntary responding* includes conditioned reactions that are not under volitional control (e.g., rumination, intrusive thinking, emotional arousal, cognitive interference, inaction). In community samples (Compas et al., 2001), engagement coping has shown correlations with lower internalizing symptoms ($r = -.39$ to $-.52$) and lower externalizing problems ($r = -.27$ to $-.37$). Disengagement coping has been correlated with higher internalizing and externalizing symptoms ($r = .18$ to $.29$). Involuntary responding also proves strongly correlated with internalizing symptoms ($r = .36$ to $.53$).

In clinical samples, structural equation models (Compas et al., 2006) have demonstrated that specific anxiety and depression symptoms can be differentially predicted by engagement and disengagement coping. In a sample of adolescents with recurrent abdominal pain, disengagement coping strongly predicted higher levels of anxiety, depression, and somatic complaints. Secondary control engagement coping (acceptance, distraction, positive thinking, cognitive restructuring) predicted lower levels of anxiety and depression symptoms and somatic complaints. Primary control engagement (problem solving, emotion regulation, emotional expression), surprisingly, did not. A series of studies with offspring of depressed parents (Jaser et al., 2005, 2007; Langrock, Compas, Keller, & Merchant, 2002) did not find significant relations between disengagement coping and anxiety or depression symptoms, but secondary control engagement coping was again significantly related to better health. Likewise, in a treatment study (Compas et al., 2010), mediation analysis demonstrated that increases in secondary control coping strategies led to subsequent change in internalizing symptoms during preventive family treatment directed at families with a parent with past depression. Coping change accounted for approximately half of the intervention effect. The differences in outcomes across these studies may reflect differences in samples (identified pediatric youth vs. offspring of depressed parents) and reporter differences (youth vs. parent report). The mixed findings for the relationship between disengagement coping and anxious and depressed symptoms may reflect the fact that the subscale entails multiple forms of disengagement, including mental and behavioral avoidance. Isolating behavioral avoidance from denial and wishful thinking may produce more consistent findings.

Behavioral Avoidance Tasks in Treatment Studies

Observing avoidant behavior may be the most direct way to identify forms of avoidance in youth with anxiety, but observational studies are relatively rare except when used as outcome measures in clinical trials (Silverman & Ollendick, 2005). Such procedures traditionally cover three main types of tasks: (1) social evaluative tasks, (2) behavioral avoidance tasks, and (3) parent–youth interaction tasks (as presented earlier). Social evaluative tasks ask the child to perform an anxiety-provoking task (e.g., reading a story aloud), after which researchers code for inhibited behaviors (e.g., speaking softly). Behavioral avoidance tasks (BATs) expose children to feared stimuli under relatively controlled and replicable conditions (e.g., approaching a container with a snake and holding it for 10 seconds). This method has primarily been used with youth with specific phobias or to assess parent–youth interactions. There is a notable lack of standardization across these tasks, and no one paradigm has been developed to translate across different kinds of fears (e.g., specific fear vs. general worry) and contexts (e.g., fear of specific object vs. social evaluation). This makes it difficult to identify general themes in this literature.

The use of behavioral observations as outcome measures in clinical trials has demonstrated support for the effectiveness of current treatments in reducing avoidant behaviors. Chu and Harrison (2007) conducted a meta-analysis of clinical trials for youth anxiety and depression that also measured behavioral processes. The majority of anxiety studies assessed some behavioral process, including avoidance. Behavioral observations were typically coded for general behavioral and social inhibition, but some included approach tasks that assessed change in specific skills targeted in treatment (e.g., social skills, avoidant solutions, speech-giving skills). Other behavioral measures included parent- or youth-report questionnaires assessing youth behavioral traits or idiographic fear ratings (e.g., fear thermometer). In these trials, cognitive and behavioral treatments (CBT) reliably produced large treatment effects (ES = 1.02) across behavioral outcomes, including BATs.

Anxiety Disorders Summary

Together, avoidance plays an identifiable and substantial role in promoting and maintaining anxiety in youth. Experimental data demonstrates that in nonclinical youth, fears and threat attitudes can be enhanced through behavioral avoidance. Likewise, behavioral avoidance is a consistent consequence of fear and threat information. How youth cope with threats and stress also determines the distress they experience: purposeful disengagement promotes internalizing distress; active approach strategies and cognitive restructuring reduce risk for distress. The family context plays a role by encouraging avoidance and accommodating youth fears. Finally, preliminary evidence suggests that successful treatment following CBT helps reduce avoidant behaviors as anxiety symptoms diminish. This suggests a potential mediating role for avoidance in alleviating anxiety.

Avoidance in Youth Depressive Disorders

The role of avoidance in depression has received much attention in adult populations but less in youth. The symptom profile of depression itself highlights the stark *lack* of behaviors during a depressive episode and implies a potential role for avoidance in the withdrawal, isolation, and anhedonia typical of this disorder. Initial behavioral theories of depression focused on the individual's inability to access or appreciate positive reinforcement (Ferster, 1973; Lewinsohn & Graf, 1973). Daily tasks or interactions with others are perceived as difficult by the depressed individual and are therefore avoided, limiting access to potentially reinforcing environments. Moreover, an individual with depression often withdraws from the social realm, simultaneously isolating and alienating him- or herself from others. Unfortunately, this avoidance and isolation only deepens depression.

Recent conceptualizations of behavioral activation therapy for depression have highlighted the role of avoidance as a response to internal distress states (Jacobson et al., 2001). In this model, avoidance is maintained in depression much like it is in anxiety: avoidant behavior is triggered by a distressing event and then is negatively reinforced by the subsequent reduction in distress even as it contributes to a number of secondary problems. Continued avoidance perpetuates a cycle of inactivity, withdrawal, and inertia that denies the child access or opportunity to contact antidepressant sources of reinforcement (Jacobson et al. 2001; Manos, Kanter, & Busch, 2010). Research directly examining avoidance processes in depression is less common than that found in the study of anxiety, but a variety of research designs have explored the role of behavioral activity, goal setting, social withdrawal and isolation, and cognitive rumination in depression.

Activity Level, Goal Striving, and Depression

Early studies of behavioral activation in adults found support for the positive relationship between activity level and mood (Lewinsohn & Graf, 1973; Lewinsohn & Libet, 1972). This research was correlational and tracked individuals' levels of activities, as well as self-reported mood, across time. A meta-analysis conducted by Cuijpers, van Straten, and Warmerdam (2007) examined 16 studies of activity scheduling in depressed adults. They found no difference in posttreatment depression measures when comparing activity scheduling (e.g., behavioral activation) to other psychological treatments (pooled $d = 0.13$). Similar investigations of mood and activity level have been conducted with youth, replicating results found with adults. Wierzbicki and Sayler (1991) found a significant, positive relationship between children's depressed mood and their amount of unpleasant activities when examining both parent and child reports of children's depression and activities in a sample of nonclinical youth. However, when exploring the relationship between children's depressed mood and pleasant activities, a significant negative correlation was found only when examining parents', not children's, reports of children's depression. Although the role of avoidance in depression was not examined directly, these findings suggest that amounts of pleasant and unpleasant activities in an individual's repertoire are related to depression. One could hypothesize that those individuals with greater depression were avoiding activities once considered pleasant or positively reinforcing, which would contribute to, if not trigger, depressive mood.

Hopko and colleagues (Hopko, Armento, Cantu, Chambers, & Lejuez, 2003) have conducted an updated replication of this research with adults using a diary-based approach to data collection, in which activities were measured in half-hour intervals for 1 week. Similar findings resulted, with a negative relationship between the amount of experienced pleasure or reward and depressive symptoms, and activity level and depressive symptoms. More recent research has explored additional measures of activity level, such as the Behavioral Activation for Depression Scale (BADS; Kanter, Mulick, Busch, Berlin, & Martell, 2007). The BADS, which assesses the frequency of activity initiation, escape, and avoidance behaviors, has been found to correlate significantly with depression symptoms in adults (Manos et al., 2010) but is only now being studied with youth samples.

A small body of research has explored motivational goals underlying both anxiety and depression in youth (Dickson & MacLeod, 2004, 2006). Goals prompting approach behaviors tend to be focused on positive outcomes in which the individual moves toward or attempts to maintain a desirable result. In comparison, goals prompting avoidance behaviors tend to be focused on negative outcomes in which the individual moves away from or inhibits an undesirable end state (Elliot, Sheldon, & Church, 1997). Dickson and MacLeod (2004) administered self-report questionnaires to adolescents, prompting them to record as many approach and avoidance goals and plans as they could generate. Prompts to assess idiographic goals included: "In the future it will be important for me to..." and "In the future it will be important for me to avoid. . .". Plans were assessed with prompts such as, "How can I accomplish this?" and "How can I avoid this?" (Dickson & MacLeod, 2004, pp. 420–421). Subsequently, participants were asked to choose their two most important approach and avoidance goals and to record their strategies for achieving their goals. Results from the study indicated that youth in the high-depression group and youth with mixed anxiety and depression recorded significantly fewer approach goals and fewer approach plans compared with controls. Additionally, they generated significantly more avoidance plans—but not more avoidance goals—than controls. In conjunction with the cognitive theory of depression, Dickson and MacLeod suggest that this lack of approach motivation may perpetuate a "depressive motivational cycle" (p. 427) that contributes to anhedonia and a limited activity repertoire, thereby limiting the youth's opportunity for positive reinforcement. Furthermore, the adolescents with high anxiety generated significantly more avoidance goals compared with the depression and control groups. The authors suggest that these differences may distinguish youth with depression from those with anxiety. The mechanism that explains why youth with depression use more avoidance plans even when they do not make it a goal to be avoidant. Further research should demonstrate direct links between avoidant goals and plans, subsequent avoidance actions, and ultimate depressed mood. Combining methodologies from this literature with the self-report and diary methods in the pleasant activities literature may allow research to progress.

Social Relations and Avoidance

Isolation, avoidance, and dysfunctional peer relations have a unique transactional relationship in youth with depression. Excessive reassurance seeking, complaining, and a negative attitude may disrupt and damage social relationships by eliciting negative responses and avoidance from peers (see Rudolph, Flynn, & Abaied, 2008). Research has also found that youth with depression exhibit a decrease in adaptive interpersonal behaviors, such as problem-solving behavior and positive statements, during interactions with family (Sheeber & Sorensen, 1998). Additionally, research exploring avoidance in the form of social withdrawal emphasizes its role in maintaining depression in youth.

Using factor analysis, Bell-Dolan, Reaven, and Peterson (1993) explored the relationship between depression in youth and various forms of social functioning. Previous research had suggested that youth with depression have a lower overall frequency of peer interactions, as well as a higher frequency of negative interactions (e.g., aggression; Altmann & Gotlib, 1988). Additional research suggested that the attempts of youth with depression to get social support might often result in rejection from peers (Peterson, Mullins, & Ridley-Johnson, 1985). Bell-Dolan and colleagues' (1993) assessment using multiple reporters (child, peer, teacher, parent) revealed that ratings of aggressive social behavior and social withdrawal were positively related to depression (R^2 = .28 to .62). Similarly, Gazelle and Rudolph (2004) showed that adolescents with anxiety and their teachers who reported high levels of peer exclusion also exhibited social avoidance and depression. Without social exclusion, youth demonstrated an increase in social approach and fewer depressive symptoms. This cross-sectional research suggests an important role of social withdrawal and isolation in intensifying depression.

Several studies employed longitudinal designs to map trajectories of depressed affect and identify unique roles of individual avoidance (withdrawal, isolation) and social exclusion from peers in predicting depression. Gazelle and Ladd (2003) established evidence for a "snowball effect" wherein initial social exclusion and isolation resulted in accelerating depressive affect and other maladjustment over time. A five-wave assessment of children in kindergarten through fourth grade demonstrated that depressive affect increased among children who were initially withdrawn and those who were initially excluded. Children who were both isolative and socially excluded displayed the greatest increases in depressed affect over time. Comparable findings come from a study of early adolescents (Oh et al., 2008), in which a trajectory of increasing withdrawal, from grades 5 through 8, was marked by high degrees of friendlessness, friendship instability, and peer exclusion.

Bukowski, Laursen, and Hoza (2010) studied the combined impact of accelerating social avoidance and peer exclusion with the moderating role of friendship as a buffer against depressed affect. Three-wave multilevel modeling of children (in grades 3–5) identified multiple unique trajectories using both sociometric (peer nomination) and peer-assessment measures. Initial social avoidance or exclusion was associated with concurrent levels of depressed affect and was antecedent to escalating trajectories of depressed affect over time. Youth identified as both avoidant and excluded showed the greatest accelerated trajectory. Interaction effects did demonstrate a buffering effect for youth who had at least one close friend or who developed a friendship over time. Future research will want to employ experimental or cross-lagged designs to establish causality, and depressed affect will need to be linked to depressive disorders, but initial evidence points to predictive roles for individual avoidance, withdrawal, and isolation in depressive symptoms. Of note, each study identified a buffering role of friendship, even among children who started as isolative or avoidant. This suggests that youth can overcome initial avoidance both with decreased individual avoidance and greater social exposure.

Cognitive Avoidance

A cognitive process that is often discussed in terms of depressive avoidance is rumination. Rumination serves to reduce an individual's engagement with his or her environment and therefore disrupts problem-solving and antidepressant activities (Jacobson et al., 2001). Moulds, Kandris, Starr, and Wong (2007) found that self-report measures of rumination and behavioral avoidance were significantly positively correlated in a sample of nonclinical undergraduate students. Behavioral activation therapy considers rumination a key treatment target and aims to clarify which emotions or stressors the individual is effectively avoiding when he or she spends time ruminating (Jacobson et al., 2001). That is, behavioral activation aims to identify the function of ruminative behavior for an individual (i.e., avoidance). Some researchers suggest that ruminating, or active complaining (a type of ruminative negative behavior), develops because it was likely successful at one point in removing the individual from an undesirable situation (Ferster, 1973). For example, rumination may help the individual feel prepared for the potential of undesired outcomes by anticipating worst-case scenarios. Moulds and colleagues propose that rumination may serve as a strategy for avoiding negative emotions associated with aversive material. Watkins and Moulds (2007) suggest that, similar to theories of the function of worry in generalized anxiety disorder, rumination may allow the individual to avoid poignant imagery or emotions. Similarly, we propose that the central depressive symptom of anhedonia is closely related to avoidance. Anhedonia, defined as a lack of interest in the majority of activities once enjoyed by the individual, may be maintained by a fear that one's own actions have no impact on potential outcomes—one's fears motivate the avoidance that manifests itself as anhedonia.

Behavioral Outcomes in Depression Treatment Studies

Behavioral outcomes are infrequently assessed in youth depression trials, but innovative assessment techniques are currently being investigated, particularly with adults (Manos et al., 2010). When behavioral outcomes have been assessed in youth treatment studies, there is cause for concern. As described earlier, Chu and Harrison (2007) conducted a meta-analysis of depression clinical trials that assessed behavioral outcomes. Only half of the identified clinical trials included a measure of a behavioral process. Measures included the assessment of pleasant activities and social skills, but behavioral observations were not used. In contrast to anxiety trials, CBT for depression did not produce reliable change (ES = 0.01) in behavioral outcomes across eight randomized clinical trials (RCTs). The results suggest that current evidence-based treatments may need to be developed further to successfully target critical behavioral processes that maintain depression in youth. Furthermore, the specific role of avoidance has not been isolated in most attempts to measure behaviors, either as a treatment outcome or a mediator of outcomes.

Depression Research Summary

A variety of design methods (youth and other report, daily diaries) have established consistent relations between depressed mood and avoidant processes, including decreased activity, limited positive events and increased negative events, social withdrawal and isolation, and cognitive rumination. Youth with depression seem to have particular difficulties in generating both approach goals and plans. However, they only seem to have problems generating avoidance plans but not avoidance goals. Social isolation in the form of individual avoidance and peer exclusion has significant concurrent and predictive power, as youth showing early signs of either have poor prognoses for future socialization and depressed mood. Still, friendship serves as a powerful buffer. Overall, behavioral variables are key to depressive mood, but avoidance processes need to be isolated in cross-sectional, longitudinal, and treatment studies.

Avoidance in Disruptive Behavior Disorders

Disruptive behavior disorders (DBDs: oppositional defiance disorder [ODD], conduct disorder [CD], and attention-deficit/hyperactivity disorder [ADHD]) are heterogeneous disorders (Burke, Loeber, Lahey, & Rathouz, 2005; Frick & Ellis, 1999) that likely include subgroups characterized by distinct patterns of behavior and etiologic mechanisms (Hinshaw, 2002). Although avoidance is not typically considered a key process underlying the emergence and maintenance of DBDs, avoidance may play a role for certain youth presenting with DBDs. In order to draw inferences about the role of avoidance in DBDs, we review several literatures, including the co-occurrence of DBDs with anxiety and depressive disorders, avoidance of task demands, and avoidant coping strategies.

DBDs and Anxiety

Anxiety and DBDs commonly co-occur, where the presence of ODD, CD, or ADHD increases chances of an anxiety disorder two to three times (Angold, Costello, & Erkanli, 1999). Evaluating comorbidity among disorders may be the best route to identifying common mechanisms (Hinshaw, 2002). Research has focused on temperament, neurology, and social information processes (Drabick, Ollendick, & Bubier, 2010), but few have looked at behavioral avoidance. The temperament literature focuses on level of emotionality and effortful control (regulatory processes). Information process research focuses on the similarity of cognitive biases among youth with anxiety and disruptive disorders as they interpret ambiguous social scenarios. However, findings from emotion regulation research may contain leads to identifying common behavioral processes in anxiety disorders and DBDs. For instance, youth showing high rates of co-occurring DBDs and anxiety tend to display reactive aggression as opposed to proactive aggression (Bubier & Drabick, 2009), where reactive aggression resembles features common to anxiety. Reactive aggression includes angry, explosive, and often emotionally dysregulated reactions to a perceived threat (Card & Little, 2006), but it is often accompanied by fear and is characterized by high levels of autonomic arousal and hypervigilance to threatening stimuli (Crick & Dodge, 1996; Hubbard et al., 2002). In a related line of research, Barry and colleagues (2000) reported that youth diagnosed with both ADHD and ODD/CD who are low on callous–unemotional (CU) personality traits show elevated levels of anxiety compared with those high on CU traits. Researchers have offered a number of reasons to explain the association between DBDs and anxiety disorders; however, the specific role of avoidance has yet to be investigated.

DBDs and Depression

High rates of comorbidity also typify depression and DBDs, such that having ODD, CD, or ADHD increases odds of depression by five to six times (Angold et al., 1999). DBDs and depression also follow a common developmental trajectory, wherein DBDs generally precede rather than follow the development of depression (Burke et al., 2005). Scant research has focused on common mechanisms, with negative affect identified as playing an important role in distinguishing ODD, CD, and depression (Burke & Loeber, 2010). Evidence for avoidance as a maintaining mechanism comes from conceptual work developed within the "failure model," described by Capaldi and Patterson (Capaldi, 1992; Patterson & Capaldi, 1990). Here, depression results from experiences of failure such as rejection by peers and aversive school experiences associated with antisocial behavior and the high levels of interpersonal conflict characteristic of DBDs. Youth with DBDs characterized by reactive aggression may be particularly likely to follow the failure model. It has been suggested that reactively aggressive youth appear to be at higher risk for social isolation, peer rejection, and social withdrawal than proactively aggressive youth (Poulin & Boivin, 2000). As with depression, because peer rejection is associated with anxiety symptoms (Bell-Dolan, Foster, & Christopher, 1995), it is possible that reactive aggression may also lead to anxiety (Bubier & Drabick, 2009). None of these authors directly imply avoidance as an etiological mechanism of DBDs, but most describe the spiraling nature of initial disruptive behavior preceding depressive disorders. In this way, avoidance may operate as a secondary process whereby avoidance of negative emotions follows an aversive experience (e.g., rejection by or conflict with peers and parents) and increases the likelihood for comorbid depression and further aggressive tendencies.

Avoidance of Task Demands as a Function of Disruptive Behavior

Task demands are a common trigger among youth with DBDs, and experimental research using functional behavioral assessment (FBA) provides evidence that escape from negative affect during task demands may maintain disruptive behavior (e.g., Hawkins & Axelrod, 2008; Moore, Anderson, & Kumar, 2005). Hawkins and Axelrod (2008) completed an experiment using FBA methods to identify the function of off-task behaviors during homework and compared the relative effectiveness of interventions to increase on-task behavior. Four teens (ages 11–16) with various DBDs in a residential treatment program participated in an alternating treatment with baseline design to assess the effects of three treatment conditions for on-task behavior, including noncontingent breaks (i.e., escape) and a differential reinforcement schedule. For three of the four participants, the most effective intervention in increasing on-task behavior during homework was providing a noncontingent break in which the student could sit alone (as opposed to having access to a preferred activity or to edibles), indicating that escape was a powerful reinforcer for on-task behavior. For the fourth participant, escape from task demands did not increase on-task behaviors the most, but it was important. Thus, noncompliant and off-task behavior were frequently maintained by escape from tasks.

In examining ADHD specifically, DuPaul, McGoey, Eckert, and VanBrakle (2001) examined task avoidance in 94 preschool children (58 with ADHD) using direct observations of four parent–child interactions in a clinic playroom, each with varying degrees of parent attention and task demand (e.g., cleaning up playroom). Youth with ADHD exhibited more than twice the level of noncompliance and more than five times the amount of inappropriate behavior than control youth when asked to complete tasks by parents. Furthermore, the authors noted that these results, coupled with the minimal group differences in interactions during low-adult-attention situations, suggest that for many youth with ADHD, escape from parent-directed tasks, assumed to be aversive to youth, is a prime motivation for noncompliant behavior.

Evidence for escape from task demands as an underlying causal mechanism of externalizing behavior also comes from research on the link between externalizing behavior and academic difficulty. For example, Arnold (1997) used direct observations of male youth in the classroom to demonstrate that youth exhibiting externalizing behaviors received less teaching than children without behavior problems and that the relationship between externalizing behaviors and academic difficulties increased with age. Arnold notes that these findings are consistent with the hypothesis that teachers may inadvertently reinforce disruptive behavior in children with academic difficulties by removing the task demands following disruptive behavior. This study focused mainly on the mediation of behavior and academic problems via attention difficulties, but escape of task demands played a prominent role. Still, future research is needed to connect emotionally motivated avoidance with escape of task demands. However, it seems plausible that youth with academic problems experience negative emotions as frustration around academic failures builds and that avoidance would seem an easier coping strategy than the alternatives (e.g., seeking help, diligent study).

Avoidant Coping, Externalizing Disorders, and Delinquency

Research on coping styles among youth with DBDs offers a more direct link between avoidance and disruptive behavior. The use of dysfunctional coping strategies, particularly avoidant coping, in response to negative emotions has been associated with engagement in risky and antisocial behaviors. As described earlier, avoidant (i.e. disengagement) coping includes most mental and behavioral efforts to remove, ignore, or distract oneself from a stressor.

In a community sample of adolescents (i.e., a sample not selected for delinquent behavior), use of avoidant coping strategies and low use of problem solving each related to delinquent behavior. Vassallo and colleagues (2002) used data from the longitudinal Australian Temperament

Project (ATP) to investigate the emergence and maintenance of antisocial behaviors between 13 and 18 years of age. Avoidant coping (e.g., drug and alcohol use) differentiated between antisocial youth and controls, with the difference becoming more pronounced over time.

Daughters and colleagues (2009) investigated the role of distress tolerance in internalizing and externalizing problems among 231 adolescents (ages 9–13). Results showed that low distress tolerance was associated with an increase in past-year alcohol use and past-year delinquent behavior in specific subgroups of youth. Results from a study of incarcerated male adolescents demonstrated that incarcerated youth who used more avoidant coping strategies were more likely to use alcohol and marijuana as a means of alleviating distress (Eftekhari, Turner, & Larimer, 2004) and that avoidant coping is used more often by adolescents in correctional facilities (Ruchkin, Eisemann, & Hägglöf, 1999) than by youth who do not engage in delinquent behaviors. Together, these studies suggest that negative reinforcement processes associated with avoidance of distressing emotions may play a role in the continued engagement in externalizing behaviors.

Avoidant coping has also been associated with reactive aggression and impulsivity (Lengua, Sandler, West, Wolchik, & Curran, 1999). Youth with DBDs who were characterized as reactively aggressive may include a subgroup of youth who engage in avoidant coping and who are at an increased risk of developing internalizing problems. Crick and Dodge (1996) investigated differences in information processing and reported that reactively aggressive children attribute hostile intent to peers and respond in an aggressive way. Such threat appraisals have been shown to predict the use of avoidant coping strategies (e.g., Lengua & Long, 2002). In addition, youth with externalizing problems often show high levels of negative emotionality (Lengua & Long, 2002), which may predispose youth to a negative appraisal-coping process that exacerbates the impact of stress on adjustment. Using structural equation modeling, Lengua and Long (2002) demonstrated that negative emotionality predicted higher levels of threat appraisals, avoidant coping, and externalizing and internalizing problems beyond the effects of negative life events. Thus the attribution errors and negative emotionality that typify the reaction style of youth with DBDs may foster increased use of avoidant responses, such as drug use and social isolation.

Disruptive Behaviors Summary

The research on DBDs is mostly circumstantial with respect to avoidance processes. Internalizing disorders typified by avoidant processes co-occur frequently with DBDs, and specific emotion regulation subtypes (e.g., reactive aggression) may point to distress-based avoidance in some disruptive youth. Escape from task demands is a consistent finding in the literature, and youth with attention and impulsivity difficulties find escape a highly reinforcing function. Coping styles also seem to indicate that youth who engage in risky and antisocial behaviors (e.g., rule breaking, substance use) often do so as a means of coping with negative affect and internal distress. This type of coping more closely parallels the type of emotional avoidance seen in anxiety and depression. Perhaps the most promising link comes from conceptual models, such as the "failure model" described by Patterson and Capaldi (1990). This model suggests that avoidant processes may influence emotional distress in youth, but only after an initial disruptive episode. When a youth engages in antisocial or aggressive behavior, the subsequent peer rejection triggers a spiral of emotional distress and avoidance of future social interaction. Still, avoidance processes need to be studied directly and need to be distinguished from alternative hypotheses (e.g., intentional behavioral avoidance distinguished from unintentional impulsive or inattentive behaviors) to clarify any role of avoidance in DBDs.

Avoidance across the Disorders: An Integration

Finding common themes for avoidance processes across youth disorders requires effort. Research for each disorder follows its own methodology, measurement, and design features. Furthermore, the focus on avoidance changes depending on disorder. In anxiety disorders, avoidance and escape are studied to understand what prevents a child from entering or escaping a feared situation and what cues (safety behaviors) are used to distract from distress. For youth with depression, the initial emotional response after exposure to a stressor may not be fear but rather self-doubt, negativity, or hopelessness. Still, avoidance plays a role in maintaining depression in that avoiding distressing scenarios (prompted by negativity and self-doubt) confirms one's poor self-efficacy and feelings of hopelessness. Reengagement becomes harder as avoidance takes hold. In both anxiety and depression, avoidance is a maladaptive behavioral response that follows an emotional response (fear, self-doubt) to a trigger. When disruptive behaviors occur, it is not clear whether a single emotional response antecedes or follows avoidance. In the case of oppositional, aggressive, or antisocial behavior, anger, anxiety, self-doubt, and disappointment are all possible when a youth perceives threat. Impulsive and inattentive behavior may occur without any definable emotional response. In these cases, avoidance may still play a role, even if it is not the core maintaining process. As described in Patterson and Capaldi's (1990) failure model, a youth may avoid situations in which he or she has failed in the past, or he or she may continue to act aggressively or impulsively due to perceived low self-efficacy. A choice to avoid the failed situation prevents corrective experiences, such as receiving positive responses from others when acting appropriately.

To unify the research agenda for studying avoidance across disorders, we propose that avoidance be investigated across a *continuum of time*. In discussing cognitive disturbance across pathology, Kendall (2012; see also Kendall et al., Chapter 8, this volume) proposed that psychological disorders could be differentiated across a continuum of time. For example, anxiety disorders are characterized by an expectation of future negative events, whereas depression is characterized by evaluations and attributions after an event occurs. We propose that avoidance plays various roles in maintaining pathology depending on when it occurs along the sequence of events. Table 5.1 illustrates the various phases of exposure to a distressing stimulus/scenario and the role that avoidance plays in maintaining pathology. For anxiety, avoidance occurs throughout the time continuum (at all phases of stressor exposure), including anticipatory anxiety, procrastination and avoidance at onset, use of safety behaviors throughout exposure, and immediate relief following termination. Avoidance at any stage of exposure to the stressor can reinforce avoidance in future exposures to the trigger. Secondary interference occurs as reinforced avoidance leads to enduring fear and anxiety and accommodations to prevent future exposures (e.g., a child receiving home schooling to prevent distress of going to school).

For youth prone to depression, avoidance also occurs throughout the continuum, but it is characterized by anhedonia, discouragement, negativity, and low self-efficacy. Avoidance is reinforced to the degree that it helps youth minimize or manage distress that is prompted by challenges. Thus avoidance in depression may be differentiated from anxiety in terms of the emotions that serve as the internal trigger for avoidance. Secondary interference surfaces as anhedonia, and withdrawal increases with "successful" avoidance.

For disruptive behaviors, avoidance may not serve maintaining functions until late in the continuum. When a youth initially aggresses in response to ambiguous situations (usually social), avoidance may not be a problem. In fact, it may be preferable for a youth to avoid, or pause, instead of aggressing in response to perceived slights. However, after aggressing in an ambiguous scenario, aggressive youth may have a number of avoidant responses that produce secondary interference. The youth may feel guilt over the aggression or may blame others. The youth may misinterpret negative outcomes as out of his or her control. Such interpretations may lead to avoidance of future similar situations. This avoidance may then maintain pathology because it prevents the youth from practicing adaptive behavioral responses (e.g., social problem solving, conflict resolution) and correcting distorted conclusions about him- or herself or the situation.

TABLE 5.1. Avoidance across a Continuum of Time Relative to Exposure to Stressor (before, during, and after trigger)

Disorder	Before trigger	Trigger onset	Intraexposure	After trigger	Secondary interference
Anxiety	*Anticipatory anxiety common. Fear and negative information antecedes avoidance. Choose to avoid situations when information is ambiguous.	*Avoidance, resistance, and procrastination are common at presentation of trigger.	*Seek safety signals (friends, parents) and use safety behaviors (isolate, safe friend).	*Relief after escape. Negative reinforcement of avoidance prompts future avoidance.	*Anticipatory anxiety about future exposures. Fear, accommodation, and avoidance of future triggers persist.
Depression	*Anticipatory distress common when effort is expected. Anhedonia and avolition are examples of avoiding demanding tasks.	*Avoidance, resistance, and procrastination are common.	*Partial engagement (isolation), rejection by others (alienation), negative behaviors toward others (criticism).	*Relief after termination of stressor. Negative evaluations prompt future avoidance.	*Increasing anhedonia and withdrawal as demands increase and self-efficacy decreases.
Disruptive behaviors	*Anticipatory distress where past failures and negative social evaluations may exist.	Misperceived threat interpretation of ambiguous situation. Typically prompts aggressive or antisocial response.	Youth aggresses.	Youth feels guilt over aggression or blames others. Misinterprets negative outcomes as out of his or her control. *Feels relief from escaping situation.	*Youth may avoid situation in the future. Avoidance prevents youth from practicing prosocial behaviors in ambiguous situations and receiving corrective information about threat interpretations. Alternatively, youth may use maladaptive coping (e.g., substance use) to manage distress.
Impulsive/ inattentive behaviors	*Anticipatory distress where past failures exist.	Perceive task demands.	*Distract, disrupt, or procrastinate impulsively or to avoid demands.	*Relief from termination of demand.	*Decreased self-efficacy following poor performance and criticism from others. Avoidance of future tasks to prevent further failure.

Note. Asterisks (*) denote phases in which avoidance may serve an important maintaining function.

104

For impulse/attention problems, avoidance may be perpetuated similarly to anxiety. Initial failure in a task produces distress and worry that is
relieved only when the youth escapes the demand. In this way, we might
understand impulsive/inattentive behavior as a form of poor distress tolerance. As demands and challenges increase, the impulsive youth escapes
to manage his or her distress over self-doubts and poor self-efficacy. The
avoidance maintains pathology as the youth loses opportunities to practice necessary skills (e.g., sustained work and focus) and distress tolerance
skills.

Conclusion

Avoidance and its variants have been researched across youth disorders,
but conclusions are difficult to draw because terminology and the specific
aspects of avoidance differ across disorders. Avoidance has been studied in terms of behavioral avoidance and escape, safety behaviors, cognitive rumination, social withdrawal and peer exclusion, avoidant coping
responses, activity level, goal setting and planning, social skills, escape
from task demands, and subtypes of emotional response styles (e.g., CU).
Assessment approaches and study designs are equally diverse, including
within- and between-participant experiments, family interaction tasks,
direct observation, cross-sectional and longitudinal questionnaires, daily
diaries, school observations, and peer-nomination assessments. The preceding review provides a summary of methods and research findings to
encourage cross-fertilization of research across diagnostic categories.
Awareness of such diversity may help inspire new approaches and questions as we adapt research methods from one disorder group to another.
Furthermore, we offered a conceptual framework to help organize the
pursuit of avoidance research across disorders. By envisioning avoidance
across a continuum of time, we might pinpoint with more accuracy the
specific function that avoidance plays in maintaining pathology and its
specific context.

REFERENCES

Abramowitz, J., Tolin, D., & Street, G. (2001). Paradoxical effects of thought sup-
pression: A meta-analysis of controlled studies. *Clinical Psychology Review, 2,*
683–703.
Altmann, E. O., & Gotlib, I. H. (1988). The social behavior of depressed children:
An observational study. *Journal of Abnormal Child Psychology, 16,* 29–44.
Angold, A., Costello, E. J., & Erkanli, A. (1999). Comorbidity. *Journal of Child
Psychology and Psychiatry, 40,* 57–87.
Arnold, D. H. (1997). Co-occurrence of externalizing behavior problems and

emergent academic difficulties in young high-risk boys: A preliminary evaluation of patterns and mechanisms. *Journal of Applied Developmental Psychology, 18,* 317–330.

Askew, C., & Field, A. P. (2007). Vicarious learning and the development of fears in childhood. *Behaviour Research and Therapy, 45,* 2616–2627.

Barrett, P. M., Fox, T., & Farrell, F. (2005). Parent–child interactions with anxious children and with their siblings: An observational study. *Behaviour Change, 22,* 220–235.

Barrett, P. M., Rapee, R. M., Dadds, M. M., & Ryan, S. M. (1996). Family enhancement of cognitive style in anxious and aggressive children. *Journal of Abnormal Child Psychology, 24,* 187–203.

Barry, C. T., Frick, P. J., DeShazo, T. M., McCoy, M. G., Ellis, M., & Loney, B. R. (2000). The importance of callous-unemotional traits for extending the concept of psychopathy to children. *Journal of Abnormal Psychology, 109,* 335–340.

Bell-Dolan, D. J., Foster, S. L., & Christopher, J. S. (1995). Girl's peer relations and internalizing problems: Are socially neglected, rejected, and withdrawn girls at risk? *Journal of Clinical Child Psychology, 24,* 463–473.

Bell-Dolan, D. J., Reaven, N. M., & Peterson, L. (1993). Depression and social functioning: A multidimensional study of the linkages. *Journal of Clinical Child Psychology, 22,* 306–315.

Bubier, J. L., & Drabick, D. A. G. (2009). Co-occurring anxiety and disruptive behavior disorders: The roles of anxious symptoms, reactive aggression, and shared risk processes. *Clinical Psychology Review, 29,* 658–669.

Bukowski, W. M., Laursen, B., & Hoza, B. (2010). The snowball effect: Friendship moderates escalations in depressed affect among avoidant and excluded children. *Development and Psychopathology, 22,* 749–757.

Burke, J. D., & Loeber, R. (2010). Oppositional defiant disorder and the explanation of comorbidity between behavioral disorders and depression. *Clinical Psychology Science and Practice, 17,* 319–326.

Burke, J. D., Loeber, R., Lahey, B. B., & Rathouz, P. J. (2005). Developmental transitions among affective and behavioral disorders in adolescent boys. *Journal of Child Psychology and Psychiatry and Allied Disciplines, 46,* 1200–1210.

Capaldi, D. M. (1992). Co-occurrence of conduct problems and depressive symptoms in early adolescent boys: II. A 2-year follow-up at grade 8. *Development and Psychopathology, 4,* 125–144.

Card, N. A., & Little, T. D. (2006). Proactive and reactive aggression in childhood and adolescence: A meta-analysis of differential relations with psychosocial adjustment. *International Journal of Behavioral Development, 30,* 466–480.

Chu, B. C., & Harrison, T. L. (2007). Disorder-specific effects of CBT for anxious and depressed youth: A meta-analysis of candidate mediators of change. *Clinical Child and Family Psychology Review, 10,* 352–372.

Compas, B. E., Boyer, M. C., Stanger, C., Colletti, R. B., Thomsen, A. H., Dufton, L. M., et al. (2006). Latent variable analysis of coping, anxiety/depression, and somatic symptoms in adolescents with chronic pain. *Journal of Consulting and Clinical Psychology, 74,* 1132–1142.

Compas, B. E., Champion, J. E., Forehand, R., Cole, D. A., Reeslund, K. L., Fear,

J., et al. (2010). Coping and parenting: Mediators of 12-month outcomes of a family group cognitive–behavioral preventive intervention with families of depressed parents. *Journal of Consulting and Clinical Psychology, 78,* 623–634.

Compas, B. E., Connor-Smith, J. K., Saltzman, H., Thomsen, A. H., & Wadsworth, M. E. (2001). Coping with stress during childhood and adolescence: Problems, progress, and potential in theory and research. *Psychological Bulletin, 127,* 87–127.

Connor-Smith, J. K., Compas, B. E., Wadsworth, M. E., Thomsen, A. H., & Saltzman, H. (2000). Responses to stress in adolescence: Measurement of coping and involuntary stress responses. *Journal of Consulting and Clinical Psychology, 68,* 976–992.

Crick, N. R., & Dodge, K. A. (1996). Social information-processing mechanisms in reactive and proactive aggression. *Child Development, 67,* 993–1002.

Cuijpers, P., van Straten, A., & Warmerdam, L. (2007). Behavioral activation treatments of depression: A meta-analysis. *Clinical Psychology Review, 27,* 318–326.

Dadds, M. M., Barrett, P. M., Rapee, R. M., & Ryan, S. M. (1996). Family process and child anxiety and aggression: An observational analysis. *Journal of Abnormal Child Psychology, 24,* 715–734.

Daughters, S. B., Reynolds, E. K., MacPherson, L., Kahler, C. W., Danielson, C. K., Zvolensky, M., et al. (2009). Distress tolerance and early adolescent externalizing and internalizing symptoms: The moderating role of gender and ethnicity. *Behaviour Research and Therapy, 47,* 198–205.

Dickson, J. M., & MacLeod, A. K. (2004). Approach and avoidance goals and plans: Their relationship to anxiety and depression. *Cognitive Therapy and Research, 28,* 415–432.

Dickson, J. M., & MacLeod, A. K. (2006). Dysphoric adolescents' causal explanations and expectancies for approach and avoidance goals. *Journal of Adolescence, 29,* 177–191.

Drabick, D. A. G., Ollendick, T. H., & Bubier, J. L. (2010). Co-occurrence of ODD and anxiety: Shared risk processes and evidence of a dual-pathway model. *Clinical Psychology, Science and Practice, 17,* 307–318.

DuPaul, G. J., McGoey, K. E., Eckert, T. L., & VanBrakle, J. (2001). Preschool children with attention-deficit/hyperactivity disorder: Impairments in behavioral, social, and school functioning. *Journal of the American Academy of Child and Adolescent Psychiatry, 40,* 508–515.

Eftekhari, A., Turner, A. P., & Larimer, M. E. (2004). Anger expression, coping, and substance use in adolescent offenders. *Addictive Behaviors, 29,* 1001–1008.

Elliot, A. J., Sheldon, K. M., & Church, M. A. (1997). Avoidance personal goals and subjective well-being. *Personality and Social Psychology Bulletin, 23,* 915–927.

Ferster, C. B. (1973). A functional analysis of depression. *American Psychologist, 28,* 857–870.

Field, A. P., & Lawson, J. (2003). Fear information and the development of fears during childhood: Effects on implicit fear responses and behavioural avoidance. *Behaviour Research and Therapy, 41,* 1277–1293.

Field, A. P., & Storksen-Coulson, H. (2007). The interaction of pathways to fear in childhood anxiety: A preliminary study. *Behaviour Research and Therapy,* 45, 3051–3059.

Fisak, B., & Grills-Taquechel, A. E. (2007). Parental modeling, reinforcement, and information transfer: Risk factors in the development of child anxiety? *Clinical Child and Family Psychology,* 10, 213–231.

Foa, E. B., Huppert, J. D., & Cahill, S. P. (2006). Emotional processing theory: An update. In B. O. Rothbaum (Ed.), *Pathological anxiety: Emotional processing in etiology and treatment* (pp. 3–24). New York: Guilford Press.

Frick, P. J., & Ellis, M. (1999). Callous-unemotional traits and subtypes of conduct disorder. *Clinical Child and Family Psychology Review,* 2, 149–168.

Gazelle, H., & Ladd, G. W. (2003). Anxious solitude and peer exclusion: A diathesis–stress model of internalizing trajectories in childhood. *Child Development,* 74, 257–278.

Gazelle, H., & Rudolph, K. D. (2004). Moving toward and away from the world: Social approach and avoidance trajectories in anxious solitary youth. *Child Development,* 75, 829–849.

Harvey, A. G., Watkins, E., Mansell, W., & Shafran, R. (2004). *Cognitive behavioral processes across psychological disorders: A transdiagnostic approach to research and treatment.* Oxford, UK: Oxford University Press.

Hawkins, R. O., & Axelrod, M. I. (2008). Increasing the on-task homework behavior of youth with behavior disorders using functional behavioral assessment. *Behavior Modification,* 32, 840–859.

Hinshaw, S. P. (2002). Process, mechanism, and explanation related to externalizing behavior in developmental psychopathology. *Journal of Abnormal Child Psychology,* 30, 431–446.

Hopko, D. R., Armento, M. E., Cantu, M. S., Chambers, L. L., & Lejuez, C. W. (2003). The use of daily diaries to assess the relations among mood state, overt behavior, and reward value of activities. *Behaviour Research and Therapy,* 41, 1137–1148.

Hubbard, J. A., Smithmyer, C. M., Ramsden, S. R., Parker, E. H., Flanagan, K. D., Dearing, K. F., et al. (2002). Observational, physiological, and self-report measures of children's anger: Relations to reactive versus proactive aggression. *Child Development,* 73, 1101–1118.

Hudson, J. L., Doyle, A. M., & Gar, N. (2009). Child and maternal influence on parenting behavior in clinically anxious children. *Journal of Clinical Child and Adolescent Psychology,* 38, 256–262.

Huijding, J., Field, A. P., De Houwer, J., Vandenbosch, K., Rinck, M., & van Oeveren, M. (2009). A behavioral route to dysfunctional representations: The effects of training approach or avoidance tendencies towards novel animals in children. *Behaviour Research and Therapy,* 47, 471–477.

Jacobson, N. S., Martell, C. R., & Dimidjian, S. (2001). Behavioral activation treatment for depression: Returning to contextual roots. *American Psychological Association,* 8, 256–270.

Jaser, S. S., Champion, J. E., Reeslund, K. L., Keller, G., Merchant, M. J., Benson, M., et al. (2007). Cross-situational coping with peer and family stressors in adolescent offspring of depressed parents. *Journal of Adolescence,* 30, 917–932.

Jaser, S. S., Langrock, A. M., Keller, G., Merchant, M. J., Benson, M. A., Reeslund, K., et al. (2005). Coping with the stress of parental depression: II. Adolescent and parent reports of coping and adjustment. *Journal of Clinical Child and Adolescent Psychology, 34,* 193–205.

Kanter, J. W., Mulick, P. S., Busch, A. M., Berlin, K. S., & Martell, C. R. (2007). The Behavioral Activation for Depression Scale (BADS): Psychometric properties and factor structure. *Journal of Psychopathology and Behavioral Assessment, 29,* 191–202.

Kendall, P. C. (2012). Anxiety disorders in youth. In P. C. Kendall (Ed.), *Child and adolescent therapy: Cognitive-behavioral procedures* (4th ed., pp. 143–189). New York: Guilford Press.

Langrock, A. M., Compas, B. E., Keller, G., & Merchant, M. J. (2002). Coping with the stress of parental depression: Parents' reports of children's coping and emotional/behavioral problems. *Journal of Clinical Child and Adolescent Psychology, 31,* 312–324.

Lengua, L. J., & Long, A. C. (2002). The role of emotionality and self-regulation in the appraisal-coping process: Tests of direct and moderating effects. *Journal of Applied Developmental Psychology, 23,* 471–493.

Lengua, L. J., Sandler, I. N., West, S. G., Wolchik, S. A., & Curran, P. J. (1999). Emotionality and self-regulation, threat appraisal, and coping in children of divorce. *Development and Psychopathology, 11,* 15–37.

Lewinsohn, P. M., & Graf, M. (1973). Pleasant activities and depression. *Journal of Consulting and Clinical Psychology, 41,* 261–268.

Lewinsohn, P. M., & Libet, J. (1972). Pleasant events, activity schedules, and depressions. *Journal of Abnormal Psychology, 79,* 291–295.

Manos, R. C., Kanter, J. W., & Busch, A. M. (2010). A critical review of assessment strategies to measure the behavioral activation model of depression. *Clinical Psychology Review, 30,* 547–561.

Moore, D. W., Anderson, A., & Kumar, K. (2005). Instructional adaptation in the management of escape-maintained behavior in a classroom. *Journal of Positive Behavior Interventions, 7,* 216–223.

Moore, P. S., Whaley, S. E., & Sigman, M. (2004). Interactions between mothers and children: Impacts of maternal and child anxiety. *Journal of Abnormal Psychology, 3,* 471–476.

Morrow, J., & Nolen-Hoeksema, S. (1990). Effects of responses to depression on the remediation of depressive affect. *Journal of Personality and Social Psychology, 58,* 519–527.

Moulds, M. L., Kandris, E., Starr, S., & Wong, A. C. (2007). The relationship between rumination, avoidance, and depression in a non-clinical sample. *Behaviour Research and Therapy, 45,* 251–261.

Nolen-Hoeksema, S., Morrow, J., & Fredrickson, B. L. (1993). Response styles and the duration of episodes of depressed mood. *Journal of Abnormal Psychology, 102,* 20–28.

Oh, W., Rubin, K. H., Bowker, J. C., Booth-LaForce, C., Rose-Kransor, L., & Laursen, B. (2008). Trajectories of social withdrawal from middle childhood to early adolescence. *Journal of Abnormal Child Psychology, 4,* 553–566.

Patterson, G. R., & Capaldi, D. M. (1990). A mediational model for boys' depressed mood. In J. Rolf, A. S. Master, D. Cicchetti, K. H. Nuechterlein, & S. Weintraub (Eds.), *Risk and protective factors in the development of psychopathology* (pp. 141–163). New York: Cambridge University Press.

Peterson, L., Mullins, L. L., & Ridley-Johnson, R. (1985). Childhood depression: Peer reactions to depression and life stress. *Journal of Abnormal Child Psychology, 13,* 597–609.

Poulin, F., & Boivin, M. (2000). Reactive and proactive aggression: Evidence of a two-factor model. *Psychological Assessment, 12,* 115–122.

Ruchkin, V. V., Eisemann, M., & Hägglöf, B. (1999). Coping styles in delinquent adolescents and controls: The role of personality and parental rearing. *Journal of Youth and Adolescence, 28,* 705–717.

Rudolph, K. D., Flynn, M., & Abaied, J. L. (2008). A developmental perspective on interpersonal theories of youth depression. In J. R. Z. Abela & B. L. Hankin (Eds.), *Handbook of depression in children and adolescents* (pp. 79–102). New York: Guilford Press.

Salkovskis, P. M. (1991). The importance of behaviour in the maintenance of anxiety and panic: A cognitive account. *Behavioural Psychotherapy, 19,* 6–19.

Schrock, M., & Woodruff-Borden, J. (2010). Parent–child interactions in anxious families. *Child and Family Behavior Therapy, 32,* 291–310.

Sheeber, L., & Sorensen, E. (1998). Family relationships of depressed adolescents: A multimethod assessment. *Journal of Clinical Child Psychology, 27,* 268–277.

Shortt, A. L., Barrett, P. M., Dadds, M. R., & Fox, T. L. (2001). The influence of family and experimental context on cognition in anxious children. *Journal of Abnormal Child Psychology, 29,* 585–596.

Silverman, W. K., & Ollendick, T. H. (2005). Evidence-based assessment of anxiety and its disorders in children and adolescents. *Journal of Clinical Child and Adolescent Psychology, 34,* 380–411.

Vassallo, S., Smart, D., Sanson, A., Dussuyer, I., McKendry, B., Tombourou, J., et al. (2002). *Patterns and precursors of adolescent antisocial behaviour: The first report.* Melbourne: Australian Institute of Family Studies and Crime Prevention.

Watkins, E., & Moulds, M. L. (2007). Reduced concreteness of rumination in depression: A pilot study. *Personality and Individual Differences, 43,* 1386–1395.

Wegner, D., Schneider, D., Carter, S., & White, T. (1987). Paradoxical effects of thought suppression. *Journal of Personality and Social Psychology, 53,* 5–13.

Whaley, S. E., Pinto, A., & Sigman, M. (1999). Characterizing interactions between anxious mothers and their children. *Journal of Consulting and Clinical Psychology, 67,* 826–836.

Wierzbicki, M., & Sayler, M. K. (1991). Depression and engagement in pleasant and unpleasant activities in normal children. *Journal of Clinical Psychology, 47,* 499–505.

CHAPTER 6

The Role of Peer Relationships in Youth Psychopathology

Annette M. La Greca and Betty S. Lai

Peer relationships play an important role in youngsters' emotional development. From early childhood on, children spend a considerable amount of time with peers, and by age 7, children spend most of their daytime hours in school or play settings with classmates and friends (La Greca & Prinstein, 1999). During adolescence, the size and diversity of youths' peer networks increase, and close friends begin to equal, and in some cases even surpass, parents as the primary source of social support (Furman, McDunn, & Young, 2009). Dating relationships also emerge and become increasingly important; in fact, by age 16, most adolescents have had a romantic relationship (Carver, Joyner, & Udry, 2003).

Successful peer relationships contribute to youngsters' emotional health, facilitate the development of social skills, and foster feelings of personal competence that are essential for adult interpersonal functioning (Hartup, 1996). Romantic relationships also have mental health benefits, as they can provide social support, enhance self-esteem, and prepare youth for adult relationships and the development of intimacy (Connolly & Goldberg, 1999; see La Greca, Davila, Landoll, & Siegel, 2011; La Greca, Davila, & Siegel, 2009).

At the same time, problematic peer relations represent a significant stressor for children and adolescents. During the school years, children who experience interpersonal difficulties with peers are at substantial risk

111

for later emotional and behavioral problems (Kupersmidt & Coie, 1990). Among adolescents, problems with peers have been identified as strong predictors of internalizing problems, such as social anxiety (La Greca & Harrison, 2005; La Greca & Lopez, 1998; Siegel, La Greca, & Harrison, 2009) and depression (Hawker & Boulton, 2000; Prinstein, Boergers, & Vernberg 2001). Moreover, romantic relationships often contribute to strong emotions for older adolescents, including feelings of anxiety, anger, jealousy, and depression (Larson, Clore, & Wood, 1999). Even the presence of a romantic relationship has been associated with symptoms of depression among adolescent girls (see La Greca et al., 2009).

This chapter focuses on peer processes that contribute to the etiology or maintenance of psychopathology in youth. To the extent that the current literature allows, we describe peer processes that have common influences across psychological disorders. In particular, we review literature that may help us to understand how peer processes are problematic across diagnostic categories and how such processes could be the target for transdiagnostic assessment and intervention.

The first main section of the chapter provides a brief overview of peer relations in youths' development to provide a context for the remainder of the chapter. This is followed in the second section by a discussion of peer-focused interpersonal stressors and a review of their associations with psychopathology in youth. The third section focuses on socialization processes that have been linked with youths' adjustment, and the final section provides a summary with recommendations for assessment and treatment.

Brief Overview of Peer Relations

A brief overview of developmental aspects of youths' peer relations may provide a useful perspective for understanding the role of peer processes in youths' psychopathology. The reader is also referred to several sources for further details (Furman et al., 2009; Kingery, Erdley, Marshall, Whitaker, & Reuter, 2010; La Greca & Landoll, 2011; La Greca & Prinstein, 1999).

Peer Acceptance/Peer Rejection

The broader peer group is important for youths'[1] social and emotional development, as it can provide a sense of *belonging and acceptance* (La

---

[1]Throughout the chapter, we use the term *youth* to refer to both children and adolescents.

Greca & Prinstein, 1999). In fact, peer relations have been evaluated along two distinct dimensions: acceptance and rejection.

Acceptance refers to the degree to which a child or adolescent is actively liked by peers, whereas *rejection* reflects peers' active dislike (Newcomb, Bukowski, & Pattee, 1993).

Studies often use peer nominations to identify *popular* youth (those high on liking and low on disliking) and *rejected* youth (those low on liking and high on disliking; e.g., Coie, Dodge, & Kupersmidt, 1990; La Greca & Stone, 1993). Popular youth often have good social and academic skills (e.g., Estell et al., 2008). In contrast, rejected youth may display interpersonal, emotional, and academic difficulties, such as aggressive or disruptive behaviors (Hartup, 1996) and internalizing problems, such as social anxiety (La Greca & Landoll, 2011; La Greca & Lopez, 1998; La Greca & Stone, 1993) and depression (see La Greca et al., 2009).

For adolescents, affiliating with a peer crowd also may represent a way of gaining peer acceptance and social status (Brown, 1990; Furman et al., 2009). Across studies, typical peer crowds include *jocks, populars, brains, burnouts,* and *alternatives* (Brown, 1990; La Greca, Prinstein, & Fetter, 2001). In addition to a sense of acceptance and belonging, peer crowds can provide opportunities for social activities, friendships, and romantic relationships (Brown, 1990; La Greca & Prinstein, 1999). Peer crowds' importance peaks in mid-adolescence and then gradually declines as close friends and romantic relationships become prominent (Brown, 1990).

Peer Victimization

Although relatively few youth are actively rejected, it is not uncommon for youth to report some degree of victimization by peers. Initially, peer victimization (PV) was examined in the context of understanding peer aggression and its impact on youth (Crick & Grotpeter, 1996). Recent work suggests that there are multiple types of PV: *overt* PV typically refers to obvious acts of physical aggression, such as hitting, pushing, or verbal threats; *relational* PV refers to social exclusion, social isolation, or other ways of manipulating friendships; and *reputational* PV reflects efforts to embarrass others or damage their reputation (Crick & Grotpeter, 1996; De Los Reyes & Prinstein, 2004; Prinstein et al., 2001; Siegel et al., 2009).

Among children, girls report more relational and less overt PV than boys (Crick & Bigbee, 1998). Adolescent boys also report more overt PV than adolescent girls, although sex differences in relational and reputational PV are less clear for adolescents (De Los Reyes & Prinstein, 2004; La Greca & Harrison, 2005; Siegel et al., 2009).

Studies have begun to examine victimization that occurs through technologies, such as social networking sites, instant messaging, or text messages (Landoll, La Greca, & Lai, 2013; Williams & Guerra, 2007). Although in its early stages, it appears that cyber victimization may be a particularly salient form of PV for adolescents (Williams & Guerra, 2007).

Close Friendships

Close friendships provide youth with intimacy, support, and companionship and can enhance self-esteem (La Greca & Prinstein, 1999). Until adolescence, close friendships occur almost exclusively between same-sex peers; however, during adolescence, other-sex close friendships become common and set the stage for romantic relationships (Kuttler, La Greca, & Prinstein, 1999). At all ages, girls are more likely than boys to have a "best friend" and to have more close friends (Parker & Asher, 1993).

Common qualities of youths' close friendships include companionship, affection, receiving help, trust, and sharing. As children transition into adolescence, intimacy (e.g., sharing private thoughts and feelings) and emotional support become increasingly important (Furman et al., 2009; La Greca & Prinstein, 1999). Friendships also can have negative aspects, such as conflict, pressure, and betrayal (Kuttler & La Greca, 2004; La Greca & Harrison, 2005). Across development, youth with better quality friendships have fewer behavioral and emotional problems and display greater social competence (see La Greca & Prinstein, 1999).

Romantic Relationships

Romantic relationships represent an important but relatively understudied aspect of adolescents' peer relations. During early adolescence, mixed-sex peer groups emerge, followed by romantically involved couples in later adolescence (Connolly & Goldberg, 1999). Although adolescent girls are more likely than boys to be romantically involved (Glickman & La Greca, 2004), both boys and girls report more positive than negative qualities in their romantic relationships (La Greca & Harrison, 2005; La Greca & Mackey, 2007). The qualities of adolescents' romantic relationships are strikingly similar to those reported in close friendships, with an additional emphasis on intimacy and sexual involvement (Kuttler & La Greca, 2004).

The occurrence and progression of adolescents' romantic relationships appears to be substantially similar across different U.S. ethnic groups (Carver et al., 2003; O'Sullivan, Cheng, Harris, & Brooks-Gunn, 2007). However, Asian and Hispanic adolescents who are involved in romantic relationships are less likely to report engaging in sexual events (e.g., intimate touching, sexual intercourse) than white or black adolescents (O'Sullivan et al., 2007).

Theoretical and Empirical Perspectives on Peer Relations' Role in Psychopathology

Several theoretical perspectives are consistent with the notion that problematic peer relations play a causal role in the development and/or maintenance of psychopathology. Relevant to this discussion are the concepts of *multifinality* (i.e., that a particular risk factor may lead to multiple psychological outcomes or disorders) and *equifinality* (i.e., that any given psychological disorder may have multiple pathways that contribute to its development; Hinshaw, 2008).

Using this framework, problematic peer relationships can be viewed as a causal risk factor that is associated with multiple problematic outcomes. In addition, problematic peer relationships may be one among a host of other causal factors, such as genetic makeup and parenting, that contribute to the development and maintenance of psychological disorders.

Problematic Peer Relationships as Significant Interpersonal Stressors

Theoretical Perspective

One way to conceptualize how peer relationships contribute to disorder in youth is to view problematic peer relationships, particularly as reflected by peer rejection and PV, as significant interpersonal stressors that lead to dysfunction. It has long been recognized that stressful life experiences pose a threat to youths' psychological well-being and contribute to poor mental health outcomes (see Grant et al., 2003).

In fact, Grant, Compas, Thurm, McMahon, and Gipson (2004) reviewed 60 prospective studies that used a wide range of methodologies to examine stressful events' association with symptoms of psychopathology in youth. The overwhelming majority of studies (88%) found that stressful events predicted *increases* in symptoms over time. Stressful events predicted increases in both internalizing and externalizing symptoms across different informants, although the associations were stronger for internalizing versus externalizing problems, and youths' reports of stressors were more strongly associated with their own reports of symptoms than were parent-reported symptoms (Grant et al., 2004). Also of interest, among studies that examined the impact of both prior and recent stressors, *recent* stressors appeared to have a greater impact on youths' mental health than prior stressors.

In the broad conceptual model of stress and psychopathology pro-posed by Grant and colleagues (2003), the authors offer several proposi-tions. These propositions include that: (1) there is *specificity* in the associa-tions between particular stressors and psychological outcomes, as well as specificity in the mediators and moderators of these associations, and (2) relations among stressors, moderators, mediators, and psychopathology are reciprocal and dynamic.

Extending this line of reasoning to interpersonal stressors, such as peer rejection and PV, one might expect that interpersonal stressors would be linked with particular psychological problems (e.g., symptoms of social anxiety) via a particular mediating process (e.g., enhanced per-ceptions of social threat; discomfort and avoidance of social situations) in the context of a particular moderating variable (e.g., female gender; see Grant et al., 2004). In turn, feelings of social anxiety might contribute to awkward or uncomfortable feelings around peers that might lead to fur-ther victimization or rejection by peers. In other words, once anxious or distressed feelings develop, these feelings may exacerbate interpersonal problems and contribute to further victimization and dysfunctional emo-tional adjustment.

Specifically, youth who experience PV may feel nervous or uncom-fortable with peers, worry about peers' reactions to them, and avoid peer-oriented social situations (La Greca, 2001; La Greca & Landoll, 2011). Once socially anxious feelings and behavioral patterns develop, they may interfere with interpersonal functioning. Youth who avoid peers may miss out on key socialization experiences that are necessary for normal social-emotional development (Coie et al., 1990); and youth who are uncom-fortable around peers may be less desirable companions, making them targets for further social exclusion (Blöte & Westenberg, 2007).

Over time, these processes could also contribute to youths' social withdrawal and depressive affect. Evidence suggests that anxiety disor-ders, including social phobia and social anxiety disorder, are a potential gateway to psychological disorders such as depression (Grant, Beck, Far-row, & Davila, 2007). In fact, social anxiety disorder shares a high degree of comorbidity with depression (Costello, Egger, & Angold, 2005). Inter-personal aspects of socially anxious behaviors, especially social avoidance, have been prospectively associated with subsequent feelings of depression (see Grant et al., 2007).

Interpersonal stressors, such as PV, also contribute to externalizing behavioral problems in youth. For example, Rudolph, Troop-Gordon, Hessel, and Schmidt (2011) followed children from early to late elemen-tary school, finding that PV in the second grade predicted children's depressive symptoms and overt aggression in the fifth grade; moreover, girls who were victimized in the second grade were likely to engage in relational aggression later on. The findings suggest that PV leads to a negative spiral wherein victimization prompts youth to retaliate, which in turn elicits negative responses from peers (e.g., rejection, further retaliation), and thus leads to further increases in aggressive behavior and also in depressive affect (see Rudolph et al., 2011). This interpretation is consistent with evidence that youth who are victimized by peers may retaliate and become aggressors (e.g., Nansel et al., 2001) and that aggression predicts subsequent peer rejection (e.g., Lansford, Malone, Dodge, Pettit, & Bates, 2010; Little & Garber, 1995) and increasing internalizing symptoms over time (Murray-Close, Ostrov, & Crick, 2007). Furthermore, a potential mechanism underlying this interplay of peer rejection/victimization and aggressive behavior is social information processing, problems with which have been strongly implicated in the development of both aggressive behavior and peer rejection (Lansford et al., 2010).

In summary, consistent with the developmental psychopathology concept of multifinality, it may be useful to conceptualize aversive peer experiences, such as peer rejection and PV, as interpersonal stressors that contribute to and maintain both internalizing and externalizing problems in youth. Note that this conceptualization of aversive peer experiences also fits well within the transdiagnostic approach to understanding mechanisms and processes that contribute to disorder and that are important to address in treatment. Next we review studies of aversive peer experiences in the development of psychopathology in youth.

Empirical Support: Peer Rejection, PV, and Internalizing Problems

In this section, we integrate and discuss both peer rejection and PV experiences in relation to internalizing problems. Note, however, that PV differs from peer rejection in that victimization focuses on negative experiences that are specifically directed toward a child or adolescent, whereas peer rejection reflects the prevailing attitudes of peers toward an individual (Lopez & DuBois, 2005). Although rejected youth experience PV, accepted youth can also be the targets of PV (Prinstein & Cillessen, 2003). Nevertheless, PV and peer rejection both are aversive, are interpersonal stressors, and are associated with youths' internalized distress.

Community Studies. Although there are multiple pathways to peer rejection (La Greca & Prinstein, 1999), peer-rejected youth are at high risk for current and future psychological difficulties (Coie et al., 1990; Parker & Asher, 1987). Community studies find that peer-rejected youth have substantial interpersonal and emotional difficulties (Coie et al., 1990; La Greca & Prinstein, 1999) and report greater social anxiety than their peers (La Greca & Lopez, 1998; La Greca & Stone, 1993), as well more depressive symptoms (Prinstein & Aikins, 2004).

Similarly, PV experiences also have an impact on youths' anxious and depressive symptoms (see meta-analysis by Hawker & Boulton, 2000). In particular, overt and relational PV experiences are strongly associated with both anxiety (especially social anxiety) and depression (e.g., Crick & Grotpeter, 1996; La Greca & Harrison, 2005; Prinstein, Borelli, Cheah, Simon, & Aikins, 2005; Siegel et al., 2009; Vernberg, 1990; Wang, Iannotti, Luk, & Nansel, 2010). Among adolescents, *relational* PV is uniquely and strongly associated with social anxiety, even when controlling for other forms of PV (La Greca & Harrison, 2005; Siegel et al., 2009). Moreover, in a study of more than 3,000 adolescents ages 15–16, Ranta, Kaltiala-Heino, Pelkonen, and Marttunen (2009) demonstrated that PV is significantly associated with adolescents' symptoms of social phobia/anxiety, regardless of their level of depressive symptoms.

Prospective Studies. Prospective studies find that peer rejection and other aversive PV experiences predict loneliness and depressive affect and, conversely, that symptoms of depression predict subsequent peer rejection and aversive peer experiences (Harrison, 2006; Little & Garber, 1995; Vernberg, 1990). For example, Little and Garber (1995) found that depressive symptoms among early adolescents predicted increases in peer rejection over a 3-month period. Vernberg (1990) evaluated early adolescents at two time points during the school year, finding that aversive peer experiences predicted increases in depressive affect over time and that initial levels of depressive symptoms also predicted increases in aversive peer experiences. Similarly, Harrison (2006) found that PV predicted increases in depressive symptoms over a 2-month period, and this relationship was stronger for adolescents who were high in rejection sensitivity (the tendency to expect, perceive, and overreact to rejection).

Prospective studies also elucidate potential pathways between PV and anxiety in youth (Siegel et al., 2009; Storch, Brassard, & Masia-Warner, 2003; Vernberg, Abwender, Ewell, & Beery, 1992). Vernberg and colleagues (1992) evaluated adolescents at three time points during a school year, assessing the quality of their peer relationships, PV experiences, and levels of social anxiety. They found that rejection and social exclusion (i.e., relational PV) predicted increases in adolescents' social anxiety over a 2-month period and increases in social avoidance and distress over the school year. Other recent work shows that relational PV leads to *increases* in adolescents' symptoms of social anxiety over time (Siegel et al., 2009) and in symptoms of social phobia (Storch et al., 2003).

In contrast, these same studies provide mixed evidence regarding the reverse pathway—whether social anxiety leads to *subsequent* PV. Two studies did not find that social anxiety led to increases in PV over the school year (Storch et al., 2003; Vernberg et al., 1992), although Siegel and colleagues (2009) did find that social anxiety predicted increases in adolescents' relational victimization over a two month period. Others have found evidence that youth who are socially anxious are treated more negatively by their classmates than are those who are not socially anxious (Blöte & Westenberg, 2007). One reason that it may be difficult to evaluate whether social anxiety leads to increases in PV is that youth with social anxiety who are victimized may learn to *avoid social situations* in order to limit their opportunities for further victimization. Studies are needed that examine the bidirectional influences of PV and social anxiety, as well as mediating and moderating variables (e.g., presence of a close friend in school).

Clinical Samples. Among youth with clinical diagnoses, studies also support associations between peer rejection, PV, and internalizing disorders. Strauss, Frame, and Forehand (1987) found that anxiety-disordered (AD) children were less well liked than non-anxiety-disordered (NAD) children. Ginsburg, La Greca, and Silverman (1998) evaluated children with simple phobia, finding that those with comorbid social phobia had significantly lower levels of peer acceptance and more negative peer interactions than those without comorbid social phobia. Relatedly, Verduin and Kendall (2008) found that AD children were significantly less liked than were NAD children, and AD children with social phobia were significantly less liked than those without social phobia; however, children with other anxiety disorders did not differ in peer liking compared with NAD youth. Clinical samples of adolescents also provide evidence that PV is associated with social anxiety. Ranta and colleagues (2009) found that adolescents who met criteria for social phobia had substantially higher rates of PV than those without social phobia.

Similarly, youth with clinical depression have interpersonal difficulties with peers, and the social behaviors of youth with depression appear to contribute to their problematic peer relations. Adolescents with depression are rejected more frequently by peers and are less popular than youth without depression (Little & Garber, 1995). Moreover, laboratory studies examining adolescents' opinions of unfamiliar peers find that adolescents with clinical depression are rated more negatively than adolescents without depression (Connolly, Geller, Marton, & Kutcher, 1992). Some studies also find a stronger relationship between peer rejection and depression for girls than for boys (e.g., Lopez & DuBois, 2005). For example, Connolly and colleagues (1992) found that peers viewed adolescent girls with depression as less skilled at making friends and less interested in getting to know others than girls without depression but that the same was not true for boys.

Summary. Evidence clearly supports a relationship between youths' aversive peer experiences, such as peer rejection and PV, and their social anxiety and depressive affect. Some associations may be stronger for girls than for boys, and for adolescents who display certain cognitive vulnerabilities (e.g., rejection sensitivity). Available findings are consistent with interpersonal theories of depression (e.g., Hammen, 1991) and with stress-diathesis perspectives on depression (e.g., Lewinsohn, Joiner, & Rohde, 2001) that emphasize the contributions of rejection experiences and interpersonal stress. Findings are also consistent with theories of social anxiety that emphasize interpersonal threat and fear of negative evaluation from others as important contributing factors (e.g., Juster & Heimberg, 1995). Further research would benefit from theory-driven studies examining underlying mechanisms and moderating variables that explain why some youth develop depressive or anxious symptoms in response to peer rejection/aversive peer experiences whereas others do not.

Empirical Support: Peer Rejection, PV, and Externalizing Problems

Many studies have demonstrated that peer rejection and PV lead to subsequent aggression and that aggressive behavior leads to both peer rejection and further PV (see Coie et al., 1990; Lansford et al., 2010; Parker & Asher, 1987). Such findings are consistent with theoretical perspectives that link interpersonal rejection with anger and aggressive behavior (Leary, Twenge, & Quinlivan, 2006).

Community Studies. Community studies find that peer-rejected youth have substantial behavioral difficulties (La Greca & Prinstein, 1999). Rejected children often demonstrate aggressive, disruptive, or inattentive behaviors (Coie et al., 1990). Similarly, PV is positively associated with externalizing behaviors (Singh & Bussey, 2011). For example, PV is positively associated with reactive aggression in elementary school-age children (Lamarche et al., 2007), and children who experience PV and are bullies are also aggressive and impulsive across elementary, middle, and high school years (O'Brennan, Bradshaw, & Sawyer, 2009). Furthermore, among 2,161 children ages 10–15 years, Singh and Bussey (2011) demonstrated that PV is significantly associated with youth's externalizing behaviors.

Prospective Studies. Peer rejection experiences predict later externalizing behavioral problems, and externalizing problems are associated with subsequent peer rejection (Laird, Jordan, Dodge, Pettit, & Bates, 2001). For example, Dodge and colleagues (2003) conducted four studies with children ages 5–12 years and demonstrated that peer rejection in grades 1–3 predicted a growth in aggressive behavior four years later (grades 5–7). In addition, peer rejection in kindergarten predicted antisocial development in the third grade among children who were disposed toward aggression in kindergarten. Furthermore, Hodges, Boivin, Vitaro, and Bukowski (1999) studied 393 children in grades 4 and 5 and found that externalizing behaviors predicted PV 1 year later and also that PV predicted increases in externalizing behaviors year later among children without a mutual best friend.

Prospective studies also reveal potential bidirectional causal pathways between peer rejection experiences, including PV, and peer aggression (Cook, Williams, Guerra, Kim, & Sadek, 2010; Dodge et al., 2003; Reijntjes et al., 2010). For example, acute peer rejection predicts aggressive behavior among youth (10–13 years) who are alienated (Reijntjes et al., 2010). Lansford and colleagues (2010) followed children from kindergarten to grade 3 and demonstrated that peer rejection not only predicts aggressive behavior but also has a direct effect on subsequent peer rejection. Considered together, these studies indicate that there are recursive, potentially escalating influences between problematic peer relationships and externalizing behaviors.

Clinical Samples. Among youth with clinical diagnoses, studies also support associations between peer rejection, PV, and externalizing disorders. For example, research has linked peer rejection and PV with attention-deficit/hyperactivity disorder (ADHD; Hoza, 2007). Mrug and colleagues (2012) followed youth with ADHD from the Multisite Treatment of ADHD study, finding that even after controlling for youths' symptoms of ADHD, disruptive and conduct-disordered behavior, and level of the relevant outcome variable at 24 months, peer rejection predicted youths' cigarette smoking, delinquency, and global impairment at 6 years postbaseline and global impairment at 8 years postbaseline. Such findings underscore the importance of addressing youths' peer functioning to improve long-term outcomes in children with ADHD.

Youth with oppositional defiant disorder (ODD) and conduct disorder (CD) also have difficulties with peer functioning (Kokkinos & Panayiotou, 2004; Miller-Johnson, Coie, Maumary-Gremaud, Bierman, & the Conduct Problems Prevention Research Group, 2002). Early peer rejection predicts conduct problems in elementary school youth (Miller-Johnson et al., 2002), and ODD and CD are associated with both PV (Kokkinos & Panayiotou, 2004) and peer rejection (Frick, 2006).

Summary. Evidence clearly supports a relationship between youths' aversive peer experiences and externalizing problems. Findings are compatible with theoretical perspectives that link interpersonal rejection with anger and aggressive behavior (Leary et al., 2006). Moreover, multiple processes may underlie these associations, including problems with social information processing (e.g., Dodge et al., 2003), poor emotion regulation (e.g., Deater-Deckard, 2001; McLaughlin, Hatzenbeuhler, Mennin, &

Nolen-Hoeksema, 2011), and deviancy training from peers who also have behavior problems (e.g., Snyder et al., 2005).

Overall, evidence strongly supports the importance of understanding youths' aversive peer experiences, especially peer rejection and PV. Attention to youths' aversive peer experiences will be an important consideration for the assessment and treatment of all youth who are seen in clinical settings.

Peer Selection and Socialization Influences: Friends and Romantic Partners

Theoretical Perspective

Homophily (Kandel, 1978a, 1978b) is another theoretical perspective that provides a useful framework for understanding the role of peer relationships in youth psychopathology. Homophily comprises the processes of "selection" (peers with similar interests and characteristics cluster together and seek one another out) and "socialization" (peers reward and reinforce similar attitudes and behaviors among group members or friends).

Consistent with the selection process, children choose friends based on similar characteristics, such as age, sex, race, and preference for certain activities (La Greca & Prinstein, 1999). By adolescence, friendship choices are based on less observable factors, such as personality, attitudes, and self-esteem (Aboud & Mendelson, 1998). Friends also "socialize" each other by supporting and reinforcing each other's behaviors and feelings (Prinstein, 2007).

Although much less well studied, similar selection and socialization processes come into play in adolescents' romantic relationships (e.g., Furman et al., 2009; Furman & Simon, 2008; Simon, Aikens, & Prinstein, 2008; Wargo, Simon, & Prinstein, 2010). For example, Simon and colleagues (2008) found that even *before* their relationship, adolescents and their partners were similar on variables such as popularity, attractiveness, and depressive symptoms. Wargo and colleagues (2010) also illustrated that romantic socialization effects occur as well, particularly for youths' cigarette use and behavioral problems.

Empirical Support for Homophily in Internalizing Problems

Selection and socialization processes have been studied predominantly with regard to externalizing behavioral problems (Bukowski, Brendgen, & Vitaro, 2007), but these processes also play a role in youths' internalizing problems. Specifically, adolescents seek friends with similar levels of internalizing problems and also display increases in internalizing symptoms over time when their close friends are high on internalizing symptoms (Deater-Deckard, 2001).

Prospective studies are especially important for understanding selection and socialization processes. In this regard, Goodwin, Mrug, Borch, and Cillessen (2012) followed adolescents from the 6th to the 11th grades, examining peer selection and socialization processes across school transitions. After each school transition, adolescents selected friends who were similar in their levels of depressive symptoms; friends also socialized adolescents to become more similar in depressive affect during the middle school years, but not during high school. Prinstein (2007) conducted an 18-month longitudinal study of "peer contagion" of depressive symptoms among 11th graders, finding that adolescents whose close friends reported high levels of internalizing symptoms showed increases in their own internalizing symptoms over time. Moreover, several variables moderated these associations. For girls, greater social anxiety was associated with greater susceptibility to friends' depressive symptom contagion; for boys, lower levels of friendship quality and higher friend popularity were associated with greater susceptibility to peer contagion.

These findings are intriguing and consistent with emerging evidence that corumination processes within friendships may contribute to adolescents' socialization of internalizing symptoms. Hankin, Stone, and Wright (2010) conducted a multiwave study of early and middle adolescents, finding that baseline corumination predicted increasing trajectories of all forms of internalizing symptoms (especially depressive symptoms and anxious arousal) but not externalizing problems. Also of interest, Dishion and Tipsord (2011) recently described how peer contagion processes are relevant to adolescent depression and identified corumination as an interactive process that may mediate these effects.

Although less well studied, evidence also suggests that homophily is relevant to understanding social anxiety in youth. Van Zalk, Van Zalk, Kerr, and Stattin (2011) recently evaluated early adolescents and their friendships, finding socially anxious youth were less popular, chose fewer friends, and tended to select friends who were socially anxious. Over time socially anxious youth and their friends influenced each other into becoming more socially anxious, and this effect was greater for girls than for boys.

Finally, homophily also comes into play in youths' romantic relationships (Furman & Simon, 2008). For example, Simon and colleagues (2008) examined peer selection processes in middle school youth, finding that adolescents and their romantic partners were similar on levels of depressive symptoms even prior to their relationship.

Empirical Support for Homophily in Externalizing Problems

Peer selection and socialization processes have long been believed to play a role in youths' externalizing problems and aggressive behavior (Hanish,

Martin, Fabes, Leonard, & Herzog, 2005). For example, Espelage, Holt, and Henkel (2003) demonstrated that early adolescent boys and girls affiliate with peers who are aggressive (i.e., bully and fight) at the same frequency and also that the peer context influenced youths' own aggressive behavior, especially for bullying. Furthermore, Snyder, Horsch, and Childs (1997) found that children affiliated with peers who were similar to themselves in their levels of aggression, although children high in aggression had difficulty establishing mutual friendships. Moreover, the amount of time children spent interacting with aggressive peers predicted increases in their own aggression levels three months later.

Although aggressive youth have friends who are also aggressive, it is not always clear whether this is due to an active selection process or to "default" selection (i.e., nonaggressive peers refuse to be friends with aggressive youth, so aggressive peers are chosen by default). Sijtsema, Lindenberg, and Veenstra (2010) evaluated these competing explanations among boys, finding that highly aggressive boys preferred peers who were not particularly high or low on aggression but ended up with friends who were aggressive, consistent with a default selection process. As these authors note, although aggressive boys prefer supportive friends, they end up in friendships with the least supportive peers.

Substantial evidence documents the importance of peer socialization of aggression and problem behaviors (e.g., substance use), even when controlling for selection effects (Gifford-Smith, Dodge, Dishion, & McCord, 2005). Dishion and Tipsord (2011) reviewed evidence that children's peer interactions contribute to increases in aggression during childhood and in serious problem behaviors (e.g., violence, drug use, delinquency) during adolescence. Peer deviancy training may be one mechanism that underlies this effect (see Dishion & Tipsord, 2011).

Although studies of romantic relationships are relatively scant, it appears that selection and socialization processes in romantic relationships also play a role in youths' problem behaviors. For example, Wargo and colleagues (2010) followed middle school youth over 11 months, assessing adolescents and their romantic partners both before and after their relationships were initiated. Findings emerged mainly for eighth graders, indicating that adolescents and their partners were initially alike on alcohol use and that over time romantic socialization effects emerged for their cigarette use and behavioral problems.

Summary

Youths' close friends and romantic relationships influence their psychological adjustment and are important to consider in clinical contexts. As growing evidence indicates, both peer selection and socialization processes play a role in youths' psychological adjustment and contribute to and maintain internalizing and externalizing problems. At the same time, there also appears to be some differentiation of internalizing versus externalizing problems. For externalizing problems, selection can apparently occur through a less active "default" peer selection process, whereas it is not yet known whether a "default" process is also at play for internalizing problems. There is also differentiation in the ways in which peer socialization occurs, with processes such as corumination playing a role in internalizing problems and deviancy training playing a role in externalizing problems.

Overall, current evidence supports the idea that natural peer processes (i.e., selection, socialization) could be viewed as transdiagnostic mechanisms that contribute to the development and maintenance of diverse psychological disorders in youth. Important directions for further research include conducting multiwave prospective studies that examine underlying mediators and moderators of the associations between peer variables and youths' dysfunction. Such work would allow for better specification of the pathways linking youths' friendships and romantic relationships with their psychological adjustment. Major challenges in this area of research are the difficulty of controlling for comorbid conditions and the difficulty of jointly modeling how changes in peer variables influence changes in psychological symptomatology over time.

Clinical Implications for Assessment and Treatment

Within a transdiagnostic framework, assessing youths' peer relationships and close friendships should be an essential component of any comprehensive assessment process. Most professionals will encounter youth with substantial social dysfunction in clinical practice, even if it is not articulated as part of the referral problem. For this reason, it is advisable to screen youth for social dysfunction early in the assessment process. When social problems are evident, a more detailed evaluation of social functioning would be indicated, and some form of social intervention should be considered as part of the overall treatment plan.

Screening and Assessment of Youths' Peer Relations

We recently provided a detailed overview of measures that assess youths' peer influences and how they can be applied in clinical situations (La Greca, Lai, Chan, & Herge, 2013; also see La Greca & Prinstein, 1999). Here we discuss the assessment processes more generally, along with the kinds of information that would be useful to planning interventions.

In terms of initial screening for youths' peer relations, it is important to determine: (1) *how youth are viewed* by peers and classmates (i.e., levels of peer acceptance/rejection), (2) *whether youth are experiencing PV*, and if so, what types and how often, (3) *whether youth have close friends or romantic attachments*, and the qualitative features of these relationships, and (4) *what youths' friends (and romantic attachments)* are like. Most of this information can initially be obtained from youth and parent reports. Identified problem areas might be followed by more detailed assessments (see La Greca et al., 2013).

Because peer relations are interactive, it will be important to understand not only youth characteristics that could contribute to problematic peer relations (e.g., poor social skills, threat perceptions, social avoidance) but also the contextual and transactional factors that could play a role in youths' peer relation difficulties (e.g., aggressive or deviant peer group, lack of school reporting procedures for PV). Interventions may need to address both the youths' characteristics and the broader peer/social context in order to be effective.

Furthermore, it is important to identify areas of strength in peer relations, such as close, supportive friendships. Support from close friends has been found to buffer the adverse impact of stress (e.g., Adams, Santo, & Bukowski, 2011; La Greca, Silverman, Lai, & Jaccard, 2010). Thus enhancing peer friendships might represent an important transdiagnostic treatment strategy for youth with diverse emotional and behavioral problems.

Transdiagnostic Treatment Issues for Peer Rejection and Victimization

When youth are rejected by peers or victimized, part of the transdiagnostic intervention strategy might be to address the broader peer context by *improving peer reputation*, as well as addressing individual concerns by *enhancing positive interaction skills* and *reducing annoying or interfering behaviors*. Negative peer reputations, once established, are difficult to alter, and enhancing youths' social skills alone has a limited impact on peer acceptance (see Spence, 2003). Furthermore, studies indicate that evidence-based interventions may be less effective with peer-rejected youth, who have been found to demonstrate significant long-term impairments (Mrug et al., 2012). On the other hand, it may be difficult to improve youths' peer reputations, even with new peers, if the interpersonal or behavioral difficulties that contributed to the problem initially (e.g., aggressive behavior, poor social skills, impulsive or avoidant behaviors) are not addressed.

There are several strategies for broadly *improving youths' peer reputations*. First, peer buddying or peer-pairing strategies encourage youth to associate with higher status or more accepted peers and have been used in evidence-based intervention programs (Beidel, Turner, & Young, 2006). In school, teachers could identify a "buddy" or well-accepted classmate who could work with target youth on classroom projects and activities. Outside of school, parents might facilitate their child's interactions with youth who are well accepted (e.g., invite them to social activities). Older youth and adolescents might be encouraged to pair up with a more accepted peer in school who can facilitate their social connectedness.

A second strategy for improving youths' peer reputations is to ensure that school policies and procedures discourage peer aggression, and especially PV and bullying. For example, teachers and peers should be encouraged to take a stand when they see youth victimizing others (see *www. stopbullying.gov*; United States Health and Human Services, 2013). School bullying intervention programs have demonstrated modest positive outcomes, although they are more likely to influence knowledge, attitudes, and self-perceptions than actual bullying behaviors (Merrell, Gueldner, Ross, & Isava, 2008).

An additional strategy, used after other strategies have been attempted, would be to change youths' classroom or school placements. For elementary school youth, this might be a change of classroom; for older youth, this might entail changing multiple classes or even changing schools. The idea is to allow the youth to start "fresh" with a new peer group. This strategy should be implemented in close consultation with school professionals, parents, and youth, to facilitate youths' transition to a new setting.

Strategies for *improving youths' positive interaction skills* might include social skills training to increase friendship initiation and to help youth develop more positive and less negative peer interaction skills. Evidence suggests that "social and emotional learning" benefits a wide range of youth and improves school adjustment (Durlak, Weissberg, Dymnicki, Taylor, & Schellinger, 2011). Interpersonal skills training is effective when the skills are socially valid and culturally sensitive to youths' social contexts, when it helps youth identify target behaviors and the rationale for behaviors, and when it includes an adequate duration of training (see Spence, 2003).

Strategies for *reducing youths' annoying or interfering behavior* will vary as a function of the diagnostic problem and may be addressed by relevant evidence-based interventions (e.g., Beidel et al, 2006; Masia-Warner, Fisher, Shrout, Rathor, & Klein, 2007). Interventions for aggressive or impulsive youth also address relevant behavioral problems, such as decreasing disruptive classroom behavior and increasing positive behaviors such as sharing (see Pelham & Fabiano, 2008).

Finally, research is needed to identify effective coping strategies for youth experiencing peer rejection and PV, as the current literature is unclear regarding effective coping strategies. For example, some research suggests that youth should disclose their experiences of PV because nondisclosure is related to feelings of loneliness (Vernberg, Ewell, Beery,

Freeman, & Abwender, 1995). Yet other research suggests that disclosure leads to feelings of powerlessness, loneliness, and hopelessness (Kochenderfer-Ladd & Skinner, 2002). In addition, problem-solving strategies are effective for nonvictimized youth, but they are not effective for youth who are frequently victimized, perhaps because these children may view situations as less controllable or more difficult to change (Kochenderfer-Ladd & Skinner, 2002).

Transdiagnostic Treatment Issues for Friendships and Other Close Peer Relations

It is important for youth to have close friends, and the characteristics of youths' friends influence youths' adjustment. Youth who lack or are limited in their close friendships may need assistance in developing friendship ties, such as by improving their interpersonal skills and by identifying appropriate (i.e., well-adjusted, nonproblematic) peers for friendships.

Strategies for improving youths' friendships may include social skills training (e.g., Beidel et al., 2006; Masia-Warner et al., 2007; Mrug et al., 2012; Mufson et al., 2004) to improve positive interaction skills. These skills are important for making and keeping friends and for dealing with the stress and conflict that inevitably arise in close peer relationships (see Ladd, 1999). Similar interpersonal skills are important for developing romantic relationships (Kuttler & La Greca, 2004; Kuttler et al., 1999).

An additional strategy for improving and developing friendship ties is to increase youths' opportunities for social interactions with potential friends (Updegraff, McHale, Crouter, & Kupanoff, 2001). Parents and teachers may identify appropriate peers and create opportunities for interaction (e.g., invite peers to play at home; encourage their child to sit with a classmate during lunch). Parents might also arrange play activities and social outings with potential friends. Enrolling youth in after-school activities (e.g., Scouts, dance, gymnastics) may increase exposure to desirable peers and foster friendships; for boys, it is associated with increased peer acceptance and greater propensity to engage in prosocial activities (Ladd & Hart, 1992). This strategy has the added advantage of developing youths' areas of strength or expertise (e.g., artistic and athletic skills) that could be highly valued by the larger peer group.

Parents have less control over adolescents' peer networks. Friendship facilitation strategies for parents of adolescents should include knowledge of adolescents' friendships. Parents may monitor social interactions (e.g., show an interest in friends, get to know friends). Parents may also include adolescents' friends in family outings and activities. Moreover, it is useful to evaluate and understand adolescents' crowd affiliations, as these affiliations reveal the kinds of pressures they experience (e.g., "brains" may feel pressured to perform well in school) and the kinds of teens available for social contacts and friendships. Also, adolescents themselves may be encouraged to find friends who are "like them" and to develop friendships.

Conclusions

In this chapter, we described how peer processes influence the development or maintenance of social and emotional problems across disorders. We described key aspects of peer relations (e.g., friendships, acceptance) and how problematic peer relations are both theoretically and empirically linked to child and adolescent disorders. Finally, we noted the importance of assessing key aspects of youths' peer functioning and offered some strategies that could be incorporated into a transdiagnostic approach to clinical intervention.

Youths' social functioning is not typically addressed in a clinical context, and, in fact, peer functioning is often relatively overlooked in comparison with other presenting problems. However, we have highlighted the fact that social problems are prevalent across numerous disorders and should always be an important consideration in treatment planning. Initial assessments may reveal problem areas in peer functioning, but they may also reveal areas of strength. Both strengths and weaknesses in peer functioning should be considered in treatment planning. Screening should also include questions about adolescents' romantic relationships, which may be a source of either stress or support (Furman et al., 2009; La Greca, Davila, Landoll, & Siegel, 2011).

Furthermore, it is imperative for clinicians and researchers to remain "conversant" and up-to-date with modern technology in order to understand how this plays a role in youths' social interactions. Technology is changing how youth communicate and socialize. For example, among youth ages 12–17, 93% use the Internet and close to three-quarters of online youth use social networking sites (Lenhart, Purcell, Smith, & Zickuhr, 2010). Clinicians and researchers need to understand how technology plays a role in youths' peer relationships and how technology may lead to the underdevelopment of important social skills (e.g., lack of "in person" communication, difficulties negotiating conflict) or miscommunication (e.g., misinterpretation of online communication due to lack of social cues).

Finally, both clinicians and researchers are encouraged to consider focusing on the broader peer contexts within which youth function. Interventions for social problems have tended to be limited to the individual or dyadic interactions of target youth (e.g., social skills training, decreasing annoying or interfering behavior). Youths' broader social-level context presents a fruitful area to target in both interventions (e.g., school bullying programs, increasing youths' interactions with peer groups outside the classroom) and in research.

REFERENCES

Aboud, F. E., & Mendelson, M. J. (1998). Determinants of friendship selection and quality: Developmental perspectives. In W. M. Bukowski, A. F. Newcomb, & W. W. Hartup (Eds.), *The company they keep: Friendships in childhood and adolescence* (pp. 87–112). New York: Cambridge University Press.

Adams, R. E., Santo, J. B., & Bukowski, W. M. (2011). The presence of a best friend buffers the effects of negative experiences. *Developmental Psychology, 47,* 1786–1791.

Beidel, D. C., Turner, S. M., & Young, B. J. (2006). Social effectiveness therapy for children: Five years later. *Behavior Therapy, 37,* 416–425.

Blöte, A. W., & Westenberg, P. M. (2007). Socially anxious adolescents' perception of treatment by classmates. *Behaviour Research and Therapy, 45,* 189–198.

Brown, B. B. (1990). Peer groups and peer cultures. In S. S. Feldman & G. R. Elliot (Eds.), *At the threshold: The developing adolescent* (pp. 171–196). Cambridge, MA: Harvard University Press.

Bukowski, W. M., Brendgen, M., & Vitaro, F. (2007). Peers and socialization: Effects on externalizing and internalizing problems. In J. E. Grusec & P. D. Hastings (Eds.), *Handbook of socialization: Theory and research* (pp. 355–381). New York: Guilford Press.

Carver, K., Joyner K., & Udry, J. R. (2003). National estimates of adolescent romantic relationships. In P. Florsheim (Ed.), *Adolescent romantic relationships and sexual behavior: Theory, research, and practical implications* (pp. 291–329). Mahwah, NJ: Erlbaum.

Coie, J. D., Dodge, K. A., & Kupersmidt, J. B. (1990). Peer group behavior and social status. In S. R. Asher & J. D. Coie (Eds.), *Peer rejection in childhood* (pp. 17–59). Cambridge, UK: Cambridge University Press.

Connolly, J., Geller, S., Marton, P., & Kutcher, S. (1992). Peer responses to social interaction with depressed adolescents. *Journal of Clinical Child Psychology, 21,* 365–370.

Connolly, J. A., & Goldberg, A. (1999). Romantic relationships in adolescence: The role of friends and peers in their emergence and development. In W. Furman, B. B. Brown, & C. Feiring (Eds.), *The development of romantic relationships in adolescence* (pp. 266–290). New York: Cambridge University Press.

Cook, C., Williams, K., Guerra, N., Kim, T., & Sadek, S. (2010). Predictors of bullying and victimization in childhood and adolescence: A meta-analytic investigation. *School Psychology Quarterly, 25,* 65–83.

Costello, E. J., Egger, H. L., & Angold, A. (2005). The developmental epidemiology of anxiety disorders: Phenomenology, prevalence, and comorbidity. *Child and Adolescent Psychiatric Clinics of North America, 14,* 631–648.

Crick, N. R., & Bigbee, M. A. (1998). Relational and overt forms of peer victimization: A multi-informant approach. *Journal of Consulting and Clinical Psychology, 66,* 337–347.

Crick, N. R., & Grotpeter, J. K. (1996). Children's treatment by peers: Victims of relational and overt aggression. *Development and Psychopathology, 8,* 367–380.

De Los Reyes, A., & Prinstein, M. J. (2004). Applying depression-distortion hypotheses to the assessment of peer victimization in adolescents. *Journal of Clinical Child and Adolescent Psychology, 33,* 325–335.

Deater-Deckard, K. (2001). Annotation: Recent research examining the role of peer relationships in the development of psychopathology. *Journal of Child Psychology and Psychiatry, 42,* 565–579.

Dishion, T. J., & Tipsord, J. M. (2011). Peer contagion in child and adolescent social and emotional development. *Annual Review of Psychology, 62,* 189–214.

Dodge, K., Lansford, J., Burks, V., Bates, J., Pettit, G., Fontaine, R., et al. (2003). Peer rejection and social information-processing factors in the development of aggressive behavior problems in children. *Child Development, 74,* 374–393.

Durlak, J., Weissberg, R., Dymnicki, A., Taylor, R., & Schellinger, K. (2011). The impact of enhancing students' social and emotional learning: A meta-analysis of school-based universal interventions. *Child Development, 82,* 405–432.

Espelage, D. L., Holt, M. K., & Henkel, R. R. (2003). Examination of peer group contextual effects on aggression during early adolescence. *Child Development, 74,* 205–220.

Estell, D. B., Jones, M. H., Pearl, R., Van Acker, R., Farmer, T. W., & Rodkin, P. C. (2008). Peer groups, popularity, and social preference: Trajectories of social functioning among students with and without learning disabilities. *Journal of Learning Disabilities, 41,* 5–14.

Frick, P. (2006). Developmental pathways to conduct disorder. *Child and Adolescent Psychiatric Clinics of North America, 15,* 311–331.

Furman, W., McDunn, C., & Young, B. (2009). The role of peer and romantic relationships in adolescent affective development. In N. Allen & L. Sheeber (Eds.), *Adolescent emotional development and the emergence of depressive disorders* (pp. 299–317). New York: Cambridge University Press.

Furman, W., & Simon, V. A. (2008). Homophily in adolescent romantic relationships. In M. J. Prinstein & K. A. Dodge (Eds.), *Understanding peer influence in children and adolescents* (pp. 203–224). New York: Guilford Press.

Gifford-Smith, M., Dodge, K., Dishion, T., & McCord, J. (2005). Peer influence in children and adolescents: Crossing the bridge from developmental to intervention science. *Journal of Abnormal Child Psychology, 33,* 255–265.

Ginsburg, G. S., La Greca, A. M., & Silverman, W. K. (1998). Social anxiety in children with anxiety disorders: Relation with social and emotional functioning. *Journal of Abnormal Child Psychology, 26*(3), 175–185.

Glickman, A. R., & La Greca, A. M. (2004). The Dating Anxiety Scale for Adolescents: Scale development and associations with adolescent functioning. *Journal of Clinical Child and Adolescent Psychology, 33,* 566–578.

Goodwin, N. P., Mrug, S., Borch, C., & Cillessen, A. H. (2012). Peer selection and socialization in adolescent depression: The role of school transitions. *Journal of Youth and Adolescence, 41,* 320–332.

Grant, D., Beck, J. G., Farrow, S. M., & Davila, J. (2007). Do interpersonal features of social anxiety influence the development of depressive symptoms? *Cognition and Emotion, 21,* 646–663.

Grant, K., Compas, B., Thurm, A., McMahon, S., & Gipson, P. (2004). Stressors and child and adolescent psychopathology: Measurement issues and prospective effects. *Journal of Clinical Child and Adolescent Psychology, 33,* 412–425.

Grant, K. E., Compas, B. E., Stuhlmacher, A., Thurm, A. E., McMahon, S., & Halpert, J. (2003). Stressors and child/adolescent psychopathology: Moving from markers to mechanisms of risk. *Psychological Bulletin, 129,* 447–466.

Hammen, C. (1991). The generation of stress in the course of unipolar depression. *Journal of Abnormal Psychology, 100,* 555–561.

Hanish, L., Martin, C., Fabes, R., Leonard, S., & Herzog, M. (2005). Exposure to externalizing peers in early childhood: Homophily and peer contagion processes. *Journal of Abnormal Child Psychology, 33,* 267–281.

Hankin, B. L., Stone, L., & Wright, P. A. (2010). Corumination, interpersonal stress generation, and internalizing symptoms: Accumulating effects and transactional influences in a multiwave study of adolescents. *Developmental Psychopathology, 22,* 217–235.

Harrison, H. M. (2006). Peer victimization and depressive symptoms in adolescence. *Dissertation Abstracts International, 67*(4), 96B. (UMI No. 3215231).

Hartup, W. W. (1996). The company they keep: Friendships and their developmental significance. *Child Development, 67,* 1–13.

Hawker, D .S. J., & Boulton, M. J. (2000). Twenty years' research on peer victimization and psychosocial maladjustment: A meta-analytic review of cross-sectional studies. *Journal of Psychology and Psychiatry, 41,* 441–455.

Hinshaw, S. P. (2008). Developmental psychopathology as a scientific discipline: Relevance to behavioral and emotional disorders of childhood and adolescence. In T. P. Beauchaine & S. P. Hinshaw (Eds.), *Child and adolescent psychopathology* (pp. 3–26). Hoboken, NJ: Wiley.

Hodges, E., Boivin, M., Vitaro, F., & Bukowski, W. (1999). The power of friendship: Protection against an escalating cycle of peer victimization. *Developmental Psychology, 35,* 94–101.

Hoza, B. (2007). Peer functioning in children with ADHD. *Ambulatory Pediatrics, 7,* 101–106.

Juster, H. R., & Heimberg, R. G. (1995). Social phobia: Longitudinal course and long-term outcome of cognitive behavioral treatment. *Psychiatric Clinics of North America, 18,* 821–842.

Kandel, D. B. (1978a). Homophily, selection, and socialization in adolescent friendships. *American Journal of Sociology, 84,* 427–436.

Kandel, D. B. (1978b). Similarity in real-life adolescent friendship pairs. *Journal of Personality and Social Psychology, 36,* 306–312.

Kingery, J., Erdley, C., Marshall, K., Whitaker, K., & Reuter, T. (2010). Peer experiences of anxious and socially withdrawn youth: An integrative review of the developmental and clinical literature. *Clinical Child and Family Psychology Review, 13,* 91–128.

Kochenderfer-Ladd, B., & Skinner, K. (2002). Children's coping strategies: Moderators of the effects of peer victimization? *Developmental Psychology, 38,* 267–278.

Kokkinos, C., & Panayiotou, G. (2004). Predicting bullying and victimization among early adolescents: Associations with disruptive behavior disorders. *Aggressive Behavior, 30,* 520–533.

Kupersmidt, J. B., & Coie, J. D. (1990). Preadolescent peer status, aggression, and school adjustment as predictors of externalizing problems in adolescence. *Child Development, 61,* 1350–1362.

Kuttler, A. F., & La Greca, A. M. (2004). Adolescents' romantic relationships: Do they help or hinder close friendships? *Journal of Adolescence, 27,* 395–414.

Kuttler, A. F., La Greca, A. M., & Prinstein, M. J. (1999). Friendship qualities and social-emotional functioning of adolescents with close, cross-sex friendships. *Journal of Research on Adolescence, 9,* 339–366.

La Greca, A. M. (2001). Friends or foes?: Peer influences on anxiety among children and adolescents. In W. K. Silverman & P. D. A. Treffers (Eds.), *Anxiety disorders in children and adolescents: Research, assessment, and intervention* (pp. 159–186). New York: Cambridge University Press.

La Greca, A. M., Davila, J., Landoll, R. R., & Siegel, R. (2011). Dating, romantic relationships and social anxiety in young people. In C. A. Alfano & D. C. Beidel (Eds.), *Social anxiety in adolescents and young adults: Translating developmental science into practice.* Washington, DC: American Psychological Association.

La Greca, A. M., Davila, J., & Siegel, R. (2009). Peer relations, friendships, and romantic relationships: Implications for the development and maintenance of depression in adolescents. In N. Allen & L. Sheeber (Eds.), *Adolescent emotional development and the emergence of depressive disorders* (pp. 318–336). New York: Cambridge University Press.

La Greca, A. M., & Harrison, H. M. (2005). Adolescent peer relations, friendships, and romantic relationships: Do they predict social anxiety and depression? *Journal of Clinical Child and Adolescent Psychology, 34,* 49–61.

La Greca, A. M., Lai, B., Chan, S., & Herge, W. (2013). Peer assessment strategies. In B. D. McLeod, A. Jensen-Doss, & T. H. Ollendick (Eds.), *Diagnostic and behavioral assessment in children and adolescents: A clinical guide* (pp. 277–315). New York: Guilford Press.

La Greca, A. M., & Landoll, R. R. (2011). Peer influences. In W. K. Silverman & A. Field (Eds.), *Anxiety disorders in children and adolescents: Research, assessment and intervention* (2nd ed., pp. 323–346). London: Cambridge University Press.

La Greca, A. M., & Lopez, N. (1998). Social anxiety among adolescents: Linkages with peer relations and friendships. *Journal of Abnormal Child Psychology, 26,* 83–94.

La Greca, A. M., & Mackey, E. (2007). Adolescents' anxiety in dating situations: The potential role of friends and romantic partners. *Journal of Clinical Child and Adolescent Psychology, 36,* 522–533.

La Greca, A. M., & Prinstein, M. J. (1999). The peer group. In W. K. Silverman & T. H. Ollendick (Eds.), *Developmental issues in the clinical treatment of children and adolescents* (pp. 171–198). Needham Heights, MA: Allyn & Bacon.

La Greca, A. M., Prinstein, M. J., & Fetter, M. D. (2001). Adolescent peer crowd affiliation: Linkages with health-risk behaviors and close friendships. *Journal of Pediatric Psychology, 26*(3), 131–143.

La Greca, A. M., Silverman, W. K., Lai, B. S., & Jaccard, J. (2010). Hurricane-related exposure experiences and stressors, other life events, and social support: Concurrent and prospective impact on children's persistent post-traumatic stress symptoms. *Journal of Consulting and Clinical Psychology, 78,* 794–805.

La Greca, A. M., & Stone, W. L. (1993). The Social Anxiety Scale for Children–Revised: Factor structure and concurrent validity. *Journal of Clinical Child Psychology, 22,* 17–27.

Ladd, G. (1999). Peer relationships and social competence during early and middle childhood. *Annual Review of Psychology, 50,* 333–359.

Ladd, G., & Hart, C. (1992). Creating informal play opportunities: Are parents' and preschooler's initiations related to children's competence with peers? *Developmental Psychology, 28,* 1179–1187.

Laird, R., Jordan, K., Dodge, K., Pettit, G., & Bates, J. (2001). Peer rejection in childhood, involvement with antisocial peers in early adolescene, and the development of externalizing behavior problems. *Developmental Psychopathology, 13,* 337–354.

Lamarche, V., Brendgen, M., Boivin, M., Vitaro, F., Dionne, G., & Perusse, D. (2007). Do friends' characteristics moderate the prospective links between peer victimization and reactive and proactive aggression? *Journal of Abnormal Child Psychology, 35,* 665–680.

Landoll, R. R., La Greca, A. M., & Lai, B. S. (2013). Aversive experiences on social networking sites: Development of the Social Networking–Peer Experiences Questionnaire. *Journal of Research on Adolescence.*

Lansford, J. E., Malone, P. S., Dodge, K. A., Pettit, G. S., & Bates, J. E. (2010). Developmental cascades of peer rejection, social information processing biases, and aggression during middle childhood. *Development and Psychopathology, 22,* 593–602.

Larson, R. W., Clore, G. L., & Wood, G. A. (1999). The emotions of romantic relationships: Do they wreak havoc on adolescents? In W. Furman, B. B. Brown, & C. Feiring (Eds.), *The development of romantic relationships in adolescence* (pp. 19–49). New York: Cambridge University Press.

Leary, M. R., Twenge, J. M., & Quinlivan, E. (2006). Interpersonal rejection as a determinant of anger and aggression. *Personality and Social Psychological Review, 10,* 111–132.

Lenhart, A., Purcell, K., Smith, A., & Zickuhr, K. (2010). Social media and mobile Internet use among teens and young adults. Retrieved February 29, 2012, from *www.pewinternet.org/trend-data-for-teens/online-activites-total.aspx.*

Lewinsohn, P. M., Joiner, T. E., Jr., & Rohde, P. (2001). Evaluation of cognitive diathesis–stress models in predicting major depressive disorder in adolescents. *Journal of Abnormal Psychology, 110,* 203–215.

Little, S. A., & Garber, J. (1995). Aggression, depression, and stressful life events predicting peer rejection in children. *Development and Psychopathology, 7,* 845–856.

Lopez, C., & DuBois, D. L. (2005). Peer victimization and rejection: Investigation of an integrative model of effects on emotional, behavioral, and academic adjustment in early adolescence. *Journal of Clinical Child and Adolescent Psychology, 34,* 25–36.

Masia-Warner, C., Fisher, P. H., Shrout, P. E., Rathor, S., & Klein, R. G. (2007).

Treating adolescents with social anxiety disorder in school: An attention control trial. *Journal of Child Psychology and Psychiatry, 48,* 676–686.

McLaughlin, K. A., Hatzenbuehler, M. L., Mennin, D. S., & Nolen-Hoeksema, S. (2011). Emotion dysregulation and adolescent psychopathology: A prospective study. *Behavior Research and Therapy, 49,* 544–554.

Merrell, K., Gueldner, B., Ross, S., & Isava, D. M. (2008). How effective are school bullying intervention programs?: A meta-analysis of intervention research. *School Psychology Quarterly, 23,* 26–42.

Miller-Johnson, S., Coie, J., Maumary-Gremaud, A., Bierman, K., & the Conduct Problems Prevention Research Group. (2002). Peer rejection and aggression and early starter models of conduct disorder. *Journal of Abnormal Child Psychology, 30,* 217–230.

Mrug, S., Molina, B. S. G., Hoza, B., Gerdes, A. C., Hinshaw, S. P., Hechtman, L., et al. (2012). Peer rejection and friendships in children with attention-deficit/hyperactivity disorder: Contributions to long-term outcomes. *Journal of Abnormal Child Psychology, 40,* 1–14.

Mufson, L., Dorta, K. P., Wickramaratne, P., Nomura, Y., Olfson, M., & Weissman, M. M. (2004). The effectiveness of interpersonal psychotherapy for depressed adolescents. *Archives of General Psychiatry, 61,* 577–584.

Murray-Close, D., Ostrov, J. M., & Crick, N. R. (2007). A short-term longitudinal study of growth of relational aggression during middle childhood: Associations with gender, friendship intimacy, and internalizing problems. *Development and Psychopathology, 19,* 187–203.

Nansel, T., Overpeck, M., Pilla, R., Ruan, W. J., Simons-Morton, B., & Scheidt, P. (2001). Bullying behaviors among U.S. youth: Prevalence and association with psychosocial adjustment. *Journal of the American Medical Association, 285,* 2094–2100.

Newcomb, A. F., Bukowski, W. M., & Pattee, L. (1993). Children's peer relations: A meta-analytic review of popular, rejected, neglected, controversial, and average sociometric status. *Psychological Bulletin, 113,* 99–128.

O'Brennan, L., Bradshaw, C. P., & Sawyer, A. L. (2009). Examining developmental differences in the socio-emotional problems among frequent bullies, victims, and bully/victims. *Psychology in the Schools, 46,* 100–115.

O'Sullivan, L. F., Cheng, M. M., Harris, K. M., & Brooks-Gunn, J. (2007). I wanna hold your hand: The progression of social, romantic and sexual events in adolescent relationships. *Perspectives on Sexual and Reproductive Health, 39,* 100–107.

Parker, J., & Asher, S. (1993). Peer relations and later personal adjustment: Are low-accepted children at risk? *Psychological Bulletin, 102,* 357–389.

Pelham, W., & Fabiano, G. (2008). Evidence-based psychosocial treatments for attention-deficit/hyperactivity disorder. *Journal of Clinical Child and Adolescent Psychology, 37,* 184–218.

Prinstein, M. J. (2007). Moderators of peer contagion: A longitudinal examination of depression socialization between adolescents and their best friends. *Journal of Clinical Child and Adolescent Psychology, 36,* 159–170.

Prinstein, M. J., & Aikins, J. W. (2004). Cognitive moderators of the longitudinal association between peer rejection and adolescent depressive symptoms. *Journal of Abnormal Child Psychology, 32,* 147–158.

Prinstein, M. J., Boergers, J., & Vernberg, E. M. (2001). Overt and relational aggression in adolescents: Social-psychological adjustment of aggressors and victims. *Journal of Clinical Child and Adolescent Psychology, 30,* 479–491.

Prinstein, M. J., Borelli, J. L., Cheah, C. S. L., Simon, V. A., & Aikins, J. W. (2005). Adolescent girls' interpersonal vulnerability to depressive symptoms: A longitudinal examination of reassurance-seeking and peer relationships. *Journal of Abnormal Psychology, 114,* 676–688.

Prinstein, M. J., & Cillessen, A. H. N. (2003). Forms and functions of adolescent peer aggression associated with high levels of peer status. *Merrill-Palmer Quarterly, 49,* 310–342.

Ranta, K., Kaltiala-Heino, R., Pelkonen, M., & Marttunen, M. (2009). Associations between peer victimization, self-reported depression and social phobia among adolescents: The role of comorbidity. *Journal of Adolescence, 32,* 77–93.

Reijntjes, A., Thomaes, S., Bushman, B., Boelen, P., de Castro, B., & Telch, M. (2010). The outcast-lash-out effect in youth: Alienation increases aggression following peer rejection. *Psychological Science, 21,* 1394–1398.

Rudolph, K., Troop-Gordon, W., Hessel, E., & Schmidt, J. (2011). A latent growth curve analysis of early and increasing peer victimization as predictors of mental health across elementary school. *Journal of Clinical Child and Adolescent Psychology, 40,* 111–122.

Siegel, R. S., La Greca, A. M., & Harrison, H. M. (2009). Peer victimization and social anxiety in adolescents: Prospective and reciprocal relationships. *Journal of Youth and Adolescence, 38,* 1096–1109.

Sijtsema, J. J., Lindenberg, S. M., & Veenstra, R. (2010). Do they get what they want or are they stuck with what they can get?: Testing homophily against default selection for friendships of highly aggressive boys: The TRAILS study. *Journal of Abnormal Child Psychology, 38,* 803–813.

Simon, V. A., Aikins, J. W., & Prinstein, M. J. (2008). Romantic partner selection and socialization during early adolescence. *Child Development, 79,* 1676–1692.

Singh, P., & Bussey, K. (2011). Peer victimization and psychological maladjustment: The mediating role of coping self-efficacy. *Journal of Research on Adolescence, 21,* 420–433.

Snyder, J., Horsch, E., & Childs, J. (1997). Peer relationships of young children: Affiliative choices and the shaping of aggressive behavior. *Journal of Child Psychology, 26,* 145–156.

Snyder, J., Schrepferman, L., Oeser, J., Patterson, G. R., Stoolmiller, M., Johnson, K., et al. (2005). Deviancy training and association with deviant peers in young children: Occurrence and contribution to early-onset conduct problems. *Speech and Language Pathology and Applied Behavior Analysis, 1,* 43–54.

Spence, S. (2003). Social skills training with children and young people: Theory, evidence, and practice. *Child and Adolescent Mental Health, 8,* 84–96.

Storch, E. A., Brassard, M. R., & Masia-Warner, C. L. (2003). The relationship of peer victimization to social anxiety and loneliness in adolescence. *Child Study Journal, 33,* 1–18.

Strauss, C. C., Frame, C. L., & Forehand, R. L. (1987). Psychosocial impairment associated with anxiety in children. *Journal of Clinical Child Psychology, 16,* 235–239.

U.S. Department of Health and Human Services. (2009). Be more than a bystander. Retrieved February 29, 2012, from *www.stopbullying.gov*.

Updegraff, K., McHale, S., Crouter, A., & Kupanoff, K. (2001). Parents' involvement in adolescents' peer relationships: A comparison of mothers' and fathers' roles. *Journal of Marriage and Family, 63*, 655–668.

Van Zalk, N., Van Zalk, M., Kerr, M., & Stattin, H. (2011). Social anxiety as a basis for friendship selection and socialization in adolescents' social networks. *Journal of Personality, 79*, 499–526.

Verduin, T. L., & Kendall, P. C. (2008). Peer perceptions and liking of children with anxiety disorders. *Journal of Abnormal Child Psychology, 36*, 459–469.

Vernberg, E., Ewell, K., Beery, S., Freeman, C., & Abwender, D. (1995). Aversive exchanges with peers and adjustment during early adolescence: Is disclosure helpful? *Child Psychiatry and Human Development, 26*, 43–59.

Vernberg, E. M. (1990). Psychological adjustment and experiences with peers during early adolescence: Reciprocal, incidental, or unidirectional relationships? *Journal of Abnormal Child Psychology, 18*, 187–198.

Vernberg, E. M., Abwender, D. A., Ewell, K. K., & Beery, S. H. (1992). Social anxiety and peer relationships in early adolescence: A prospective analysis. *Journal of Clinical Child Psychology, 21*, 189–196.

Wang, J. J., Iannotti, R. J., Luk, J. W., & Nansel, T. R. (2010). Co-occurrence of victimization from five subtypes of bullying: Physical, verbal, social exclusion, spreading rumors, and cyber. *Journal of Pediatric Psychology, 35*, 1103–1112.

Wargo, A. J., Simon, V. A., & Prinstein, M. J. (2010). Romantic partner selection and socialization of young adolescents' substance use and behavior problems. *Journal of Adolescence, 33*, 813–826.

Williams, K. R., & Guerra, N. G. (2007). Prevalence and predictors of Internet bullying. *Journal of Adolescent Health, 41*, S14–S21.

CHAPTER 7

Mindful Parenting
in the Development and Maintenance
of Youth Psychopathology

Justin D. Smith and Thomas J. Dishion

Transdiagnostic models of family process focus on the shared dynamics, functions, and structure of interaction patterns related to various forms of youth psychopathology. The promise of a transdiagnostic approach lies in the development of prevention and intervention strategies that address multiple adjustment difficulties in children and adolescents (Chu, 2012; Dishion & Stormshak, 2007). In this chapter we propose *mindful parenting* as a superordinate construct that describes parents' efforts to self-regulate their own emotions, needs, and automatic reaction patterns in the interest of promoting the short- and long-term well-being of their children. While developing interventions for families, our research team at the Child and Family Center has organized family management into three broad domains: positive behavior support, healthy limit setting and parental monitoring, and family relationship building (Dishion, Storm-shak, & Kavanagh, 2012). In this chapter we have organized our discussion of mindful parenting into a brief review of these domains as they apply to the concept of mindful parenting in transdiagnostic models of youth psychopathology. The chapter culminates with a critical analysis of the current state of research in this area and with proposed future directions for empirical inquiry.

The Concept of Mindful Parenting

Mindful parenting extends the concept of mindfulness (Kabat-Zinn, 2003) to describe a parent's ability to be aware, to self-regulate, and to navigate the interpersonal issues (self and other) in parenting (Kabat-Zinn & Kabat-Zinn, 1997; Steinberg, 2004). Being proactive and monitoring children and adolescents is certainly a core aspect of mindful parenting, as is being aware of and compassionate about the short- and long-term needs of youth. It is likely that over time all cultures derived unique strategies for effective parenting, and therefore the instantiation of mindful parenting is likely to vary depending on socioeconomic and cultural context.

The model of mindful parenting put forth by Duncan, Coatsworth, and Greenberg (2009) posits that "parents who can remain aware and accepting of their child's needs through the use of mindfulness practices can create a family context that allows for more enduring satisfaction and enjoyment in the parent–child relationship" (p. 256). Mindful parenting, therefore, fosters higher quality relationships within families. Dishion and colleagues (2011) present a model of mindful parenting that further differentiates the parenting skills and intrafamilial processes involved, the elements of which are discussed in the remainder of this chapter and depicted in Figure 7.1. We believe positive behavior support, parents' healthy limit setting, and family relationship building comprise a testable latent construct of mindful parenting.

The core skills and processes involved in mindful parenting are a transdiagnostic mechanism, the lack of which contributes to the development, amplification, and maintenance of youth psychopathology.

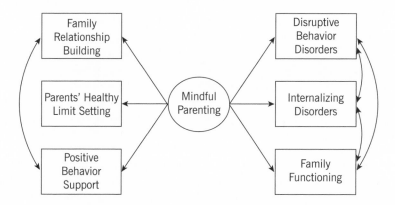

FIGURE 7.1. The elements of mindful parenting and the relationship to psychopathology and family functioning.

Conversely, Dumas (2005) proposed that fostering everyday mindful parenting practices can improve the effectiveness of interventions targeting parenting practices, suggesting that they are likely to be a mechanism of change for various disorder classes. To date, mindfulness-based parenting interventions have been shown to be effective for improving family functioning, parenting practices, parenting satisfaction, and mindful parenting skills (see Coatsworth, Duncan, Greenberg, & Nix, 2010).

Parental Reactivity and Youth Psychopathology

It is assumed that all forms of youth psychopathology are multidetermined and have significant genetic and environmental roots (e.g., Rutter, 2006). A multilevel analysis of psychopathology suggests that gene, brain, and environment work together to shape underlying mechanisms that in turn form typical and atypical development (Cicchetti, 1993, 2008). Of interest, however, is the ubiquity of parenting processes that can amplify genetic vulnerabilities. From a relationship perspective of developmental psychopathology, evidence is clear that a key dimension of the environment is reactive and conflictual close relationships (Beach et al., 2006). Parent reactivity is intrinsic to parent–child conflict but can also be an essential aspect of neglect. Parents who are consumed by the concerns of their personal life can neglect or ignore the needs of their children. Often, neglect and conflict go hand in hand: cycles of neglect can lead to severe conflict once a conduct problem is fully developed (Dishion & Patterson, 2006).

Parent reactivity is implicated in the development and amplification of all forms of youth psychopathology, including disruptive behavior disorders (e.g., Frick & Loney, 2002; Johnston & Mash, 2001; Patterson, 1982; Smith & Farrington, 2004), unipolar and bipolar depression (e.g., Alloy, Abramson, Smith, Gibb, & Neeren, 2006; Goodman & Gotlib, 1999; Radke-Yarrow, Ricters, & Wilson, 1988; for a review, see Restifo & Bogels, 2009; Sheeber & Sorenson, 1998), substance abuse disorders (e.g., Dishion, Capaldi, & Yoerger, 1999; Liddle & Dakof, 1995), attention-deficit/hyperactivity disorder (ADHD; e.g., Lindahl, 1998), borderline personality disorder (Crowell, Beauchaine, & Lenzenweger, 2008), and schizophrenia (Asarnow & Kernan, 2008; Doane, Goldstein, Miklowitz, & Falloon, 1986; Falloon et al., 1985). Addressing fractured, conflictual familial relationships is central to attachment (Bowlby, 1980) and to social learning theories (Patterson, 1982; Patterson, Reid, & Dishion, 1992) with regard to development of psychopathology in children and adolescents.

The literature about parenting is vast, and a thorough discussion of the conceptual and measurement issues underlying a science of parenting is beyond the scope of this chapter. It is likely that much of the debate about which parenting constructs are the most important to children's development may actually be related to problems of measurement (Dishion, Burraston, & Li, 2003). The literature regarding parenting practices is challenging to integrate, given inconsistent measurement practices and construct definitions, which we discuss in greater detail later in this chapter, but there is ample evidence to support the assertion that family processes are basic mechanisms involved in the etiology of common youth mental health disorders and can therefore be the targets of family-based transdiagnostic interventions.

We discuss the concept of mindful parenting as it applies to family management practices, a term originally introduced by Patterson and colleagues (1992). The key features of family management are parents' efforts to monitor and attend to children's behavior and whereabouts, to consider what is being learned (or conditioned) in a situation, and to respond patiently and with a vision for the future that integrates compassion for the child with beneficence for the child and family. Such an approach to parenting requires motivated awareness, self-regulation, and vigilance about the present, similar to the concept of mindfulness often used in psychology and associated with a state of mind cultivated in meditation. The key that links the concept of individual mindfulness with family management is attention to the present detail and responding out of awareness rather than from emotional reactivity. It is not surprising that parenting, a process that accounts for successful education of youth and maintenance of peaceful community, would require a set of skills also found useful for establishing and maintaining psychological well-being. To activate mindful parenting, focus is shifted to the interpersonal interaction dynamics of one's family, including those among adult partners and especially those that involve parents and children.

Our model of mindful parenting incorporates three key parenting processes that have been empirically demonstrated to be tied to the development and maintenance of youth psychopathology: (1) positive behavior support, which involves paying attention to children's positive behavior, proactively setting up situations for children's success and enjoyment, and being responsively contingent when noticing positive behavior; (2) healthy limit setting, which includes parents' efforts to proactively structure children's lives to ensure that they are supervised by adults and to safeguard them from potential risks and dangers; and (3) family relationship building, which consists of daily efforts to communicate with family members in such a way as to increase mutual understanding and compassion and to solve problems peacefully, considering each family member's point of view. Unlike with individual mindfulness, mindful parenting involves focusing attention on parent–child transactions rather than on the self.

Positive Behavior Support

Positive behavior support is a prevalent and effective behavior management principle that emphasizes the use of nonaversive, reinforcing adult–child interactions (e.g., Horner & Carr, 1997; Sugai, Horner, & Sprague, 1999). A core aspect of parenting is to be attentive to children's efforts, to be aware of their "zones of proximal development," and to acknowledge, reinforce, and support their prosocial efforts. Positive behavior support includes parenting behaviors such as warmth, praise, positive reinforcement, and monitoring. Integral to positive behavior support and to all parenting practices is to proactively offer children opportunities to be successful and to provide learning opportunities and situations that are rewarding and that minimize conflict and negative interactions (Gardner, 1987). At the foundation of positive behavior support is parents' willingness to make effective requests of their children or adolescents and to reinforce positive child behaviors consistent with those requests. The literature describing the relationship between positive behavior support and related parenting constructs and later development of problem behaviors during childhood and adolescence is quite robust. Although an exhaustive review of this topic is well beyond the scope of this chapter, following are mentions of notable studies and conceptual models of positive behavior support that have emanated from research conducted at the Child and Family Center and its affiliates. Shaw and Gross (2008) found that negative and neglectful parenting practices of children at 2 years old are prognostic of later problem behaviors (e.g., interpersonal aggression, violent crime). Lack of warmth and positive involvement during early childhood is associated with later problem behaviors (e.g., Gardner, Sonuga-Barke, & Sayal, 1999; Gardner, Ward, Burton, & Wilson, 2003; Kashdan et al., 2004; Stormshak, Bierman, McMahon, & Lengua, 2000). Similarly, lack of parental involvement and inconsistent discipline practices have been implicated in the etiology of disruptive behavior disorders in youth (Connor, 2002).

The literature also provides empirical findings regarding the relationship between positive behavior support and unipolar and bipolar depression. Given its close link to the immediate family context, depression in youth ought to be associated with family functioning (Stark, Swearer, Kurowski, Sommer, & Bowen, 1996). Cicchetti and Toth (1998) proposed that the quality of caregiving an infant receives contributes to variations in neurobiological growth and development of the infant's brain, which results in greater risk for developing depressive symptoms later in life. Parenting practices are associated with the later development of depressive disorders (e.g., Garber, Robinson, & Valentiner, 1997; Kim & Ge, 2000) and with the co-occurrence of depression and conduct problems (Ge, Best, Conger, & Simons, 1996). Connell and Dishion (2008) found that levels of adolescent depression were significantly diminished as a result of an intervention aimed at increasing positive behavior support to reduce externalizing behavior problems. The reduction in depression that has been found to occur with these interventions seems to be a collateral benefit of having improved positive behavior support within the family. Another example of this phenomenon comes from a study by Shaw, Connell, Dishion, Wilson, and Gardner (2009), who found that improvements in positive parenting were associated with reductions in the caregiver's depressive symptoms. Other collateral benefits of increasing positive behavior support can also be found in the intervention literature. For example, Lunkenheimer and colleagues (2008) found an indirect effect between improved positive behavior support and child language development and inhibitory control. A growing body of evidence supports the assertion that positive behavior support is a transdiagnostic mechanism associated with a host of important child and adolescent mental health indicators and multiple disorder classes, including anxiety, externalizing behaviors, and depression (e.g., Wood, McLeod, Sigman, Hwang, & Chu, 2003).

Mindful parenting is fundamental to positive behavior support strategies. Mindful parents demonstrate compassion for their child by being aware of the positive impact of reinforcing desired behaviors regardless of the child's competing emotions or demands for attention at the time. In many cases, this approach requires that parents actively inhibit more automatic responses when they feel the child is not listening or is purposely defying family rules and expectations. Becoming more aware of one's emotional reactions to the child and how this awareness can subsequently lead to specific, improved responses is a defining behavior of the mindful parent and a core skill promoted in traditional mindfulness practices.

Parental Healthy Limit Setting

The core component of healthy limit setting is monitoring children's behavior and whereabouts and safeguarding one's children. *Parental monitoring* is a term coined by Gerald Patterson in the 1980s (Patterson, 1982; Patterson & Stouthamer-Loeber, 1984) to denote parents' overall involvement with their children and their direct and indirect knowledge of their children's safety, behavior, feelings, experiences, and whereabouts (for a review, see Dishion & McMahon, 1998). Lack of parental monitoring of adolescents has been shown to be highly predictive of externalizing behavior problems in boys and in girls (Fosco, Stormshak, Dishion, & Winter, 2012; Kerr & Stattin, 2000) and is a known correlate of aggression and antisocial behaviors in children (Connor, 2002). Internalizing problems are also associated with the absence of monitoring: Kim and Ge (2000) found that increased use of parental monitoring and inductive reasoning practices reduced the risk of youth depression. DiClemente and colleagues (2001) found that adolescents who perceived less parental monitoring were more likely to endorse engaging in risky sexual behaviors and to test positive for a sexually transmitted disease. They also found that less monitoring was associated with greater rates of substance use, which is consistent with the findings of other researchers (e.g., Chilcoat & Anthony, 1996; Kiesner, Poulin, & Dishion, 2010; Lac & Crano, 2009; Tobler & Komro, 2010). In a similar vein, Caruthers, Van Ryzin, and Dishion (in press) found that improving parental monitoring by implementing a brief intervention during early adolescence resulted in less high-risk sexual behaviors reported during early adulthood. Brody (2003) found that changes in monitoring were related to changes in child externalizing behaviors over time. He also found that children with difficult temperaments (e.g., low levels of self-regulation) benefited most from parental monitoring. That is, the relationship between difficult temperament and externalizing behavior was weaker in well-monitored homes.

Contemporary parent and family intervention models that target parental monitoring also help parents take constructive action in the form of setting healthy limits. Externalizing and internalizing problems occur at a much higher rate when youth experience inconsistent and harsh parental discipline practices (Connor, 2002; Garber et al., 1997) and negative, physically aggressive punishment strategies (Kashdan et al., 2004; Stormshak et al., 2000). Monitoring might have particularly important implications for high-risk youth. Increasing parental monitoring has been found to prevent early-onset substance abuse by high-risk adolescents (Dishion, Nelson, & Kavanagh, 2003). In a longitudinal study, Laird, Criss, Pettit, Dodge, and Bates (2008) found that better parental monitoring attenuated the relationship between the influence of a deviant peer group and adolescent delinquent behaviors. The collective empirical knowledge regarding the relationship between parental monitoring and various youth mental health and behavioral problems indicates that monitoring plays a prominent role in the development of these problems and could prove to be a robust mechanism of change in parenting and family-based interventions. To a large extent, mindful parenting contributes to parental monitoring practices. Parents who are more mindful are likely to appreciate the positive, long-term outcomes of monitoring their children and setting healthy limits, even though these practices can be a source of parent–child disagreement at a time when a less mindful parent might feel compelled to retract a limit he or she had set.

Family Relationship Building

The literature is quite clear that poor family relationships lead to increased incidence rates of youth psychopathology. Conflict is inevitable in close relationships, and the way in which it is resolved determines the course of a relationship. A parent's emotional reactivity is one of the best predictors of poor resolution of conflict (Forgatch, 1989). The coercion model is one way to understand problematic family relationship dynamics (Patterson et al., 1992). Coercive parenting practices have been linked to the development and maintenance of nearly all common disorders of youth (Cummings, Davies, & Campbell, 2000). The coercive-parenting model continues to guide several parenting interventions for a variety of youth disorders and is supported by several cross-sectional and longitudinal studies (see Campbell & Patterson, 1995, for a review). The first step a parent takes in the coercion cycle is to react emotionally to the behavior of the child. When a behavior upsets parents, they may react in a variety of ways: they may completely avoid discussing the situation and be angry, do something to hurt the youth (e.g., yelling, hitting, name calling), or make requests or demands that are unclear, blaming, or unrealistic and that lead to more conflict. In turn, the child's behavior continues or even escalates, depending on parents' reactions. When parents take a mindful approach, they may be able to disrupt the destructive cycle of negativity and disengagement that at times becomes automatic for some parent–child dyads (Dishion, Burraston, & Li, 2003). Ongoing involvement in coercive interactions segues to poorer quality parent–child relationships, and the youth can develop clinical-level problem behaviors or maintain those behaviors that are already reinforcing the cycle of coercion in the family (Patterson et al., 1992).

Conflict can be inherent in the coercion cycle. Familial conflict has been implicated in the development of unipolar and bipolar depression (e.g., Du Rocher Schudlich, Youngstrom, Calabrese, & Findling, 2008; Geller et al., 2002; Sheeber, Hops, Alpert, Davis, & Andrews, 1997; Sheeber & Sorenson, 1998), substance use (e.g., Repetti, Taylor, & Seeman, 2002), schizophrenia (Asarnow & Kernan, 2008), borderline personality disorder (e.g., Weaver & Clum, 1993), and conduct problems (e.g., Bank, Burraston, & Snyder, 2004; Garcia, Shaw, Winslow, & Yaggi, 2000; Rubin, Burgess, Dwyer, & Hastings, 2003). Conflict reciprocally influences the other elements of mindful parenting; for example, parents in conflict-filled relationships with their youth may be more likely to disengage, which can contribute to less parental monitoring and greater risk for youth conduct or substance use problems (Dishion, Nelson, & Bullock, 2004). Similarly, conflict contributes to poorer relationships between youth and caregivers, which inhibits caregivers' ability to effectively set healthy limits. Barnes, Brown, Krusemark, Campbell, and Rogge (2007) found that more mindful individuals were more likely to respond constructively to stress in interpersonal relationships. Increased use of problem-solving skills in the presence of stress and conflict can disrupt the coercion cycle and result in better outcomes for the child and the family. These findings suggest that increasing parents' capacity for mindful parenting is likely to be a key in the treatment of youth psychopathology when conflict, poor relationships, and a lack of positive behavior support pervade the family system.

Mindful Parenting as a Mechanism of Change in Family-Based Intervention

The significance of improved family functioning as a mechanism of change with respect to youth problems is a long-held, core assumption among family systems theorists (e.g., Henggeler & Borduin, 1990; Mann, Borduin, Henggeler, & Blaske, 1990; Sholevar, 2003), yet the literature provides relatively few empirical findings to support this assumption (e.g., Kazdin, 2005; Kazdin & Nock, 2003; Shirk & Russell, 1996; Weisz, Huey, & Weersing, 1998). Identifying common mechanisms of change is perhaps the key to developing effective transdiagnostic treatment approaches for youth psychopathology. Yet to date, the evidence from disorder-specific treatment models that target family processes is somewhat mixed, even though clinicians and researchers generally believe in the importance of including caregivers and families in the treatment of youth psychiatric disorders. Despite this belief, the paucity of studies that include parents in treatment, let alone include them as agents of change, has been noted in recent reviews (Diamond & Josephson, 2005; Restifo & Bogels, 2009; Sander & McCarty, 2005). For example, the family is involved in any capacity in less than one-third (32%) of treatments for youth depression (Sander & McCarty, 2005). Likewise, only 11% of studies reviewed by Weisz, McCarty, and Valeri (2006) included the family in treatment as agents of change.

Literature that identifies family processes as mechanisms of change in the treatment of youth psychopathology is limited, yet encouraging. Family processes have been shown empirically to mediate the relationship between treatment and outcome in family-based interventions for conduct problems in youth (e.g., Barlow & Stewart-Brown, 2000; Dishion et al., 2008; Woolfenden, Williams, & Peat, 2009), substance abuse disorders (e.g., Liddle, 2004; Liddle & Dakof, 1994), attention-deficit/ hyperactivity disorder (e.g., Pelham, Wheeler, & Chronis, 1998), schizophrenia (e.g., McFarlane, Dixon, Lukens, & Lucksted, 2002; Pharoah, Mari, Rathbone, & Wong, 2010), and anxiety disorders (e.g., Ginsburg & Schlossberg, 2002). The literature about disruptive behavior disorders is the most robust in this regard. Many empirically supported treatments for disruptive behavior in youth target multiple levels, most commonly the child and parent but at times the family as a whole (e.g., Compton et al., 2004; Loeber, Burke, & Pardini, 2009; Pardini, 2008). The most successful treatment models typically include intervention components for both the child and the parents (see Pardini, 2008, for a review), and interventions focused exclusively on the child are not promising (Burke, Loeber, & Birmaher, 2002). Parenting practices, specifically those elements that make up our mindful parenting construct, have been implicated as mechanisms of change in family interventions for disruptive behavior disorders (e.g., Dishion, Nelson, & Kavanagh, 2003; Dishion, Patterson, & Kavanaugh, 1992; Dishion et al., 2008; Gardner, Burton, & Klimes, 2006; Gardner, Shaw, Dishion, Burton, & Supplee, 2007; Huey, Henggeler, Brondino, & Pickrel, 2000; Mann et al., 1990; Smith, Dishion, Moore, Shaw, & Wilson, 2013; Smith, Dishion, Shaw, & Wilson, in press; Stoolmiller, Duncan, Bank, & Patterson, 1993). However, treatments for other common youth disorders often disregard the family and seldom target family processes as mechanisms of change.

A relatively strong relationship exists between mindfulness, its related processes, and psychopathology (see Aldao, Nolen-Hoeksema, & Schweizer, 2010, for a review). This connection has generated a number of interventions that target parent and youth mindfulness as a mechanism of change. Mindfulness-based interventions for children and adolescents have an inherently intrapsychic focus as opposed to the interpersonal focus of mindfulness-based interventions for parents, which emphasize mindfulness in the context of interactions and relationships within the family. Empirical evidence suggests that mindfulness-based interventions are effective for reducing individual psychopathology and improving family functioning in youth (e.g., Burke, 2010; Lee, Semple, Rosa, & Miller, 2008; Singh, Singh, et al., 2010) and in parents (Cohen & Semple, 2010; Dumas, 2005; Singh, Lancioni, et al., 2010). The preliminary success of these mindfulness-based family interventions suggests that mindful parenting is likely to be an important mechanism of change in family-based intervention approaches for various disorder classes and problematic family relationships.

Future Research on Family Processes as Transdiagnostic Mechanisms of Change

As transdiagnostic interventions become more prevalent in the child and adolescent behavioral arena, the need to better understand common family processes that contribute to youth problems will increase. To meet this need, these processes must be more effectively targeted by intervention and prevention efforts. Intervention scientists would do well to draw on the developmental and family process literature as they design and test treatment protocols for youth disorders. This approach is particularly apt for transdiagnostic treatments, which target common processes in an effort to address complex symptom presentations. If intervention scientists are to benefit from this research, epidemiologists and developmental scientists must broaden the scope of their work beyond single disorders and disorder classes to include developmental models of comorbid disorders and common symptom profiles.

Construct and measurement issues are one of the challenges inherent in establishing a research agenda for family processes and youth psychopathology. As an example, measures of mindful parenting are needed that are not culturally narrow. A mixed-method approach grounded in observation is well suited to the problem of conceptualizing and measuring mindful parenting (Dishion & Patterson, 1999). The first step is to conduct cross-cultural studies that document the instantiation of mindful parenting in a variety of cultural and socioeconomic settings. Classic work by Whiting is an example of this approach (Whiting & Edwards, 1988), as is the early work of Ainsworth (1989). The second step is to develop measures that would capture the core dimension of mindful parenting by using both observational measurement and self-report methods (interview, questionnaire, etc.). This step involves measuring other domains of parenting, such as positive behavior support, healthy limit setting and monitoring, and relationship building. With respect to validity, one must determine whether the mindful parenting measure can be differentiated from other core dimensions of parenting and whether a superordinate factor model fits the data. The third and final step would be to design systematic intervention studies that attempt to increase mindful parenting to determine whether it can be addressed in prevention and intervention studies and to identify the extent to which youth benefit from parents' increased mindfulness. It is possible that for some families, increasing awareness and consciousness under some circumstances could increase irritability and negativity, and therefore conflict. Additional research is needed to better understand these relationships.

Currently, the literature contains a number of self-report measures of constructs that are likely related to mindful parenting practices, such as the parent's general mindfulness (e.g., Brown & Ryan, 2003) and experiential avoidance and acceptance of emotions (Cheron, Ehrenreich, & Pincus, 2009). Self-report measures probably tap a parent's capacity for mindful parenting, but not necessarily mindful parenting behaviors. Our mindful parenting construct is measured solely by observable parenting practices and family interactions that demonstrate the act of mindful parenting. Examining the convergent validity between our construct and other measures and measurement methods (i.e., self-report) is a necessary step in understanding the link between a parent's capacity for mindfulness and the ability to put this aptitude into practice in the context of his or her family.

One exciting potential direction is to develop a program of research on the neuroscience of parenting. Not directly observable in most measurement paradigms is the degree of intersubjectivity between a parent and child (Vygotsky, 1986). Intersubjectivity is the shared understanding between the parent and child about the interpersonal underpinnings of the relationship, mutual attachment and compassion, and values and norms. Much of self-regulation is enacted or entrained in the daily interactions of close family members and is only barely available to conscious recall (Bargh & Williams, 2006). At times, self-regulation in families becomes conscious and effortful (e.g., Posner & Rothbart, 2000); however, these occurrences are likely to be only a fraction of the interpersonal dynamics that form the substrate of regulation in a close relationship.

Given that much of self-regulation involves analysis of neurocognitive processing over very short periods of time, there is a sense that affective neuroscience provides the scientific tools for understanding individual differences in parents' ability to regulate emotion in the service of interacting positively with their children (Amodio, 2011). Moreover, much of the action–reaction dynamic in parent–child interaction goes unseen in that parents and youth mutually self-regulate, for example when they work toward cooperation and comfort during times of stress. Although the concept of "internalization" has been key to socialization theories (Grusec & Goodnow, 1994; Hoffman, 1991; Kochanska, 2002), it has never been measured as a process. Paradoxically, mindful parenting may be best understood as an intricately developed unconscious process by which conscious self-regulation is required only to make minor changes in the course of the relationship interaction.

Understanding the measurement strategies and interpersonal dynamics of mindful parenting will lead the way to understanding the ways in which these parenting behaviors lead to change. In the family intervention literature, greater attention must be given to family-based mechanisms of change. More exploration of the proposed mechanisms of change in family treatment would provide a stronger empirical understanding of which treatment processes are actually contributing to observed improvements (Pinsof & Wynne, 2000). As we put forth in this chapter, there is evidence that the elements of mindful parenting are potentially key elements of family change processes. Innovative research designs capable of providing the necessary support for these parenting elements as mechanisms of change are needed. Developing transdiagnostic treatment models for youth psychopathology before strong evidence of common change mechanisms is gathered may be somewhat hasty. However, in the current health care and economic climates the need is greater than ever to develop cost-effective, evidence-supported treatment approaches for children and adolescents. Transdiagnostic intervention approaches certainly have a place in this changing landscape.

ACKNOWLEDGMENTS

Research support for Justin D. Smith was provided by Research Training Grant No. MH20012 from the National Institute of Mental Health, awarded to Elizabeth Stormshak. Research support for Thomas J. Dishion was provided by Grant No. DA07031 from the National Institute on Drug Abuse. We gratefully acknowledge Cheryl Mikkola for her editorial support.

REFERENCES

Ainsworth, M. S. (1989). Attachments beyond infancy. *American Psychologist, 44*, 709–716.

Aldao, A., Nolen-Hoeksema, S., & Schweizer, S. (2010). Emotion-regulation strategies across psychopathology: A meta-analytic review. *Clinical Psychology Review, 30*, 217–237.

Alloy, L. B., Abramson, L. Y., Smith, J. M., Gibb, B. E., & Neeren, A. M. (2006). Role of parenting and maltreatment histories in unipolar and bipolar mood disorders: Mediation by cognitive vulnerability to depression. *Clinical Child and Family Psychology Review, 9*, 23–64.

Amodio, D. M. (2011). Self-regulation in intergroup relations: A social neuroscience framework. In A. Todorov, S. T. Fiske, & D. A. Prentice (Eds.), *Social neuroscience: Toward understanding the underpinning of the social mind* (pp. 101–122). Oxford, UK: Oxford University Press.

Asarnow, R. F., & Kernan, C. L. (2008). Childhood schizophrenia. In T. P. Beauchaine & S. P. Hinshaw (Eds.), *Child and adolescent psychopathology* (pp. 614–642). New York: Wiley.

Bank, L., Burraston, B., & Snyder, J. (2004). Sibling conflict and ineffective parenting as predictors of adolescent boys' antisocial behavior and peer difficulties: Additive and interactional effects. *Journal of Research on Adolescence, 14*, 99–125.

Bargh, J. A., & Williams, E. L. (2006). The automaticity of social life. *Current Directions in Psychological Science, 15*, 1–4.

Barlow, J., & Stewart-Brown, S. (2000). Behavior problems and group-based parent education programs. *Journal of Developmental and Behavioral Pediatrics, 21*, 356–370.

Barnes, S., Brown, K. W., Krusemark, E., Campbell, W. K., & Rogge, R. D. (2007). The role of mindfulness in romantic relationship satisfaction and responses to relationship stress. *Journal of Marital and Family Therapy, 33*, 482–500.

Beach, S. R. H., Wamboldt, M. Z., Kaslow, N. J., Heyman, R. E., First, M. B., Underwood, L. G., et al. (Eds.). (2006). *Relational processes and DSM-V: Neuroscience, assessment, prevention, and treatment*. Washington, DC: American Psychiatric Association.

Bowlby, J. (1980). *Attachment and loss: Vol. 3. Loss: Sadness and depression*. New York: Basic Books.

Brody, G. H. (2003). *Parental monitoring: Action and reaction*. Mahwah, NJ: Erlbaum.

Brown, K. W., & Ryan, R. M. (2003). The benefits of being present: Mindfulness and its role in psychological well-being. *Journal of Personality and Social Psychology, 84*, 822–848.

Burke, C. A. (2010). Mindfulness-based approaches with children and adolescents: A preliminary review of current research in an emergent field. *Journal of Child and Family Studies, 19*, 133–144.

Burke, J. D., Loeber, R., & Birmaher, B. (2002). Oppositional defiant and conduct disorder: A review of the past 10 years. Part II. *Journal of the American Academy of Child and Adolescent Psychiatry, 41*, 1275–1293.

Campbell, T. L., & Patterson, J. M. (1995). The effectiveness of family interventions in the treatment of physical illness. *Journal of Marital and Family Therapy, 21*, 545–584.

Caruthers, A. S., Van Ryzin, M. J., & Dishion, T. J. (in press). Preventing high-risk sexual behavior in early adulthood with family interventions in adolescence: Outcomes and developmental processes. *Prevention Science.*

Cheron, D. M., Ehrenreich, J. T., & Pincus, D. (2009). Assessment of parental experiential avoidance in a clinical sample of children with anxiety disorders. *Child Psychiatry and Human Development, 40*, 383–403.

Chilcoat, H. D., & Anthony, J. C. (1996). Impact of parent monitoring on initiation of drug use through late childhood. *Journal of the American Academy of Child and Adolescent Psychiatry, 35*, 91–100.

Chu, B. C. (2012). Translating transdiagnostic approaches to children and adolescents. *Cognitive and Behavioral Practice, 19*, 1–4

Cicchetti, D. V. (1993). Developmental psychopathology: Reactions, reflections, projections. *Developmental Review, 13*, 471–502.

Cicchetti, D. V. (2008). Multi-level analysis perspective on research and development and psychopathology. In T. P. Beauchaine & S. P. Hinshaw (Eds.), *Child and adolescent psychopathology* (pp. 27–57). New York: Wiley.

Cicchetti, D. V., & Toth, S. L. (1998). The development of depression in children and adolescents. *American Psychologist, 53*, 221–241.

Coatsworth, J. D., Duncan, L., Greenberg, M., & Nix, R. (2010). Changing parent's mindfulness, child management skills and relationship quality with their youth: Results from a randomized pilot intervention trial. *Journal of Child and Family Studies, 19*, 203–217.

Cohen, J. A. S., & Semple, R. J. (2010). Mindful parenting: A call for research. *Journal of Child and Family Studies, 19*, 145–151.

Compton, S. N., March, J. S., Brent, D., Albano, A. M., Weersing, V. R., & Curry, J. (2004). Cognitive-behavioral psychotherapy for anxiety and depressive disorders in children and adolescents: An evidence-based medicine review. *Journal of the American Academy of Child and Adolescent Psychiatry, 43*, 930–959.

Connell, A. M., & Dishion, T. J. (2008). Reducing depression among at-risk early adolescents: Three-year effects of a family-centered intervention embedded within schools. *Journal of Family Psychology, 22*, 574–585.

Connor, D. F. (2002). *Aggression and antisocial behavior in children and adolescents: Research and treatment.* New York: Guilford Press.

Crowell, S. E., Kaufman, E. A., & Lenzenweger, M. F. (2013). The development of borderline personality disorder and self-inflicted injury. In T. P. Beauchaine & S. P. Hinshaw (Eds.), *Child and adolescent psychopathology* (2nd ed., pp. 577–609). Hoboken, NJ: Wiley.

Cummings, E. M., Davies, P. T., & Campbell, S. B. (2000). *Developmental psychopathology and family process: Theory, research, and clinical implications.* New York: Guilford Press.

Diamond, G. S., & Josephson, A. (2005). Family-based treatment research: A 10-year update. *Journal of the American Academy of Child and Adolescent Psychiatry, 44,* 872–887.

DiClemente, R. J., Wingood, G. M., Crosby, R., Sionean, C., Cobb, B. K., Harrington, K., et al. (2001). Parental monitoring: Association with adolescents' risk behaviors. *Pediatrics, 107,* 1363–1368.

Dishion, T. J., Burraston, B., & Li, F. (2003). Family management practices: Research design and measurement issues. In Z. Sloboda & W. J. Bukoski (Eds.), *Handbook for drug abuse prevention: Theory, science, and practice* (pp. 587–607). New York: Plenum Press.

Dishion, T. J., Capaldi, D. M., & Yoerger, K. (1999). Middle childhood antecedents to progression in male adolescent substance use: An ecological analysis of risk and protection. *Journal of Adolescent Research, 14,* 175–205.

Dishion, T. J., & McMahon, R. J. (1998). Parental monitoring and the prevention of child and adolescent problem behavior: A conceptual and empirical formulation. *Clinical Child and Family Psychology Review, 1,* 61–75.

Dishion, T. J., Nelson, S. E., & Bullock, B. M. (2004). Premature adolescent autonomy: Parent disengagement and deviant peer process in the amplification of problem behavior. *Journal of Adolescence, 27,* 515–530.

Dishion, T. J., Nelson, S. E., & Kavanagh, K. (2003). The Family Check-Up for high-risk adolescents: Preventing early-onset substance use by parent monitoring. *Behavior Therapy, 34,* 553–571.

Dishion, T. J., & Patterson, G. R. (1999). Model-building in developmental psychopathology: A pragmatic approach to understanding and intervention. *Journal of Clinical Child Psychology, 28,* 502–512.

Dishion, T. J., & Patterson, G. R. (2006). The development and ecology of antisocial behavior in children and adolescents. In D. Cicchetti & D. J. Cohen (Eds.), *Developmental psychopathology: Vol. 3. Risk, disorder, and adaptation* (pp. 503–541). Hoboken, NJ: Wiley.

Dishion, T. J., Patterson, G. R., & Kavanaugh, K. (1992). An experimental test of the coercion model: Linking theory, measurement, and intervention. In J. McCord & R. Tremblay (Eds.), *Preventing antisocial behavior: Interventions from birth through adolescence* (pp. 253–282). New York: Guilford Press.

Dishion, T. J., Shaw, D. S., Connell, A., Gardner, F. E. M., Weaver, C., & Wilson, M. (2008). The Family Check-Up with high-risk indigent families: Preventing problem behavior by increasing parents' positive behavior support in early childhood. *Child Development, 79,* 1395–1414.

Dishion, T. J., & Stormshak, E. A. (2007). *Intervening in children's lives: An ecological, family-centered approach to mental health care.* Washington, DC: American Psychological Association.

Dishion, T. J., Stormshak, E. A., & Kavanagh, K. (2011). *Everyday parenting: A professional's guide to building family management skills.* Champaign, IL: Research Press.

Doane, J., Goldstein, M. J., Miklowitz, D. J., & Fallon, I. R. H. (1986). The impact of individual and family treatment on the affective climate of families of schizophrenics. *British Journal of Psychiatry, 148*, 279–287.

Du Rocher Schudlich, T., Youngstrom, E., Calabrese, J., & Findling, R. (2008). The role of family functioning in bipolar disorder in families. *Journal of Abnormal Child Psychology, 36*, 849–863.

Dumas, J. E. (2005). Mindfulness-based parent training: Strategies to lessen the grip of automaticity in families with disruptive children. *Journal of Clinical Child and Adolescent Psychology, 34*, 779–791.

Duncan, L. G., Coatsworth, J. D., & Greenberg, M. T. (2009). A model of mindful parenting: Implications for parent–child relationships and prevention research. *Clinical Child and Family Psychology Review, 12*, 255–270.

Falloon, I. R., Boyd, J. L., McGill, C. W., Williamson, M., Razani, J., Moss, H. B., et al. (1985). Family management in the prevention of morbidity of schizophrenia: Clinical outcome of a two-year longitudinal study. *Archives of General Psychiatry, 42*, 887–896.

Forgatch, M. S. (1989). Patterns and outcome in family problem solving: The disrupting effect of negative emotion. *Journal of Marriage and the Family, 51*, 115–124.

Fosco, G. M., Stormshak, E. A., Dishion, T. J., & Winter, C. (2012). Family relationships and parental monitoring during middle school as predictors of early adolescent problem behavior. *Journal of Clinical Child and Adolescent Psychology, 41*, 202–213.

Frick, P. J., & Loney, B. R. (2002). Understanding the association between parent and child antisocial behavior. In R. J. McMahon & R. D. Peters (Eds.), *The effects of parental dysfunction on children* (pp. 105–126). New York: Plenum Press.

Garber, J., Robinson, N. S., & Valentiner, D. (1997). The relation between parenting and adolescent depression: Self-worth as a mediator. *Journal of Adolescent Research, 12*, 12–33.

Garcia, M., Shaw, D. S., Winslow, E. B., & Yaggi, K. (2000). Destructive sibling conflict and the development of conduct problems in young boys. *Developmental Psychology, 36*, 44–53.

Gardner, F. E. M. (1987). Positive interaction between mothers and conduct-problem children: Is there training for harmony as well as fighting? *Journal of Abnormal Child Psychology, 15*, 283–293.

Gardner, F. E. M., Burton, J., & Klimes, I. (2006). Randomised controlled trial of a parenting intervention in the voluntary sector for reducing child conduct problems: Outcomes and mechanisms of change. *Journal of Child Psychology and Psychiatry, 47*, 1123–1132.

Gardner, F. E. M., Shaw, D. S., Dishion, T. J., Burton, J., & Supplee, L. (2007). Randomised prevention trial for early conduct problems: Effects on proactive parenting and links to toddler disruptive behavior. *Journal of Family Psychology, 21*, 398–406.

Gardner, F. E. M., Sonuga-Barke, E., & Sayal, K. (1999). Parents anticipating misbehaviour: An observational study of strategies parents use to prevent conflict with behaviour problem children. *Journal of Child Psychology and Psychiatry, 40*, 1184–1196.

Gardner, F. E. M., Ward, S., Burton, J., & Wilson, C. (2003). The role of mother–child joint play in the early development of children's conduct problems: A longitudinal observational study. *Social Development, 12*, 361–379.

Ge, X., Best, K. M., Conger, R. D., & Simons, R. L. (1996). Parenting behaviors and the occurrence and co-occurrence of adolescent depressive symptoms and conduct problems. *Developmental Psychology, 32*, 717–731.

Geller, B., Craney, J. L., Bolhofner, K., Nickelsburg, M. J., Williams, M., & Zimerman, B. (2002). Two-year prospective follow-up of children with a prepubertal and early adolescent bipolar disorder phenotype. *American Journal of Psychiatry, 159*, 927–933.

Ginsburg, G. S., & Schlossberg, M. (2002). Family-based treatment of childhood anxiety disorders. *International Review of Psychiatry, 14*, 143–154.

Goodman, S. H., & Gotlib, I. H. (1999). Risk for psychopathology in the children of depressed mothers: A developmental model for understanding mechanisms of transmission. *Psychological Review, 106*, 458–490.

Grusec, J. E., & Goodnow, J. J. (1994). Impact of parental discipline methods on child's internalization of values: A reconceptualization of current points of view. *Developmental Psychology, 30*, 4–19.

Henggeler, S. W., & Borduin, C. M. (1990). *Family therapy and beyond: A multisystemic approach to treating the behavior problems of children and adolescents.* Pacific Grove, CA: Brooks/Cole.

Hoffman, L. W. (1991). The influence of the family environment on personality: Accounting for sibling differences. *Psychological Bulletin, 110*, 187–203.

Horner, R. H., & Carr, E. G. (1997). Behavioral support for students with severe disabilities: Functional assessment and comprehensive intervention. *Journal of Special Education, 31*, 84–109.

Huey, S. J., Jr., Henggeler, S. W., Brondino, M. J., & Pickrel, S. G. (2000). Mechanisms of change in multisystemic therapy: Reducing delinquent behavior through therapist adherence and improved family and peer functioning. *Journal of Consulting and Clinical Psychology, 68*, 451–467.

Johnston, C., & Mash, E. J. (2001). Families of children with attention-deficit/hyperactivity disorder: Review and recommendations for future research. *Clinical Child and Family Psychology Review, 4*, 183–207.

Kabat-Zinn, J. (2003). Mindfulness-based interventions in context: Past, present, and future. *Clinical Psychology: Science and Practice, 10*, 144–156.

Kabat-Zinn, M., & Kabat-Zinn, J. (1997). *Everyday blessings: The inner work of mindful parenting.* New York: Hyperion.

Kashdan, T. B., Jacob, R., Pelham, W., Lang, A. R., Hoza, B., Blumenthal, J. D., et al. (2004). Depression and anxiety in parents of children with ADHD and varying levels of oppositional defiant behaviors: Modeling relationships with family functioning. *Journal of Clinical Child and Adolescent Psychology, 33*, 169–181.

Kazdin, A. E. (2005). Treatment outcomes, common factors, and continued neglect of mechanisms of change. *Clinical Psychology: Science and Practice, 12*, 184–188.

Kazdin, A. E., & Nock, M. K. (2003). Delineating mechanisms of change in child and adolescent therapy: Methodological issues and research recommendations. *Journal of Child Psychology and Psychiatry, 44*, 1116–1129.

Kerr, M., & Stattin, H. (2000). What parents know, how they know it, and several forms of adolescent adjustment: Further support for a reinterpretation of monitoring. *Developmental Psychology, 36,* 366–380.

Kiesner, J., Poulin, F., & Dishion, T. J. (2010). Adolescent substance use with friends: Moderating and mediating effects of parental monitoring and peer activity contexts. *Merrill-Palmer Quarterly, 56,* 529–556.

Kim, S. Y., & Ge, X. (2000). Parenting practices and adolescent depressive symptoms in Chinese American families. *Journal of Family Psychology, 14,* 420–435.

Kochanska, G. (2002). Committed compliance, moral self, and internalization: A mediational model. *Developmental Psychology, 38,* 339–351.

Lac, A., & Crano, W. D. (2009). Monitoring matters: Meta-analytic review reveals the reliable linkage of parent monitoring with adolescent marijuana use. *Perspectives on Psychological Science, 4,* 578–586.

Laird, R. D., Criss, M. M., Pettit, G. S., Dodge, K. A., & Bates, J. E. (2008). Parents monitoring knowledge attenuates the link between antisocial friends and adolescent delinquent behavior. *Journal of Abnormal Child Psychology, 36,* 299–310.

Lee, J., Semple, R. J., Rosa, D., & Miller, L. (2008). Mindfulness-based cognitive therapy for children: Results of a pilot study. *Journal of Cognitive Psychotherapy, 22,* 15–28.

Liddle, H. A. (2004). Family-based therapies for adolescent alcohol and drug use: Research contributions and future research needs. *Addiction, 99,* 76–92.

Liddle, H. A., & Dakof, G. (1995). Family-based treatment for adolescent drug use: State of the science. In E. Rahdert & D. Czechowicz (Eds.), *Adolescent drug abuse: Clinical assessment and therapeutic interventions* (NIDA Research Monograph). Rockville, MD: National Institute on Drug Abuse.

Lindahl, K. M. (1998). Family process variables and children's disruptive behavior problems. *Journal of Family Psychology, 12,* 420–436.

Loeber, R., Burke, J. D., & Pardini, D. A. (2009). Perspectives on oppositional defiant disorder, conduct disorder, and psychopathic features. *Journal of Child Psychology and Psychiatry, 50,* 133–142.

Lunkenheimer, E. S., Dishion, T. J., Shaw, D. S., Connell, A. M., Gardner, F. E. M., Wilson, M. N., et al. (2008). Collateral benefits of the Family Check-Up on early childhood school readiness: Indirect effects of parents' positive behavior support. *Developmental Psychology, 44,* 1737–1752.

Mann, B. J., Borduin, C. M., Henggeler, S. W., & Blaske, D. M. (1990). An investigation of systemic conceptualizations of parent–child coalitions and symptom change. *Journal of Consulting and Clinical Psychology, 58,* 336–344.

McFarlane, W. R., Dixon, L., Lukens, E., & Lucksted, A. (2002). Severe mental illness. In D. H. Sprenkle (Ed.), *Effectiveness research in marriage and family therapy* (pp. 255–298). Alexandria, VA: American Association for Marriage and Family Therapy.

Pardini, D. A. (2008). Empirically supported treatments for conduct disorders in children and adolescents. In J. A. Trafton & W. Gordon (Eds.), *Best practices in the behavioral management of disorders of infancy, childhood and adolescence* (pp. 290–321). Los Altos, CA: Institute for Brain Potential.

Patterson, G. R. (1982). *Coercive family process.* Eugene, OR: Castalia.

Patterson, G. R., Reid, J. B., & Dishion, T. J. (1992). *Antisocial boys.* Eugene, OR: Castalia.

Patterson, G. R., & Stouthamer-Loeber, M. (1984). The correlation of family management practices and delinquency. *Child Development, 55,* 1299–1307.

Pelham, W. E., Wheeler, T., & Chronis, A. (1998). Empirically supported psychosocial treatments for attention deficit hyperactivity disorder. *Journal of Clinical Child Psychology, 27,* 190–205.

Pharoah, F., Mari, J. J., Rathbone, J., & Wong, W. (2010). Family intervention for schizophrenia. *Cochrane Database of Systematic Reviews,* Issue 2 (Article No. CD000088), DOI: 10.1002/14651858.CD000088.pub3.

Pinsof, W. M., & Wynne, L. C. (2000). Toward progress research: Closing the gap between family therapy practice and research. *Journal of Marital and Family Therapy, 26,* 1–8.

Posner, M. I., & Rothbart, M. K. (2000). Developing mechanisms of self-regulation. *Development and Psychopathology, 12,* 427–441.

Radke-Yarrow, M., Ricters, J., & Wilson, W. E. (1988). Child development in a network of relationships. In R. Hinde & J. Stevenson-Hinde (Eds.), *Individuals in a network of relationships* (pp. 48–67). Cambridge, UK: Cambridge University Press.

Repetti, R. L., Taylor, S. E., & Seeman, T. E. (2002). Risky families: Family social environments and the mental and physical health of offspring. *Psychological Bulletin, 128,* 330–366.

Restifo, K., & Bogels, S. (2009). Family processes in the development of youth depression: Translating the evidence to treatment. *Clinical Psychology Review, 29,* 294–316.

Rubin, K. H., Burgess, K. B., Dwyer, K. M., & Hastings, P. D. (2003). Predicting preschoolers' externalizing behaviors from toddler temperament, conflict, and maternal negativity. *Developmental Psychology, 39,* 164–176.

Rutter, M. (2006). *Genes and behavior: Nature–nurture interplay explained.* Malden, MA: Blackwell.

Sander, J. B., & McCarty, C. A. (2005). Youth depression in the family context: Familial risk factors and models of treatment. *Clinical Child and Family Psychology Review, 8,* 203–219.

Shaw, D. S., Connell, A., Dishion, T. J., Wilson, M. N., & Gardner, F. E. M. (2009). Improvements in maternal depression as a mediator of intervention effects on early childhood problem behavior. *Development and Psychopathology, 21,* 417–439.

Shaw, D. S., & Gross, H. (2008). What we have learned about early childhood and the development of delinquency. In A. Lieberman (Ed.), *The long view of crime: A synthesis of longitudinal research: Part II* (pp. 79–127). New York: Springer.

Sheeber, L., Hops, H., Alpert, A., Davis, B., & Andrews, J. (1997). Family support and conflict: Prospective relations to adolescent depression. *Journal of Abnormal Child Psychology, 25,* 333–344.

Sheeber, L., & Sorenson, E. (1998). Family relationships of depressed adolescents: A multimethod assessment. *Journal of Clinical Child Psychology, 27,* 268–277.

Shirk, S. R., & Russell, R. L. (1996). *Change processes in child psychotherapy: Revitalizing treatment and research.* New York: Guilford Press.

Sholevar, G. P. (2003). Family theory and therapy: An overview. In G. P. Sholevar & L. D. Schwoeri (Eds.), *Textbook of family and couples therapy: Clinical applications* (pp. 3–28). Washington, DC: American Psychiatric Association.

Singh, N. N., Lancioni, G. E., Winton, A. S. W., Singh, J., Singh, A. N., Adkins, A. D., et al. (2010). Training in mindful caregiving transfers to parent–child interactions. *Journal of Child and Family Studies, 19,* 167–174.

Singh, N. N., Singh, A. N., Lancioni, G. E., Singh, J., Winton, A. S. W., & Adkins, A. D. (2010). Mindfulness training for parents and their children with ADHD increases the children's compliance. *Journal of Child and Family Studies, 19,* 157–166.

Smith, C., & Farrington, D. (2004). Continuities in antisocial behavior and parenting across three generations. *Journal of Child Psychology and Psychiatry, 45,* 230–247.

Smith, J. D., Dishion, T. J., Moore, K. J., Shaw, D. S., & Wilson, M. N. (2013). Video feedback in the Family Check-Up: Indirect effects on observed parent–child coercive interactions. *Journal of Clinical Child and Adolescent Psychology, 42*(3), 405–417.

Smith, J. D., Dishion, T. J., Shaw, D. S., & Wilson, M. N. (in press). Indirect effects of fidelity to the Family Check-Up on changes in parenting and early childhood problem behaviors. *Journal of Consulting and Clinical Psychology.*

Stark, K. D., Swearer, S., Kurowski, C., Sommer, D., & Bowen, B. (1996). Targeting the child and the family: A holistic approach to treating child and adolescent depressive disorders. In E. D. Hibbs & P. S. Jensen (Eds.), *Psychosocial treatments for child and adolescent disorders: Empirically based strategies for clinical practice* (pp. 207–238). Washington, DC: American Psychological Association.

Steinberg, L. (2004). *The 10 basic principles of good parenting.* New York: Simon & Schuster.

Stoolmiller, M., Duncan, T., Bank, L., & Patterson, G. R. (1993). Some problems and solutions in the study of change: Significant patterns of client resistance. *Journal of Consulting and Clinical Psychology, 61,* 920–928.

Stormshak, E. A., Bierman, K. L., McMahon, R. J., & Lengua, L. J. (2000). Parenting practices and child disruptive behavior problems in early elementary school. *Journal of Clinical Child Psychology, 29,* 17–29.

Sugai, G., Horner, R. H., & Sprague, J. R. (1999). Functional-assessment-based behavior support planning: Research to practice to research. *Behavior Disorders, 24,* 253–257.

Tobler, A. L., & Komro, K. A. (2010). Trajectories of parental monitoring and communication and effects on drug use among urban young adolescents. *Journal of Adolescent Health, 46,* 560–568.

Vygotsky, L. (1986). *Thought and language.* Cambridge, MA: MIT Press.

Weaver, T. L., & Clum, G. A. (1993). Early family environments and traumatic experiences associated with borderline personality disorder. *Journal of Consulting and Clinical Psychology, 61,* 1068–1075.

Weisz, J. R., Huey, S. J., Jr., & Weersing, V. R. (1998). Psychotherapy outcome research with children and adolescents: The state of the art. In T. H. Ollendick & R. J. Prinz (Eds.), *Advances in clinical child psychology* (pp. 49–91). New York: Plenum Press.

Weisz, J. R., McCarty, C. A., & Valeri, S. M. (2006). Effects of psychotherapy for depression in children and adolescents: A meta-analysis. *Psychological Bulletin, 132,* 132–149.

Whiting, B. B., & Edwards, C. P. (1988). *Children of different worlds: The formation of social behavior.* Cambridge, MA: Harvard University Press.

Wood, J. J., McLeod, B. D., Sigman, M., Hwang, W., & Chu, B. C. (2003). Parenting and childhood anxiety: Theory, empirical findings, and future directions. *Journal of Child Psychology and Psychiatry, 44,* 134–151.

Woolfenden, S., Williams, K. J., & Peat, J. (2009). Family and parenting interventions in children and adolescents with conduct disorder and delinquency aged 10–17. *Cochrane Database of Systematic Reviews,* Issue 2 (Article No. CD003015), DOI: 10.1002/14651858.CD003015.

PART III

Transdiagnostic Conceptualizations of Traditional Individual Therapies for Youth

C H A P T E R 8

Cognitive-Behavioral Therapy with Children and Adolescents

Philip C. Kendall, Kelly A. O'Neil Rodriguez, Marianne A. Villabø,
Kristin D. Martinsen, Kevin D. Stark, and Kelly Banneyer

Cognitive-behavioral therapy (CBT) has been applied to and evaluated for a wide variety of mental health problems seen in children and adolescents. With early roots in behaviorism (see Benjamin et al., 2011), CBT has evolved into an integrative approach with developmental, social, family, and of course cognitive and behavioral influences (Kendall, 2012b). In many ways, the results of research evaluations and clinical applications have guided the emergence of today's CBT. With widespread application and favorable research evaluations (Kazdin & Weisz, 2010), CBT merits its status as an empirically supported treatment.

Despite the fact that most evaluations and supportive outcomes have to do with CBT applied to specific identified disorders, the guiding theory behind CBT with youth (Kendall, 2012c) has more general applicability. In keeping with the theme of this volume, the strategies that constitute CBT show similarities across targeted disorders and may be appropriate for transdiagnostic application. For the purpose of considering the transdiagnostic application of CBT with youth, consider the following overview regarding the diathesis–stress model and the several anxiety and depressive disorders.

From the CBT perspective it is hypothesized that anxiety and depressive disorders arise from a combination of a diathesis that, in the presence of stress, leads to the expression of anxiety, depression, or both disorders.

There is no single common diathesis that explains the development of either disorder; rather, it is recognized that the diathesis may differ across youngsters. The diathesis could be faulty core beliefs, a deficit in information-processing abilities, a disturbance in brain structure or functioning, failure to develop emotion regulation strategies, a deficit in problem solving, a lack of interpersonal skills, or a combination. The diathesis may develop from a genetic predisposition, a faulty learning history, a trauma history, or a combination of these and other influences. The stress may be acute, traumatic, or chronic and may stem from such factors as economic disadvantage, violence, parental psychopathology, health concerns, interpersonal conflict or rejection, loss of a parent, moves, poor academic performance, and so forth. In short, there is no single diathesis or stress.

The stressful environment provides the context within which diatheses form and is a necessary ingredient for the expression of disorder. For example, having a parent who has an anxiety disorder could provide the genetic predisposition. In addition, the parent with anxiety would likely fail to model effective emotion regulation and problem solving and would express or model his or her own fears, which might then be internalized into the child's belief system. Such parental expressions of worry as "That's dangerous!" or "You'll fail and embarrass yourself" would contribute to the stressful environment. Thus the child would possess biological and psychological diatheses that would be experienced within the context of the stressful environment. The diathesis–stress model can be taken a step further and, with minor adjustments to the terms used, be an apt description of the core of a depressive disorder.

The cognitive-behavioral model includes an emphasis on a disturbance in the individual's cognitive processing. Core beliefs, sometimes referred to as core schema or self-schema, direct the attention, focus, content, and processing of information. A core belief that is active in anxiety disorders is one in which the individual perceives him- or herself as vulnerable to social and/or physical threat or danger (Beck, Emery, & Greenberg, 2005). This core belief leads the individual to be hypervigilant and to expect and perceive danger in situations that are ambiguous or not truly threatening. The cognitive disturbance in various psychological disorders can be differentiated along a continuum of time (Kendall, 2012a). Anxiety disorders are characterized by *an expectation* that there is a possibility that something bad is going to happen and that the person does not have the capacity to prevent it from happening or to moderate its emotional impact. This expectation occurs before the event. In contrast, core beliefs associated with depressive disorders are linked to notions such as "I'm unlovable," "I'm worthless," and/or "I'm helpless" (Beck & Alford, 2008). When undesirable things happen, the child with depression makes interpretations after the event about its causes (e.g., "it happened because I am unlovable or worthless") and about the future (e.g., "it is going to happen again because I am helpless to change it"). Thus the cognitive disturbance associated with depression happens after the event has occurred—as an *attribution*. Stated more strongly, an individual with anxiety anticipates that undesirable events *might* occur and that he or she can't handle them, whereas the individual with depression attributes previous undesirable events to some flaw in him- or herself that is thought to be permanent and therefore believes that the undesirable event is going to occur again in the future. Key to the cognitive-behavioral model, these cognitive disturbances then lead to, or at least contribute to, disturbances in emotion and emotion regulation, interpersonal relationships, and the failure to engage in problem solving. In an unfortunate cycle, the individual's disturbance in cognitive processing (inaccurate processing of information in the environment) provides what is mistaken for evidence that strengthens the faulty belief system.

Central to the transdiagnostic perspective is the idea that both anxiety and depressive disorders share common features. They are characterized by disturbance in cognition, affect regulation, problem solving, coping skills, and neurochemical functioning. Children with these disorders are immersed in a stressful environment that supports the aforementioned disturbances. Given this model, it would make sense that the treatment procedures used for these disorders share many common strategies and features.

Cognitive-behavioral therapy programs for depressive and anxiety disorders have many treatment components in common, and the order of presentation of the components during therapy for youth with either disorder follows a similar and logical progression. In fact, the treatment programs for depression (e.g., Brent et al., 1997; Clarke, Rohde, Lewinsohn, Hops, & Seeley, 1999; March, 2004; Stark, Stapleton, Fisher, Arora, & Krumholtz, 2011) and anxiety disorders (e.g., Barrett, 2004; Kendall, Hudson, Gosch, Flannery-Schroeder, & Suveg, 2008) are more similar than they are different. Treatments for depressive and anxiety disorders share the following major treatment components: (1) psychoeducation, (2) coping skills training, (3) problem-solving training, (4) cognitive restructuring, and (5) behavioral strategies. Thus they have features that suggest a transdiagnostic approach, although this is not to imply that targeted CBT treatments for depressive disorders and for anxiety disorders are automatically transdiagnostic, or simply interchangeable, or that providing therapy for one child with an internalizing disorder is equivalent to providing therapy for another child with another internalizing disorder. The intervention plan for each child has to be individualized based on characteristics of the child, severity and duration of the disorder, presence of comorbidity, environmental stressors and supports, nature of the youngster's skills deficits and cognitive distortions, and other variables.

This idiographic approach is important to CBT, as it has its roots in behavior therapy (Mahoney & Arnkoff, 1978).

Efficacy of CBT across Childhood Disorders

The number of controlled evaluations of various child therapies has increased greatly over recent decades, and at the same time the quality of the research has improved (Kazdin & Weisz, 2010; Kendall & Comer, 2012). Data from a meta-analysis summarizing evidence from the National Institute of Clinical Excellence in the United Kingdom and other systematic reviews conclude that the best evidence is for the use of CBT for children and adolescents with generalized anxiety, depression, obsessive–compulsive disorder (OCD) and posttraumatic stress disorder (PTSD; Solomando, Kendall, & Whittington, 2008). With regard to externalizing disorders, the researchers found support for the use of CBT to treat preschool children with attention-deficit/hyperactivity disorder (ADHD) and for a media-based CBT to treat general behavioral problems in children.

Looking specifically at anxiety disorders in children, authors of meta-analyses have concluded that there is substantial evidence for using CBT for childhood anxiety (Cartwright-Hatton, Roberts, Chitsabesan, Fothergill, & Harrington, 2004). Chambless and Ollendick (2001) classified CBT and CBT plus family anxiety management as "probably efficacious" treatments. Ishikawa, Okajima, Matsuoka, and Sakano (2007) included 20 studies in their meta-analysis of treatment for childhood anxiety disorders and reported an effect size of 0.68, which is within the medium (0.50) to large (0.80) effect. The effect size remained between medium and large at 12-month follow-up, and the effect held at 2-year follow-up. Although treatment effects at a university setting were superior to treatment effects in other settings, the effect size in clinical settings was medium in magnitude, and there was little difference in effect size between group and individual CBT. Consistent with earlier reports (Barmish & Kendall, 2005), the effects of including parents in treatment for child anxiety remained unclear. The researchers concluded at that time that CBT can be considered an effective treatment for childhood anxiety. Since these reports, at least two large outcome evaluations can be added to the amassed data. In both (Kendall, Hudson, et al., 2008; Walkup et al., 2008), CBT was found to be effective in the treatment of childhood anxiety disorders such as generalized anxiety disorder, social phobia, and separation anxiety disorder. In Kendall, Hudson, and colleagues' (2008) report, individual and family CBT were found to be effective and superior to a family education and support treatment. In Walkup and colleagues' (2008) report, CBT produced a 60% positive response rate, comparable to medication.

In addition, the combination of CBT and medication produced a superior response rate (80%), all better than a pill placebo treatment.

Focusing on childhood depression, Weisz, McCarty, and Valeri (2006) reported that whereas earlier meta-analyses indicated large effect sizes of therapy, more recent meta-analyses indicate that the treatment benefit for childhood depression is more modest. Their meta-analysis identified a mean effect of 0.34 (small–medium range). However, it is important to keep in mind that the change is significantly different from zero and that these are reliable treatment effects. Watanabe, Hunot, Omori, Churchill, and Furukawa (2007) examined the clinical benefit of psychotherapies in youth with depression and concluded in their systematic review of 27 studies that therapy is an effective treatment for depression in children and adolescents, with the largest body of evidence supporting the use of CBT.

Conceptual Background of Transdiagnostic CBT

CBT was originally conceived (e.g., Beck, 1976; Ellis, 1963; Mahoney, 1974; Meichenbaum, 1977) as a broad paradigm for treating psychological disorders. The general principles of CBT are transdiagnostic in the sense that the broad paradigm of CBT can be applied to individuals with a wide range of diagnoses.

In part due to external pressures, CBT has been viewed as a disorder-specific approach (Mansell, Harvey, Watkins, & Shafran, 2009). Disorder-specific treatment protocols for a variety of childhood disorders, including anxiety and depression, have been developed over the last decades (e.g., Barrett, 2004; Kendall & Hedtke, 2006; Stark et al. 2007). These treatments and other versions of CBT have been found to be efficacious, yet some children do not improve, and for others treatment effects fade after termination (Weisz et al., 2006). The observation that anxiety and depression often co-occur (Achenbach, 1990; Angold, Costello, & Erkani, 1999; Brady & Kendall, 1992, along with evidence of a generalized treatment response, may indicate that common processes underlie these disorders (Weisz et al, 2006; Wilamowska et al., 2010). According to Barlow, Allen, and Choate (2004), such commonalities may suggest the possibility of treating anxiety and depression with a unified approach. Such an argument follows from the observation that numerous disorder-specific treatment manuals share similar components and that the need for clinicians to learn multiple manuals may be an obstacle to the dissemination of evidence-based treatments (Wilamowska et al., 2010).

A treatment that targets multiple disorders has been proposed as a complementary approach to disorder-specific treatments (Mansell et al., 2009). Such a transdiagnostic approach hypothesizes that "there is a range of cognitive and/or behavioral processes shared across psychological disorders that causally contribute to the development and/or maintenance of symptoms" (Mansell et al., 2009). A transdiagnostic treatment can be made available to individuals with co-occurring/overlapping diagnoses. In line with this view, McEvoy, Nathan, and Norton (2008) define transdiagnostic treatments as "those that apply to the same underlying treatment principles across mental disorders, without tailoring the protocol to specific diagnosis." We propose that a transdiagnostic model is *a treatment that is flexible enough to simultaneously address multiple problems at a time using principles and strategies that target transdiagnostic mechanisms of change.* From the CBT perspective, targets of change include disturbances in cognitive processing, emotion regulation, problem solving, and so forth. Common treatment strategies can be directed toward the targets of change, although the specific content and ways of implementing these strategies will vary across disorders and children.

The tripartite model for emotional disorders (Clark & Watson, 1991) can serve as a starting point for considering possible common processes or transdiagnostic mechanisms for change. Here the core dimensions of temperament/personality, neuroticism/negative affectivity, and extraversion/positive affectivity were suggested to explain the onset, overlap, and maintenance of anxiety *and* depression (Wilamowska et al., 2010). Research supports negative affect as a risk factor for the development of both anxious and depressive disorders, and low positive affect has been linked to depression, as well as to social phobia (Trosper, Buzzella, Bennett, & Ehrenreich, 2009). Trosper and colleagues' (2009) review also pointed out that physiological hyperarousal is another process that has been found to be significantly associated with panic and separation anxiety, as well as depression. They also pointed out that there may be common processes underlying poor emotion regulation in children with internalizing disorders, as youth with both anxiety and depression tend to overestimate the intensity and duration of negative emotions when confronted with certain events (Trosper et al., 2009). Avoidance and social withdrawal are then often used as a coping strategy. They suggest that individuals both with anxiety and with depression have an implicit bias toward negative cues, with children with anxiety giving priority to threatening information and children with depression selectively attending to negative stimuli. The same review described studies indicating that children with depression and those with anxiety have a weakness in the ability to reappraise challenging events and that that difficulty with emotion expression has been shown to predict both anxious and depressive symptoms. Several processes thus seem to be shared between children and adolescents with emotional disorders. Barlow and colleagues (2004) have, based on similar reasoning, suggested that three fundamental therapeutic components are central to the treatment of emotional disorders:

(1) altering antecedent cognitive reappraisals, (2) preventing emotional avoidance, and (3) facilitating action tendencies not associated with emotion that is dysregulated.

Treatment principles within the basic CBT model are not disorder-specific but can be adapted and applied to clients presenting with multiple disorders and problems. In the approach to case conceptualization, a personal portrait of the child is created (Friedberg & McClure, 2002). The case conceptualization can take different forms (Beck, 1995; Friedberg & McClure, 2002), but CBT formulations will emphasize connecting thoughts, feelings, and behavior with a focus on precipitating and maintaining factors. Developmental history, cultural context, cognitive variables such as different levels of cognitions, and behavioral antecedents and consequences are taken into consideration as they influence the presenting problem. Such a case formulation involves generating and testing hypotheses as the therapist seeks to understand the factors that are contributing to and maintaining the problem. Such a CBT case conceptualization is not locked to a specific diagnosis: the diagnostic classification is only part of the case conceptualization (Friedberg & McClure, 2002).

A sound therapeutic alliance is a necessary component of CBT (Beck, 1995). Although the basic therapeutic qualities of empathy and warmth must be in place, the therapist in CBT should also assume a posture that emphasizes collaboration and active participation. The attitude of the therapist has been described (Kendall, 2012c) as that of a consultant or collaborator who does not have all the answers; a diagnostician who integrates data in a way that goes beyond the verbal reports of the client; or a coach or educator who observes the client's performance and gives feedback with regard to the client's strengths and weaknesses. Although a sound therapeutic alliance is important in all therapeutic relations, it might be argued that a good alliance is even more important, but also more complex, when working with children and adolescents. Children have rarely referred themselves for therapy, and the child might not recognize his or her problems. Keeping the child engaged in the therapeutic work and encouraging the child to view the process as teamwork might therefore be important. Collaboration and active participation, another core feature of CBT, may thus enhance the therapeutic alliance, whereas forcing the child to discuss difficult topics or behaving too formally may weaken the alliance (Creed & Kendall, 2005). Furthermore, the therapist must also form a therapeutic alliance with the parents, and research indicates that parent alliance may predict treatment continuation (Hawley & Weisz, 2005).

CBT with children and adolescents is goal oriented and problem focused. The ability to recognize and address problems is an important skill for children to learn (Kendall & Hedtke, 2006). Children encounter different problems at different stages in their development, and children with anxiety or depression seem to be less skilled than typical controls with regard to problem solving (Gosch, Flannery-Schroeder, Mauro, & Compton, 2006). Their solutions in challenging situations (avoidance for children with anxiety and social withdrawal for children with depression) reduce distress in the short term but make it more difficult to achieve their goals and achieve positive development in the long term. A problem-solving focus may therefore be relevant to children with both anxiety and depression and is found in empirically supported disorder-specific treatments for these disorders (Kendall & Hedke, 2006, Stark et al., 2007).

Although the cognitive therapist may spend some time examining the past, the more common approach is to focus on problems as they present themselves in the here and now (Beck, 1995). This principle suits children well, as their mental capacity may necessitate a less abstract and more concrete approach. Learning coping skills in relation to actual situations may help children attend better and may increase their motivation (Friedberg & McClure, 2002). Integrating knowledge from the educational field, Shelby and Berk (2009) recommend that CBT therapists incorporate experiential and play-based strategies in order to teach children standard CBT interventions, as this may contribute to stronger treatment effects, greater enjoyment in the therapeutic process, and greater benefits for children with lower cognitive capacities. This necessitates a here-and-now approach and is not specific to a particular disorder.

Another core principle in CBT as outlined by Beck (1995) is that CBT is educative and aims to teach the client to be his or her own therapist. Child CBT emphasizes the importance of teaching the child to understand his or her problems in relation to the CBT model. By understanding how emotions, feelings, thoughts, and behavior are connected to and influence each other (Friedberg, McClure, & Garcia, 2009), complex problems may become more intelligible to the child. For example, a central component in CBT for anxiety involves educating the child about the basic model of anxiety, including typical somatic reactions, how somatic reactions may be related to current problems, and general affective education. Children with psychological problems tend to be less skilled in understanding and differentiating between emotions (Suveg, Kendall, Comer, & Robin, 2006); thus psychoeducation may facilitate change in children with both anxiety and depression. Psychoeducation can also be provided for parents and helps to facilitate a common understanding of the disorder and treatment across clients, their families, and therapists (Friedberg et al., 2009).

Although the length of different protocols may vary, child CBT aims to be time limited. The different protocols are usually between 12 and 20 sessions (e.g., 16 sessions in the Coping Cat program, 20 sessions in the ACTION program). The program developers usually encourage flexible use, as some children may need more time to master some treatment components (Kendall, Gosch, Furr, & Sood, 2008).

Therapy sessions follow a standard structure in CBT. Structure makes the process understandable, enhances efficiency, and makes the sessions predictable (Beck, 1995). The common session structure includes a brief mood check and homework review that functions as a bridge from the previous session, collaborative agenda setting for the day's session, working together on the chosen agenda, and agreeing on suitable homework before closing the session with a summary and feedback. Although this session structure is used with children and adolescents as well, Friedberg and McClure (2002) suggest that the therapist has to be more flexible and juggle different treatment components when working with children. The topics on the agenda need to be presented in a developmentally sensitive way, and a creative approach is important.

A transdiagnostic CBT approach would be a treatment flexible enough to simultaneously address multiple problems using principles and strategies that target transdiagnostic mechanisms of change, including disturbances in cognitive processing, emotion regulation, and problem solving. Several core principles of CBT should be central to the transdiagnostic CBT approach in order to facilitate the use of specific treatment strategies that target transdiagnostic mechanisms of change. Strong case conceptualization and therapeutic alliance are also consistent with a transdiagnostic CBT approach. Transdiagnostic CBT approaches would be goal oriented and problem focused—the aim being to teach coping skills for use in the present time. Similarly, transdiagnostic CBT approaches would be time limited and structured as in targeted CBT, with the inclusion of psychoeducation. With these core principles of transdiagnostic CBT in mind, specific treatment strategies are described next.

Treatment Techniques for Transdiagnostic CBT

Several CBT strategies are applicable transdiagnostically: they can be tailored to target underlying mechanisms that are disorder specific or shared across disorders. Let's consider a few of the CBT strategies to illustrate their transdiagnostic application. A central aspect of CBT that crosses disorders is the use of psychoeducation to help the youth understand the connection between thoughts, feelings, and actions. The therapist would be able to use the "triangle" heuristic across disorders in order to help the child understand the reciprocal relationship between thoughts, emotions, and behavior and how cognitive-behavioral treatment strategies can be used to intervene at points on the triangle. However, the information provided about the nature and impact of the disorder would be disorder specific.

Coping skills training for children who are experiencing depressive and anxiety disorders is designed to help them regulate strong emotions. Thus children who are experiencing either disorder could be taught a variety of coping skills for modifying affect. For example, cognitive restructuring, problem solving, and behavioral activation are coping skills that can help children regulate their emotions, regardless of diagnosis. Children experiencing depressive and/or anxiety disorders could be taught the same set of coping skills to help them manage stress and improve their moods. However, the targets of the coping skills would vary across disorders, as would the strategies emphasized.

Negative self-talk or maladaptive automatic thoughts are considered to be a maintaining mechanism in many psychological disorders (although the content of negative thoughts differs among disorders). In anxiety, self-talk is typically anticipatory and future oriented and revolves around one's own vulnerability to perceived threats in a situation, which are often exaggerated. Self-talk in depression, on the other hand, is past oriented and commonly involves loss or feelings of worthlessness and hopelessness following an event. Such self-talk contributes to and enhances anxious or depressed feelings. Self-talk has been examined and found to be a mediator of treatment change for both anxiety (Kendall & Treadwell, 2007) and depression (Kaufman, Rohde, Seeley, Clarke, & Stice, 2005). Negative self-talk often becomes the target of cognitive restructuring (as reduced negative thinking mediates improvement), but the goal is not to remove all negative thinking; a healthier ratio between negative and positive self-talk, for anxiety and depression, is the preferred goal.

The same generic cognitive restructuring strategies (identifying negative thoughts, triggers, and their consequences) may be used when treating depressive and anxiety disorders, but they are directed at different maladaptive thoughts and beliefs. Cognitive restructuring strategies would be used to help children with depression learn that they are lovable, worthy, and efficacious, for example. In contrast, cognitive restructuring would be used to help youth with anxiety learn that they are safe in feared but nonthreatening situations and would give them confidence in their ability to manage their experiences of anxiety. This can mean examining expectations about what will happen in a situation ("I will make a fool of myself; everyone will laugh at me") and realizing how such self-talk contributes to unwanted anxious feelings. Modifying distorted perceptions and interpretations and replacing unhelpful self-talk with more rational alternatives enables the youth with anxiety or depression to actively cope. Cognitive restructuring may work by reducing negative self-talk, shifting the balance between negative and positive self-talk, or by modifying underlying beliefs.

Problem solving (D'Zurilla & Goldfried, 1971; Nezu, Nezu, & McMurran, 2009) is another CBT strategy that has transdiagnostic applicability.

Problem solving within a CBT framework involves identifying the child's problems, coming up with a range of possible (or impossible) ways to address the problem, considering their emotional and behavioral consequences, and testing them out in real life. The versatility of problem solving makes it especially useful for a vast array of symptoms, behaviors, and challenges that face the child. Many youth with depression struggle with procrastination, which feeds into their feelings of worthlessness. Problem solving helps youth to generate new and creative ways of approaching a task, possibly breaking it down into smaller steps in order to make it more manageable. The process of coming up with new ways of handling old problems breaks down dysfunctional behavior patterns, enables the youth to feel he or she can accomplish more, and improves self-esteem. Youth with anxiety avoid situations. A teen with social phobia may stay home from the school dance because he doesn't know who will be there and he dare not dance for fear of embarrassing himself. Problem solving can help him think of plans for going to the dance that are less intimidating and maximize the likelihood that the experience will be a success. Through collaboration, the teen chooses a solution to be tested and practiced in role plays with the therapist before trying it out in real life. The collaborative nature of problem solving empowers the youth and helps him feel more in control. Problem solving is indeed transdiagnostic. It is not restricted to internalizing problems but applies to externalizing problems as well (e.g., parents who can problem-solve how to handle an oppositional child). Parents and teens can problem-solve together.

CBT treatment of several childhood disorders involves some form of an exposure task. The purpose of exposures is to give the youth new learning experiences in situations that typically cause distress and to have the youth process these experiences in an adaptive manner. The way exposure tasks are implemented requires that they be individualized to the particular youth and to the identified disorder. For children with anxiety, exposure tasks provide the child with an opportunity to approach, tolerate, and cope with anxiety-provoking situations (and without avoidance). They often learn that the feared outcome actually did not happen. In addition, they habituate to the anxious arousal that triggered avoidance. That is, when confronted with a feared situation, the youth experiences an increase in anxiety, and the response is usually to try to avoid the situation in order to reduce anxiety symptoms. However, during an exposure task, the youth perseveres in the situation, often applying specific coping skills, until the level of anxiety decreases. Social activities may be used to produce changes in an anxious child's beliefs about him- or herself in relation to others, such as with a child who is experiencing social anxiety.

With children with depression, coping skills training targets elevating desirable affect as a way of managing undesirable emotions. The most powerful way to do this is typically through the use of behavioral activation in the form of engaging in fun and distracting activities that increase the child's activity level. Behavioral activation plays an important role in breaking the cycle of depressed mood, hopelessness, and avoidance of certain activities. Thus expending energy and engaging in social activities are effective strategies. Engagement in social activities of a supportive nature is comforting and reassuring. Such planned activities, which allow the child with depression to learn that she can regulate her mood and find acceptance among others, are used to build the belief that the child is lovable and worthy of friendships. Children with depression typically have a selective bias attending to negative stimuli. In processing an experience (after the fact) with the therapist, the youth can learn to correct misperceptions and even identify cues from others that they are liked. The use of strenuous activities such as exercise is also a useful coping strategy, as it elevates the mood of youth with depression and reduces tension among youngsters with anxiety.

The aforementioned primary treatment components are embedded within the self-control skills of self-monitoring, self-evaluation, and self-reinforcement. In other words, the child is taught to attend to his or her internal bodily reactions and thoughts and to use specific reactions and thoughts as cues that he or she is experiencing an unpleasant emotion. Recognition of an unpleasant emotion serves as the stimulus for coping with the experience and for problem solving to eliminate the stressor and/or for using cognitive restructuring to change the thoughts that trigger the unpleasant affect. This process involves self-monitoring of emotional experience and thoughts, as well as self-evaluation of affect to determine whether it represents an undesirable state. Self-reward is used when the child experiences satisfaction or thinks "I did a great job of catching the increase in the pain!" The content of the self-control skills (i.e., what is self-monitored) varies across children and disorders. Contingent reinforcement, albeit a simple concept, is a powerful CBT strategy. Many youth with psychological disorders have very high standards for themselves (youth with anxiety) or feel that they never get things right (youth with depression). Teaching youth to reward themselves for effort, not necessarily for succeeding or doing something perfectly, plays an important role in increasing the client's self-esteem and reducing unwanted emotional distress.

In sum, several treatment strategies commonly used in targeted CBT are applicable within the transdiagnostic CBT approach. Cognitive restructuring can be used to change maladaptive thoughts and beliefs, which may vary in content based on the specific disorder. Problem solving is transdiagnostic, as it increases flexibility and promotes independent coping for youth with a wide range of disorders. Finally, exposure tasks and behavioral activation are treatment strategies that promote both the approach to previously avoided situations and engagement in activities inconsistent with dysregulated affect (e.g., anxiety or depression). Each of these transdiagnostic CBT treatment components is embedded within self-control skills (self-monitoring, self-evaluation, self-reward). Each transdiagnostic CBT treatment strategy targets a transdiagnostic mechanism of change, such as disturbances in cognitions and emotion regulation. Psychological disorders with shared disturbances may be particularly good candidates for a transdiagnostic CBT approach, as is discussed next.

Target Disorders for the Transdiagnostic CBT Approach

Candidate target disorders for transdiagnostic CBT approaches may be identified on the basis of shared etiology, high co-occurrence rates, similar structure and response rates for single-target treatments, comorbidity effects on treatment response, and "secondary" effects of single-target treatments for other disorders. For example, anxiety and depressive disorders are diagnostic classes naturally treated by transdiagnostic CBT approaches, as they meet several of these potential criteria. Anxiety and depression are highly comorbid in youth (Angold et al., 1999) and share etiological factors (Axelson & Birmaher, 2001). Single-target CBT protocols for anxiety and depressive disorders in youth (e.g., Coping Cat—Kendall & Hedtke, 2006; ACTION—Stark et al., 2007) have similar treatment structures, strategies, and response rates (Kendall et al., 2008; Stark et al., 2011). Although some studies have found little effect of comorbidities on treatment outcomes for child anxiety disorders (e.g., Kendall, Brady, & Verduin, 2001; Rapee, 2003), other research suggests comorbid depressive disorders (Berman, Weems, Silverman, & Kurtines, 2000) and co-occurring depressive symptoms (O'Neil & Kendall, 2012) predict less favorable treatment response to CBT for anxiety disorders in youth. Likewise, comorbid anxiety disorders predict less favorable treatment outcome for adolescent depression treatment (Brent et al., 1998), although this finding is not consistent across studies (e.g., Stark et al., 2011). Additionally, single-target CBT for child anxiety reduces co-occurring depressive symptoms (Suveg et al., 2009). Similarly, single-target CBT for child depression also reduces co-occurring anxiety symptoms and disorders (Stark et al., 2011). Thus anxiety and depressive disorders in youth are diagnostic classes that meet many of the potential criteria for the transdiagnostic CBT approach in youth.

The externalizing disorders, including disruptive behavior disorders and ADHD, may also be naturally treated with the transdiagnostic CBT approach. ADHD and the disruptive behavior disorders (oppositional defiant disorder, conduct disorder) are highly comorbid (Jensen, Marin, & Cantwell, 1997) and may share etiological or maintaining factors

(Tuvblad, Zheng, Raine, & Baker, 2009). Single-target CBT protocols for ADHD and the disruptive behavior disorders (e.g., behavioral parent training—Anastopoulos & Farley, 2003; Incredible Years—Webster-Stratton & Reid, 2003; problem-solving skills training—Kazdin, 2003) share similar treatment structures, strategies, and response rates (Eyberg, Nelson, & Boggs, 2008; Pelham & Fabiano, 2008).

Eating disorders may also meet many of the potential criteria for a transdiagnostic CBT approach. Although eating disorders are a single diagnostic class, anorexia nervosa has typically been treated with single-target treatments (e.g., family-based treatment—Lock, Le Grange, Agras, & Dare, 2001) distinct from those for bulimia nervosa and eating disorder—not otherwise specified (e.g., family-based treatment—Le Grange & Lock, 2007; CBT for bulimia nervosa—Schmidt, 2009). However, the potential shared etiological and maintaining factors for the eating disorders (e.g., Fairburn, Cooper, & Shafran, 2003) suggest that they may also be successfully treated with a transdiagnostic CBT approach.

Other diagnostic classes may be harder to accommodate within the transdiagnostic CBT approach. Disorders with distinct etiological or maintaining factors, low co-occurrence rates with other disorders, or poor treatment response rates for CBT may be more effectively treated with single-target treatments that focus on the specific techniques effective with those conditions. For example, autism spectrum disorders, substance use disorders, and bipolar disorder are conditions that are likely outside the broad limits of the transdiagnostic CBT approach.

Example Transdiagnostic CBT Applications

Efforts to develop transdiagnostic CBT treatments for anxiety and depressive disorders are under way among several research groups (e.g., Chu, Colognori, Weissman, & Bannon, 2009; Ehrenreich, Goldstein, Wright, & Barlow, 2009; Ehrenreich-May & Bilek, 2011; Kendall, Stark, Martinsen, O'Neil, & Arora, 2013; Weersing, Gonzalez, Campo, & Lucas, 2008). Researchers have begun to develop transdiagnostic protocols for anxiety and depressive disorders in children and adolescents in various settings, including primary care, schools, and traditional outpatient clinics.

In one initial effort, Weersing and colleagues (2008) developed a brief transdiagnostic treatment for anxiety and depression for implementation in the primary care setting. The eight-session treatment combines the core components of both CBT for childhood anxiety (exposure) and CBT for childhood depression (behavioral activation) into an integrated core technique of "graded engagement." The first four sessions focus on building skills: psychoeducation, relaxation and coping with negative affect, problem solving, and goal setting. Three sessions are devoted to graded engagement in increasing anxiety-provoking or effort-requiring situations. The final session addresses relapse prevention techniques.

Weersing and colleagues conducted a pilot study of this integrated treatment. Participants were 45 youth ages 7–17 years with an anxiety disorder, a depressive disorder, or comorbid anxiety and depressive disorders. Youth received integrated brief behavioral therapy for their anxiety or depression in the pediatric primary care setting. The authors reported on the clinical outcomes of two participants in the pilot study. Both participants presented with comorbid anxiety and depressive disorders and received a course of integrated brief behavioral therapy. In terms of outcomes, both participants experienced reduction in both anxiety and depressive symptoms and were rated as "much improved" at posttreatment and as "very much improved" at 6-month follow-up on the Clinical Global Impression Scale. This pilot study provides initial support for an integrated brief behavioral treatment for youth anxiety and depressive disorders in the primary care setting, although additional research is necessary to examine this treatment in controlled and randomized trials.

Other researchers are conducting similar research in different settings. Chu and colleagues (2009) reported on a pilot study of group behavioral activation therapy for youth with anxiety and depression, implemented in the school setting. The group behavioral activation therapy combined adult behavioral activation protocols with exposure for anxiety. The 10-session program includes core components of psychoeducation, functional analysis, problem solving, and graded exposures or behavioral tasks. Imaginal or in vivo exposures to anxiety-provoking situations and behavioral tasks such as role plays begin in session 3, with the aim of at least one group member engaging in a practice during each session. The program was piloted with a group of five seventh- and eighth-grade students ages 12–14 years over the course of 13 weeks. Each participant met criteria for both an anxiety and a depressive disorder. Of the five students, four completed the group treatment. Of those four, three students no longer meet criteria for their principal or secondary diagnosis following treatment. Parent and child reports also indicated improvement in anxiety and depressive symptoms. Results are promising regarding the feasibility of implementing this integrated group treatment for youth anxiety and depression in the school setting. Further research with controlled and randomized designs is warranted in order to investigate the efficacy of this transdiagnostic treatment.

Ehrenreich and colleagues (2009) developed an emotion-focused unified treatment protocol for anxiety and depressive disorders in adolescence for use in the traditional outpatient clinic setting. The protocol aims to address the commonalities among the emotional disorders and the role of emotion dysregulation in these disorders. The treatment protocol was based on the adult version of a unified protocol that involved the major components of antecedent cognitive reappraisal, preventing emotional avoidance and encouraging action tendencies that are not associated with the dysregulated emotion (Barlow et al., 2004). A pilot study with three participants provided initial support for this treatment and resulted in modifications to the protocol. In the modified version of the protocol, emotion regulation skills such as strategies for preventing emotional avoidance and cognitive appraisal and reappraisal are taught. In the second half of treatment, adolescents engage in individualized emotion exposure activity, and the emotion regulation skills are reinforced. A randomized controlled trial is currently being conducted with the modified version of the protocol. Although further research is necessary to examine the efficacy of this unified protocol, the initial results lend further support to transdiagnostic interventions for internalizing disorders in youth.

Ehrenreich-May and Bilek (2011) have also developed a downward extension of the unified protocol for school-age youth, Emotion Detectives. Emotion Detectives is a 15-session group CBT protocol for youth ages 7–12 with a principal anxiety disorder and co-occurring depressive disorders. Parent and child groups meet concurrently to learn skills linked to the three core strategies of the unified protocol. This transdiagnostic treatment for school-age youth is currently being investigated in an open trial.

Finally, Kendall and colleagues (2013) have developed a transdiagnostic CBT application for youth ages 8–12 with anxiety and/or depressive symptoms. EMOTION: A Coping Kids' Program for Managing Anxiety and Depression is a 20-session group treatment that integrates core components of effective single-target treatments for anxiety and depression in youth (Coping Cat—Kendall & Hedtke, 2006; ACTION—Stark et al., 2007). The program is designed for implementation in the school or outpatient setting and includes an eight-session parent group component. This transdiagnostic protocol is being piloted in the school setting in Norway. Although further investigation of this treatment is clearly required, EMOTION represents yet another promising transdiagnostic CBT approach to treating anxiety and depression in youth.

There is a relative paucity of transdiagnostic CBT applications outside of the internalizing disorders. For example, although many CBT protocols for the externalizing disorders may often have been used transdiagnostically in real-world practice, to our knowledge none of these interventions have been explicitly framed or tested as transdiagnostic CBT applications. Additionally, there are no known transdiagnostic CBT protocols for eating disorders in youth. However, transdiagnostic CBT applications for eating disorders in adults have been developed (Fairburn, Cooper, Shafran, & Wilson, 2008) and evaluated (Fairburn et al., 2009).

Future Directions

It is an exciting time for child therapy: there are treatments that have been developed and evaluated, and the results are supportive and encouraging. Despite the advances, there is need and room for improvement. Efforts to develop and evaluate transdiagnostic treatments are one avenue worthy of effort and research, and the CBT perspective offers and holds promise.

To achieve the desired improved treatment effects, further treatment development and evaluation will be required. Specifically, randomized clinical trials (Kendall & Comer, 2012) will be needed to examine the efficacy and breadth of transdiagnostic CBT (e.g., transdiagnostic treatments compared with single-target treatments). Transdiagnostic CBT treatments for anxiety and depressive disorders in youth are perhaps the most developed applications to date (e.g., Ehrenreich et al., 2009) and would be prime for such evaluation.

Future treatment development and evaluation is needed to investigate whether other diagnostic classes (e.g., disruptive disorders, eating disorders) may also be treated with transdiagnostic CBT. The comorbidities among externalizing disorders may lend themselves to a comparable transdiagnostic treatment. Such investigations will be important in the overall test of transdiagnostic CBT for psychological disorders in youth.

REFERENCES

Achenbach, T. (1990). "Comorbidity" in child and adolescent psychiatry: Categorical and quantitative perspectives. *Journal of Child and Adolescent Psychopharmacology, 1,* 271–278.

Anastopoulos, A. D., & Farley, S. E. (2003). A cognitive-behavioral training program for parents of children with attention-deficit/hyperactivity disorder. In A. E. Kazdin & J. R. Weisz (Eds.), *Evidence-based psychotherapies for children and adolescents* (pp. 187–203), New York: Guilford Press.

Angold, A., Costello, E. J., & Erkanli, A. (1999). Comorbidity. *Journal of Child Psychology and Psychiatry, 40,* 57–87.

Axelson, D. A., & Birmaher, B. (2001). Relations between anxiety and depressive disorders in childhood and adolescence. *Depression and Anxiety, 14,* 67–78.

Barlow, D. H., Allen, L. A., & Choate, M. L. (2004). Toward a unified treatment for emotional disorders. *Behavior Therapy, 35,* 205–230.

Barmish, A. J., & Kendall, P. C. (2005). Should parents be co-clients in cognitive-behavioral therapy for anxious youth? *Journal of Clinical Child and Adolescent Psychology, 34,* 569–581.

Barrett, P. M. (2004). *Friends for life: Group leader's manual.* Brisbane: Australian Academic Press.

Beck, A. T. (1976). *Cognitive therapy and the emotional disorders.* New York: Meridian.

Beck, A. T., & Alford, B. A. (2008). *Depression: Causes and treatment.* Philadelphia: University of Pennsylvania Press.

Beck, A. T., Emery, G., & Greenberg, R. L. (2005). *Anxiety disorders and phobias: A cognitive perspective.* New York: Basic Books.

Beck, J. S. (1995). *Cognitive therapy: Basics and beyond.* New York: Guilford Press.

Benjamin, C., Puleo, C., Settipani, C., Brodman, D., Edmunds, J., Cummings, C., et al. (2011). History of cognitive-behavioral therapy (CBT) in youth. *Child and Adolescent Psychiatric Clinics of North America, 20,* 179–189.

Berman, S. L., Weems, C. F., Silverman, W. K., & Kurtines, W. M. (2000). Predictors of outcome in exposure-based cognitive and behavioral treatments for phobic and anxiety disorders in children. *Behavior Therapy, 31,* 713–731.

Brady, E. U., & Kendall, P. C. (1992). Comorbidity of anxiety and depression in children and adolescents. *Psychological Bulletin, 111,* 244–255.

Brent, D. A., Holder, D., Kolko, D., Birmaher, B., Baugher, M., Roth, C., et al. (1997). A clinical psychotherapy trial for adolescent depression comparing cognitive, family, and supportive therapy. *Archives of General Psychiatry, 54,* 877–885.

Brent, D. A., Kolko, D. J., Birmaher, B., Baugher, M., Bridge, J., Roth, C., et al. (1998). Predictors of treatment efficacy in a clinical trial of three psychosocial treatments for adolescent depression. *Journal of American Academy of Child and Adolescent Psychiatry, 37,* 906–914.

Cartwright-Hatton, S., Roberts, C., Chitsabesan, P., Fothergill, C., & Harrington, R. (2004). Systematic review of the efficacy of cognitive behavior therapies for childhood and adolescent anxiety disorders. *British Journal of Clinical Psychology, 43,* 421–436.

Chambless, D. L., & Ollendick, T. H. (2001). Empirically supported psychological interventions: Controversies and evidence. *Annual Review of Psychology, 52,* 685–716.

Chu, B. C., Colognori, D., Weissman, A. S., & Bannon, K. (2009). An initial description and pilot of group behavioral activation therapy for anxious and depressed youth. *Cognitive and Behavioral Practice, 16,* 408–419.

Clark, L. A., & Watson, D. (1991). Tripartite model of anxiety and depression: Evidence and taxonomic implications. *Journal of Abnormal Psychology, 100,* 316–336.

Clarke, G. N., Rohde, P., Lewinsohn, P. M., Hops, H., & Seeley, J. R. (1999). Cognitive-behavioral treatment of adolescent depression: Efficacy of acute group treatment and booster sessions. *Journal of the American Academy of Child and Adolescent Psychiatry, 38,* 272–279.

Creed, T. A., & Kendall, P. C. (2005). Therapist alliance-building behavior within a cognitive-behavioral treatment for anxiety in youth. *Journal of Consulting and Clinical Psychology, 73,* 498–505.

D'Zurilla, T. J., & Goldfried, M. R. (1971). Problem solving and behavior modification. *Journal of Abnormal Psychology, 78,* 107–126.

Ehrenreich, J. T., Goldstein, C. R., Wright, L. R., & Barlow, D. H. (2009). Development of a unified protocol for the treatment of emotional disorders in youth. *Child and Family Behavior Therapy, 31,* 20–37.

Ehrenreich-May, J., & Bilek, E. L. (2011). The development of a transdiagnostic, cognitive behavioral group intervention for childhood anxiety disorders and co-occurring depression symptoms. *Cognitive and Behavioral Practice, 19,* 41–55.

Ellis, A. (1963). *Rational-emotive psychotherapy.* New York: Institute for Rational-Emotive Therapy.

Eyberg, S. M., Nelson, M. M., & Boggs, S. R. (2008). Evidence-based psychosocial treatments for children and adolescents with disruptive behavior. *Journal of Clinical Child and Adolescent Psychology, 37,* 215–237.

Fairburn, C. G., Cooper, Z., Doll, H. A., O'Connor, M. E., Bohn, K., Hawker, D. M., et al. (2009). Transdiagnostic cognitive behavioral therapy for patients with eating disorders: A two-site trial with 60-week follow-up. *American Journal of Psychiatry, 166,* 311–319.

Fairburn, C. G., Cooper, Z., & Shafran, R. (2003). Cognitive behavior therapy for eating disorders: A "transdiagnostic" theory and treatment. *Behaviour Research and Therapy, 41,* 509–528.

Fairburn, C. G., Cooper, Z., Shafran, R., & Wilson, G. T. (2008). Eating disorders: A transdiagnostic protocol. In D. H. Barlow (Ed.), *Clinical handbook of psychological disorders: A step-by-step treatment manual* (pp. 578–614). New York: Guilford Press.

Friedberg, R. D., & McClure J. M. (2002). *Clinical practice of cognitive therapy with children and adolescents: The nuts and bolts.* New York: Guilford Press.

Friedberg, R. D., McClure, J. M., & Garcia, J. H. (2009). *Cognitive therapy techniques for children and adolescents: Tools for enhancing practice.* New York: Guilford Press.

Gosch, E. A., Flannery-Schroeder, E., Mauro, C. F., & Compton, S. N. (2006). Principles of cognitive-behavioral therapy for anxiety disorders in children. *Journal of Cognitive Psychotherapy: An International Quarterly, 20,* 247–262.

Hawley, K., & Weisz, J. (2005). Youth versus parent working alliance in usual clinical care: Distinctive associations with retention, satisfaction, and treatment outcome. *Journal of Clinical Child and Adolescent Psychology, 34,* 117–128.

Ishikawa, S., Okajima, I., Matsuoka, H., & Sakano, Y. (2007). Cognitive behavioral therapy for anxiety disorders in children and adolescents: A meta-analysis. *Child and Adolescent Mental Health, 12,* 164–172.

Jensen, P. S., Martin, D., & Cantwell, D. P. (1997). Comorbidity in ADHD: Implications for research, practice, and DSM-V. *Journal of the American Academy of Child and Adolescent Psychiatry, 36,* 1065–1079.

Kaufman, N. K., Rohde, P., Seeley, J. R., Clarke, G. N., & Stice, E. (2005). Potential mediators of cognitive-behavioral therapy for adolescents with comorbid depression and conduct disorder. *Journal of Consulting and Clinical Psychology, 73,* 38–46.

Kazdin, A. E. (2003). Problem-solving skills training and parent management training for conduct disorder. In A. E. Kazdin & J. R. Weisz (Eds.), *Evidence-based psychotherapies for children and adolescents* (pp. 241–262). New York: Guilford Press.

Kazdin, A. E., & Weisz, J. R. (2010). Introduction: Context, background and goals. In J. R. Weisz & A. E. Kazdin (Eds.) *Evidence-based psychotherapies for children and adolescents* (pp. 3–9). New York: Guilford Press.

Kendall, P. C. (2012a). Anxiety disorders in youth. In P. C. Kendall (Ed.), *Child and adolescent therapy: Cognitive-behavioral procedures* (4th ed., pp. 143–189). New York: Guilford Press.

Kendall, P. C. (Ed.). (2012b). *Child and adolescent therapy: Cognitive-behavioral procedures* (4th ed.). New York: Guilford Press.

Kendall, P. C. (2012c). Guiding theory for therapy with children and adolescents. In P. C. Kendall (Ed.), *Child and adolescent therapy: Cognitive-behavioral procedures* (4th ed., pp. 3–24). New York: Guilford Press.

Kendall, P. C., Brady, E. U., & Verduin, T. L. (2001). Comorbidity in childhood anxiety disorders and treatment outcome. *Journal of the American Academy of Child and Adolescent Psychiatry, 40,* 787–794.

Kendall, P. C., & Comer, J. S. (2012). Research methods in clinical psychology. In D. H. Barlow (Ed.), *Oxford handbook of clinical psychology* (pp. 52–75). New York: Oxford University Press.

Kendall, P. C., Gosch, E., Furr, J. M., & Sood, E. (2008). Flexibility within fidelity. *Journal of the American Academy of Child and Adolescent Psychiatry, 47,* 987–993.

Kendall, P. C., & Hedtke, K. (2006). *Cognitive-behavioral therapy for anxious children: Therapist manual* (3rd ed.). Ardmore, PA: Workbook Publishing.

Kendall, P. C., Hudson, J. L., Gosch, E., Flannery-Schroeder, E., & Suveg, C. (2008). Cognitive-behavioral therapy for anxiety disordered youth: A randomized clinical trial evaluating child and family modalities. *Journal of Consulting and Clinical Psychology, 76,* 282–297.

Kendall, P. C., Stark, K. D., Martinsen, K., Rodriguez, K., & Arora, P. (2013). *Group leader manual for EMOTION: "Coping kids" managing anxiety and depression.* Ardmore, PA: Workbook Publishing.

Kendall, P. C., & Treadwell, K. R. H. (2007). The role of self-statements as a mediator in treatment for youth with anxiety disorders. *Journal of Consulting and Clinical Psychology, 75,* 380–389.

Le Grange, D., & Lock, J. (2007). *Treating bulimia in adolescents: A family-based approach.* New York: Guilford Press.

Lock, J., Le Grange, D., Agras, W. S., & Dare, C. (2001). *Treatment manual for anorexia nervosa: A family-based approach.* New York: Guilford Press.

Mahoney, M. J. (1974). *Cognition and behavior modification.* Cambridge, MA: Ballinger.

Mahoney, M. J., & Arnkoff, D. (1978). Cognitive and self-control therapies. In S. L. Garfield & A. E. Bergin (Eds.), *Handbook of psychotherapy and behavior change: An empirical analysis* (pp. 689–722). New York: Wiley.

Mansell, W., Harvey, A., Watkins, E., & Shafran, R. (2009). Conceptual foundations of the transdiagnostic approach to CBT. *Journal of Cognitive Psychotherapy: An International Quarterly, 23,* 6–19.

March, J. (2004). The treatment for adolescents with depression study (TADS): Short-term effectiveness and safety outcomes. *Journal of the American Medical Association, 292,* 807–820.

McEvoy, P. M., Nathan, P., & Norton, P. J. (2008). Efficacy of transdiagnostic treatments: A review of published outcome studies and future research directions. *Journal of Cognitive Psychotherapy: An International Quarterly, 23,* 20–33.

Meichenbaum, D. (1977). *Cognitive behavior modification.* New York: Plenum Press.

Nezu, A. M., Nezu, C. M., & McMurran, M. (2009). Problem-solving therapy. In

W. T. O'Donohue & J. E. Fisher (Eds.), *General principles and empirically supported techniques of cognitive behavior therapy* (pp. 500–505). Hoboken, NJ: Wiley.

O'Neil, K. A., & Kendall, P. C. (2012). Role of comorbid depression and co-occurring depressive symptoms in outcomes for anxiety-disordered youth treated with cognitive-behavioral therapy. *Child and Family Behavior Therapy, 34*, 197–209.

Pelham, W. E., & Fabiano, G. A. (2008). Evidence-based psychosocial treatments for attention-deficit/hyperactivity disorder. *Journal of Clinical Child and Adolescent Psychology, 37*, 184–214.

Rapee, R. M. (2003). The influence of comorbidity on treatment outcome for children and adolescents with anxiety disorders. *Behaviour Research and Therapy, 41*, 105–112.

Schmidt, U. (2009). Cognitive behavioral approaches in adolescent anorexia and bulimia nervosa. *Child and Adolescent Psychiatric Clinics of North America, 18*, 147–158.

Shelby, J. S., & Berk, M. S. (2009). Play therapy, pedagogy, and CBT: An argument for interdisciplinary synthesis. In A. A. Drewes (Ed.), *Blending play therapy with cognitive behavioral therapy: Evidence-based and other effective treatments and techniques* (pp. 17–40). New York: Wiley.

Solomando, A. M., Kendall, T., & Whittington, C. J. (2008). Cognitive behavioral therapy for children and adolescents. *Current Opinion in Psychiatry, 21*, 332–337.

Stark, K. D., Simpson, J., Schnoebelen, S., Hargrave, J., Molnar, J., & Glen, R. (2007). *Treating depressed youth: Therapist manual for 'ACTION.'* Ardmore, PA: Workbook Publishing.

Stark, K. D., Stapleton, L., Fisher, M., Arora, P., & Krumholtz, (2011). *The treatment of depressed 9 to 13 year old girls: Relative efficacy of ACTION, ACTION with parent training, and a minimal contact control condition.* Manuscript submitted for publication.

Suveg, C., Hudson, J. L., Brewer, G., Flannery-Schroeder, E., Gosch, E., & Kendall, P. C. (2009). Cognitive-behavioral therapy for anxiety-disordered youth: Secondary outcomes from a randomized clinical trial evaluating child and family modalities. *Journal of Anxiety Disorders, 23*, 341–349.

Suveg, C., Kendall, P. C., Comer, J. S., & Robin, J. (2006). Emotion-focused cognitive-behavioral therapy for anxious youth: A multiple-baseline evaluation. *Journal of Contemporary Psychotherapy, 36*, 77–85.

Trosper, S. E., Buzzella, B. A., Bennett, S. M., & Ehrenreich, J. T. (2009). Emotion regulation in youth with emotional disorders: Implications for a unified treatment approach. *Clinical Child and Family Psychology Review, 12*, 234–254.

Tuvblad, C., Zheng, M., Raine, A., & Baker, L. A. (2009). A common genetic factor explains the covariation among ADHD, ODD, and CD symptoms in 9–10-year-old boys and girls. *Journal of Abnormal Child Psychology, 37*, 153–167.

Walkup, J. T., Albano, A. M., Piacentini, J., Birmaher, B., Compton, S., Sherrill, J. T., et al. (2008). Cognitive behavioral therapy, sertraline, or a combination in childhood anxiety. *New England Journal of Medicine, 359*, 2753–2766.

Watanabe, N., Hunot, V., Omori, I. M., Churchill, R., & Furukawa, T. A. (2007).

Psychotherapy for depression among children and adolescents: A systematic review. *Acta Psychiatrica Scandanavia, 116,* 84–95.

Webster-Stratton, C., & Reid, M. (2003). The Incredible Years parents, teachers, and children training series: A multifaceted treatment approach for young children with conduct problems. In A. E. Kazdin & J. R. Weisz (Eds.), *Evidence-based psychotherapies for children and adolescents* (pp. 224–240). New York: Guilford Press.

Weersing, V. R., Gonzalez, A., Campo, J. V., & Lucas, A. N. (2008). Brief behavioral therapy for pediatric anxiety and depression: Piloting an integrated treatment approach. *Cognitive and Behavioral Practice, 15,* 126–139.

Weisz, J. R., McCarty, C. A., & Valeri, A. M. (2006). Effects of psychotherapy for depression in children and adolescents: A meta-analysis. *Psychological Bulletin, 132,* 132–149.

Wilamowska, Z. A., Thompson-Hollands, J., Fairholme, C. P., Ellard, K. K., Farchione, T. J., & Barlow, D. H. (2010). Conceptual background, development, and preliminary data from the unified protocol for transdiagnostic treatment of emotional disorders. *Depression and Anxiety, 27,* 882–890.

CHAPTER 9

Interpersonal Psychotherapy for Youth Depression and Anxiety

Jami F. Young, Laura Mufson, and Jessica S. Benas

This chapter provides a description of interpersonal psychotherapy (IPT) and its adaptation for adolescents (IPT-A), summarizes the efficacy research on IPT for depression and other disorders, and provides a rationale for considering IPT as a transdiagnostic therapy model. As discussed in further detail in the chapter, IPT and IPT-A were developed specifically to treat depression. However, the underlying theory of IPT—that psychological distress occurs in the context of interpersonal relationships—is applicable to a broader array of psychiatric conditions, suggesting the transdiagnostic potential of this approach. Given the high rates of comorbidity between depression and anxiety and the interpersonal factors that contribute to the onset and maintenance of these disorders, this chapter focuses specifically on the potential of IPT-A as a transdiagnostic approach for youth depression and anxiety.

Description of the Treatment Model

IPT is a brief, time-limited intervention that was initially developed in the late 1960s for the treatment of adult depression (Weissman, Markowitz, & Klerman, 2000). Since that time, IPT has been adapted for the treatment of adolescent depression (Mufson, Dorta, Moreau, & Weissman, 2004) and for use with a number of other psychiatric conditions, including eating disorders (Fairburn, Jones, Peveler, Hope, & O'Connor, 1993; Wilfley et al., 2002), bipolar disorder (Frank et al., 2005), and anxiety disorders (e.g., Bleiberg & Markowitz, 2005; Krupnick et al., 2008; Lipsitz, Markow-itz, Cherry, & Fyer, 1999; Lipsitz et al., 2006; Talbot & Gamble, 2008). IPT stems from the work of interpersonal theorists who believed that psychi-atric problems arise from and are perpetuated by problematic patterns of interpersonal interactions (Meyer, 1957; Sullivan, 1953). In addition, IPT has its roots in Bowlby's attachment theory, specifically its emphasis on the importance of relational bonds for mental health (Bowlby, 1977). IPT is based on the premise that the quality of interpersonal relationships can cause, maintain, or buffer against depression. As such, treatment focuses on improving relationships as a mechanism to improve depressive symp-toms.

IPT-A is an outpatient treatment designed for adolescents with mild to moderate depression severity. The typical course of treatment in IPT-A is 12–15 sessions over 12 weeks. IPT-A is divided into three phases of treat-ment: the initial phase (sessions 1–4), the middle phase (sessions 5–9), and the termination phase (sessions 10–12). If treatment is extended to 15 sessions, the additional sessions typically take place in the middle phase. Although IPT-A is an individual treatment, parents are encouraged to be involved in all phases of treatment. Ideally, parents attend one session in each phase of IPT-A to be educated about the treatment approach and to support the adolescent's interpersonal work. IPT-A is an active, structured treatment. Throughout treatment, both the therapist and the adolescent play an active role in the sessions, and the sessions remain focused on the interpersonal nature of the depression. To facilitate this focus, each session begins with a brief assessment of the adolescent's depressive symp-toms. The therapist notes any changes that occurred over the course of the week and links symptom and mood changes to interpersonal events.

Initial Phase of Treatment

During the initial phase of IPT-A, the therapist assesses the adolescent's depressive symptoms, provides psychoeducation about depression and the focus of IPT-A, explores the adolescent's significant relationships with family members and peers, and identifies the problem area that will be the focus of the remainder of treatment. As part of psychoeducation in IPT-A, the therapist assigns the adolescent the limited sick role. Like some-one with a medical illness, adolescents with depression may not be able to do as many things or do things as well as they did before the depression developed. The therapist encourages the adolescent to do as many of his or her usual activities as possible while recognizing and accepting that the performance may be affected. The parent is also educated about the limited sick role to decrease blame and encourage the adolescent's activi-ties in a supportive manner.

One of the core strategies in IPT-A is the interpersonal inventory, which is completed during the initial phase of treatment. The interpersonal inventory is a detailed assessment of the adolescent's important relationships. The goal of the inventory is to identify the relationships or interpersonal patterns that are most closely related to the adolescent's depression. First, the therapist asks the adolescent to identify important people in his or her life using a closeness circle, a series of concentric circles that help to categorize the relationships by levels of closeness to the adolescent. Next, the therapist asks detailed questions about each relationship, including frequency of contact, positive and negative aspects of the relationship, areas of conflict in the relationship and how such conflict is resolved, and aspects of the relationship the adolescent would like to change. On the basis of the interpersonal inventory, the adolescent and therapist choose one of the four interpersonal problem areas to focus on in treatment: *grief, interpersonal role disputes, role transitions*, or *interpersonal deficits* (see Mufson, Dorta, Moreau, & Weissman, 2004, for more details on IPT-A). During the formulation, the therapist explains the connection between the depressive symptoms and the adolescent's interpersonal difficulties and how these difficulties fit into the framework of the specified problem area.

Grief is the identified problem area if the adolescent is experiencing a depressive episode in response to the death of a significant other. The death can be recent, or it may be a more delayed or pathological grief reaction. IPT-A helps the adolescent mourn the loss of the deceased, while encouraging the adolescent to strengthen and develop other relationships. An interpersonal role dispute exists when there are disagreements over an adolescent's expected role within a particular relationship, such as with a parent or peer. IPT-A helps the adolescent modify maladaptive communication patterns and/or unrealistic expectations about the relationship that contribute to the dispute. Role transitions are the relationship changes that occur when an adolescent progresses from one social role to another, such as transitioning to high school, moving to a new town, or adjusting to the divorce of his or her parents. During IPT-A, the adolescent and therapist discuss the gains and losses associated with the transition, and the therapist helps the adolescent develop skills that are necessary to successfully manage the new role. Finally, the identified problem area is interpersonal deficits when an adolescent lacks the social skills needed to have close relationships with family and peers and thus is socially isolated, which often both triggers and maintains the depression. The goal of treatment is to help the adolescent develop the skills needed to have more satisfying interpersonal relationships.

Middle Phase of Treatment

During the middle phase of IPT-A, the therapist and adolescent discuss the problem area in greater detail, focusing on the identification and implementation of communication and problem-solving skills that can improve the adolescent's relationships. Although the specific strategies differ for the various problem areas, a number of techniques are frequently used in the middle phase of IPT-A. These techniques, including *expression of affect, clarification of expectations for relationships, communication analysis, decision analysis, interpersonal problem solving, role playing,* and *work-at-home assignments,* tend to be used across all four problem areas. Communication analysis is an in-depth analysis of a specific interaction that occurred between an adolescent and another person. The goal of communication analysis is to help the adolescent understand the impact of his or her words and nonverbal communication on others and how modifying aspects of the communication can lead to changes in the interaction and associated feelings. This is typically followed by a discussion of specific communication strategies that are relevant to the problem area, such as acknowledging the other person's point of view to defuse an argument and having different solutions in mind so a compromise can be met. After the therapist and adolescent identify more adaptive communication strategies, it is helpful to role-play the communication using these techniques.

Once the adolescent and therapist have a better understanding of the interpersonal problem, including any communication issues, it is useful to conduct a decision analysis to determine the best course of action. This includes identifying a problematic interpersonal situation, encouraging the adolescent to generate solutions, evaluating the pros and cons of each solution, selecting a solution to try first, and role-playing the interaction needed for the chosen solution. Decision analysis helps the adolescent develop interpersonal problem-solving skills that he or she can use within and outside of session. Role playing is a key technique used in the middle phase of IPT-A that helps the adolescent practice new interpersonal skills and techniques that he or she can apply to important relationships. Following the role-play practice in session, the adolescent is often assigned "work at home," or an interpersonal experiment to have the practiced conversation on his or her own, outside of the session. This at-home conversation would then be reviewed in detail in the following session. Throughout the middle phase, the therapist links improvement in the adolescent's mood and depressive symptoms to his or her improved communication and decision making in important relationships.

Termination Phase of Treatment

The goals of the termination phase of IPT-A are to clarify warning symptoms of future depressive episodes, to identify successful strategies used in the middle phase, to foster generalization of skills to future situations, to emphasize mastery of new interpersonal skills, and to discuss the need for further treatment. During the termination sessions, the therapist and adolescent review the adolescent's progress, especially regarding the identified problem area. Changes in interpersonal relationships are linked to improved mood and decreased symptoms. The therapist and adolescent highlight which strategies have been most helpful, and the therapist emphasizes the importance of continued implementation of these strategies after termination. The conclusion of the relationship with the therapist also needs to be addressed during the final sessions of IPT-A, as well as a plan of action if the depression recurs.

Evidence of Efficacy

Treatment for Adult Depression

IPT has been evaluated in numerous studies as both an acute treatment (Elkin et al., 1989; Luty et al., 2007; Sloane, Stapes, & Schneider, 1985; Weissman et al., 1979) and a maintenance treatment (Frank et al., 1990, 2007; Klerman, DiMascio, Weissman, Prusoff, & Paykel, 1974; Reynolds et al., 1999, 2010; Weissman, Klerman, Paykel, Prusoff, & Hanson, 1974) for adult and geriatric depression. Within the adult depression literature, IPT has been compared with both medication (Elkin et al., 1989; Frank et al., 1990; Klerman et al., 1974; Reynolds et al., 1999, 2010; Sloane et al., 1985; Weissman et al., 1979) and cognitive-behavioral treatment (Elkin et al., 1989, 1995; Luty et al., 2007) and has compared favorably with both. Based on these various studies, IPT is considered a well-established treatment for adult depression (Chambless et al., 1998), with meta-analyses supporting the efficacy of IPT for adult depression relative to other psychotherapies (Cuijpers, van Straten, Andersson, & van Oppen, 2008; Cuijpers et al., 2011).

Treatment for Other Adult Disorders

In order to consider the transdiagnostic properties of IPT-A, it is beneficial to review the application of the adult model of IPT to other populations. Although IPT has been adapted for a number of diagnoses, we focus specifically on eating disorders and anxiety disorders, as these disorders seem most plausible to include in a transdiagnostic IPT treatment. Interpersonal psychotherapy has empirical support as a treatment for adults with bulimia nervosa (Agras, Walsh, Fairburn, Wilson, & Kraemer, 2000; Fairburn et al., 1991, 1993) and binge eating disorder (Wilfley et al., 1993, 2002; Wilson, Wilfley, Agras & Bryson, 2010), in both individual (Agras et al., 2000; Fairburn et al., 1991, 1993; Wilson et al., 2010) and group formats (Wilfley et al., 1993, 2002). IPT for eating disorders posits that the development of eating pathology occurs in an interpersonal context and that difficulties in relationships can contribute to and/or maintain the disordered eating behavior. Therefore, a treatment such as IPT that focuses on altering the interpersonal relationships or patterns that are contributing to or maintaining the eating problem can be effective in decreasing problematic eating behaviors (Wilfley, Frank, Welch, Spurrell, & Rounsaville, 1998).

More recently, attempts have been made to adapt IPT for the treatment of various anxiety disorders, including social anxiety (Borge et al., 2008; Lipsitz et al., 1999, 2008; Stangier, Schramm, Heidenreich, Berger, & Clark, 2011), panic disorder (Cyranowski et al., 2005; Lipsitz et al., 2006), and posttraumatic stress disorder (PTSD) (Bleiberg & Markowitz, 2005; Campanini et al., 2010; Krupnick et al., 2008; Talbot et al., 2005). These adaptations are based on the premise that anxiety disorders develop within an interpersonal context, with interpersonal functioning and interpersonal events affecting the development of the disorder and interpersonal difficulties arising as a consequence of the anxiety (see Weissman et al., 2000, for further discussion). The IPT adaptations for anxiety disorders are in differing phases of development and testing. Although preliminary data suggest that these adaptations are effective at reducing anxiety, IPT is currently not a first-line treatment for adult anxiety disorders. For instance, a recent randomized controlled trial comparing IPT and cognitive therapy for social anxiety disorder found that both treatments led to significantly greater improvements than a wait-list control condition but that cognitive therapy performed significantly better than IPT (Stangier et al., 2011).

Treatment for Adolescent Depression

Research has shown IPT-A to be an efficacious treatment for adolescent depression. Several randomized controlled clinical trials of IPT-A have been conducted, and two separate investigator teams have demonstrated its efficacy (Mufson, Dorta, Wickramaratne, et al., 2004; Mufson, Weissman, Moreau, & Garfinkel, 1999; Rosselló & Bernal, 1999; Rosselló, Bernal, & Rivera-Medina, 2008). In an initial study of IPT-A, significantly more adolescents in IPT-A met recovery criteria for major depression than adolescents in clinical monitoring. IPT-A adolescents also reported a significant decrease in depressive symptoms and increased social functioning and problem-solving skills as compared with adolescents in clinical monitoring (Mufson et al., 1999). Rosselló and Bernal (1999) and Rosselló and colleagues (2008) have examined a different adaptation of IPT designed specifically for depressed adolescents in Puerto Rico. In these studies, adolescents receiving IPT experienced reductions in depression symptoms, increases in self-esteem, and improvements in social functioning.

In addition to the efficacy trials, there is also evidence of the effectiveness of IPT-A when delivered by community clinicians (Mufson, Dorta, Wickramaratne, et al., 2004). Clinicians in several school-based health clinics were trained to deliver IPT-A. Adolescents in these schools with depression were randomized to receive either treatment as usual (which consisted of supportive, individual counseling) or IPT-A as delivered by school-based clinicians. Adolescents who received IPT-A, as compared with adolescents who received treatment as usual, demonstrated a greater decrease in depression symptoms and depression severity, greater overall functioning, and significantly better social functioning.

Treatment for Other Childhood Disorders

Although adaptations of IPT for childhood disorders lag behind those cited in the adult literature, there is some evidence from the depression treatment studies that IPT-A may also lead to reductions in anxiety. Young, Mufson, and Davies (2006b) examined outcomes of adolescents with comorbid depression and anxiety who received IPT-A or treatment as usual in the IPT-A effectiveness study (Mufson, Dorta, Wickramaratne, et al., 2004). For those adolescents with a likely anxiety disorder at baseline, approximately half no longer had an anxiety diagnosis at the end of treatment. Although treatment condition was not a significant predictor of composite anxiety symptoms postintervention, treatment condition did predict improvement in generalized anxiety disorder (GAD) symptoms. Adolescents were more likely to show improvement in their GAD symptoms if they received IPT-A. These findings suggest that IPT-A may be particularly effective for GAD, which is increasingly being recognized as having a large interpersonal component (Borkovec, Newman, Pincus, & Lytle, 2002; Roemer, Molina, & Borkovec, 1997).

A number of adaptations of IPT-A have been developed in the past several years. We highlight those adaptations that are particularly relevant to the conceptualization of IPT-A as a transdiagnostic approach. Young and Mufson (2003) developed interpersonal psychotherapy—adolescent skills training (IPT-AST), a group preventive intervention for adolescents with subthreshold symptoms of depression. In two studies, adolescents in IPT-AST reported significantly fewer depressive symptoms, better overall functioning, and fewer depression diagnoses than adolescents who received usual school counseling (SC) both after intervention and at a 6-month follow-up (Young, Mufson, & Davies, 2006a; Young, Mufson, & Gallop, 2010). Recent analyses suggest that IPT-AST is also effective at reducing anxiety symptoms. Using pooled data from the two randomized trials of IPT-AST, Young and colleagues (2012) found that adolescents who received IPT-AST reported significantly greater reductions in total anxiety symptoms, generalized anxiety symptoms, and panic/somatic symptoms during the course of the intervention than adolescents who received SC.

The findings for generalized anxiety symptoms replicate those found in studies of IPT-A (Young et al., 2006b) and suggest that interventions based on IPT may be particularly effective for adolescents with depression and generalized anxiety, whether it be elevated symptoms or comorbid diagnoses. Notably, change in rates of social anxiety symptoms did not differ by intervention condition. Adolescents in both conditions showed small reductions in social anxiety symptoms during the intervention. These findings suggest that IPT-AST, although effective at addressing anxiety more generally, is less effective at specifically targeting social anxiety symptoms. IPT-AST targets interpersonal relationships in general, but less time is spent helping adolescents confront their social anxieties in between sessions than may be needed to engender a significant reduction in social anxiety.

Tanofsky-Kraff and colleagues (2007) adapted the IPT-AST manual for the prevention of inappropriate weight gain (IPT-WG) in female adolescents who are overweight. IPT-WG posits that interpersonal events are linked to both negative affect and loss of control of eating. As such, the group intervention focuses on increasing interpersonal skills and improving relationships with the aim of reducing binge and loss of control of eating (Tanofsky-Kraff et al., 2007). A pilot study compared IPT-WG with a standard-of-care health education group. The results from this study suggest that IPT-WG is feasible and acceptable to adolescent girls. In addition, among girls with loss of control of eating at study onset, those in IPT-WG experienced greater reductions in loss-of-control episodes than those in health education (Tanofsky-Kraff et al., 2010). A large randomized controlled trial of IPT-WG for overweight girls is ongoing.

Use of IPT-A as a Transdiagnostic Approach

However, the underlying theory of IPT—that psychological distress occurs in the context of interpersonal relationships—is applicable to a broader array of psychiatric conditions. Across these various conditions, IPT endorses a biopsychosocial model of illness. IPT posits that an individual has a unique biological vulnerability that interacts with the environment in multiple ways to manifest itself in different disorders. The social environment is composed of one's significant interpersonal relationships, which can play a large role in the onset and maintenance of various disorders. Depending on the underlying biological vulnerability or an individual's unique interpersonal environment, different types of psychopathology may emerge. A large body of research has identified interpersonal factors that contribute to and/or maintain different disorders. Given the focus of this chapter on youth depression and anxiety, we summarize the interpersonal risk-factor literature for these disorders in a later section.

The applicability of IPT beyond depression is reflected in the large number of adaptations of IPT for various disorders. Although each adaptation of IPT is somewhat different, all of these adaptations share the essential elements of IPT. These essential elements include the interpersonal inventory, the interpersonal problem areas, the interpersonal formulation, and a focus on the client's current interpersonal relationships (Stuart, Robertson, & O'Hara, 2006). It is these key IPT strategies that are thought to lead to improvements in the interpersonal problem and to increased social support and resolved psychiatric symptoms. Therefore, there is growing support for considering IPT-A's potential as a transdiagnostic approach for various psychiatric conditions via the common mechanism of improving interpersonal relationships. As Stuart and colleagues (2006) argue, the interpersonal problem areas are universally applicable across diagnoses and developmental levels, which is one of IPT's greatest assets as a treatment approach. Moreover, the interpersonal problem areas have been demonstrated to be applicable to other cultures as well, which is also suggestive of its transdiagnostic potential (e.g., Bolton et al., 2003; Verdeli et al., 2003, 2008).

For which conditions is IPT-A a relevant treatment approach in its current format? As with many other transdiagnostic approaches, it seems best to start by considering whether IPT-A can be conceptualized as a transdiagnostic approach for internalizing disorders. As outlined by Barlow, Allen, and Choate (2004) originally and by others subsequently, there is a justification for targeting depression and anxiety in a single treatment given the similar etiology, overlap in symptoms, comorbidity, and treatment effects on comorbid symptomatology (Ehrenreich, Goldstein, Wright, & Barlow, 2009; Garber & Weersing, 2010). The findings outlined earlier that IPT-A and IPT-AST led to reductions in both depression and anxiety symptoms and disorders support the consideration of IPT-A as a transdiagnostic approach for internalizing disorders. The transdiagnostic approaches for youth depression and anxiety that have been developed to date primarily target cognitive biases and/or avoidance processes that are thought to be common across internalizing disorders (Chu, Colognori, Weissman, & Bannon, 2009; Chu, Merson, Zandberg, & Areizaga, 2012; Ehrenreich et al., 2009; Weersing, Gonzalez, Campo, & Lucas, 2008).

IPT-A offers a unique transdiagnostic approach in its focus instead on the interpersonal factors thought to contribute to and maintain depression and anxiety. Research suggests that individuals with depression and anxiety experience more stressful life events than individuals without a disorder (Goodyer & Altham 1991; Rapee & Szollos, 2002). Individuals with depression may act in ways that elicit stress and conflict in their relationships (e.g., Hammen, 1991; Rudolph et al., 2000), and the same may be true for individuals with anxiety disorders. As a result of their negative self-perceptions about their own social competencies or their heightened sense of "felt insecurity," adolescents with anxiety experience social withdrawal and peer rejection that can exacerbate and maintain their anxious symptoms (Bosquet & Egeland, 2006). There is also growing evidence that maladaptive interpersonal problems play an important role in many of the anxiety disorders, in particular GAD (e.g., Newman & Erickson, 2010; Roemer et al., 1997) and social anxiety disorder (e.g., Festa & Ginsburg, 2011; Gazelle & Ladd, 2003; Kingery, Erdley, Marshall, Whitaker, & Reuter, 2010). Consequently, IPT-A, with its focus on interpersonal problem areas and improving communication and affect management within relationships, is well suited to address these interpersonal deficits that contribute to and maintain anxiety.

An additional reason that IPT-A would be relevant for childhood anxiety disorders, as well as depression, is the recognition that parenting behaviors play a role in both types of internalizing disorders (for reviews, see McLeod, Weisz, & Wood, 2007; McLeod, Wood, & Weisz, 2007) and that insecure attachment is a vulnerability for both depression and anxiety (Cassidy, Lichenstein-Phelps, Sibrava, Thomas, & Borkovec, 2009; Davila, Ramsay, Stroud, & Steinberg, 2005). There is growing discussion of the significance of early attachment difficulties, specifically that insecure attachment histories with primary caregivers place children at risk for social anxiety and may increase their risk for subsequent anxiety disorders, as well as depression (Bosquet & Egeland, 2006). Given IPT-A's focus on improving the adolescent–parent relationship and its roots in attachment theory, IPT-A may be well suited to address these interpersonal risk factors of anxiety. Finally, IPT-A focuses on improving social support, which may be a generalized protective factor for depression and anxiety (Dozois, Seeds, & Collins, 2009).

Core Aspects of IPT-A in a Transdiagnostic Approach

IPT-A's focus on the link between relationships, affect management, and depression may apply to other disorders, such as anxiety. The core IPT-A constructs that enable this transdiagnostic work include the interpersonal inventory, the problem area formulation, the four interpersonal problem areas, and the focus on current interpersonal relationships. The core strategies and techniques of IPT-A that would be maintained in the transdiagnostic conceptualization include identification and expression of affect, management of affect through communication strategies, understanding the link between interpersonal difficulties and mood changes, and improving communication and problem-solving skills. These techniques are thought to be transdiagnostic because of the impact they have on improving relationships, which in turn can result in a decrease in both depressive and anxious symptoms. These symptom improvements will also contribute to improved relationships due to the reciprocal linkage between symptoms and relationships. The proposed transdiagnostic model of interpersonal psychotherapy for adolescents with anxiety and depression is depicted in Figure 9.1.

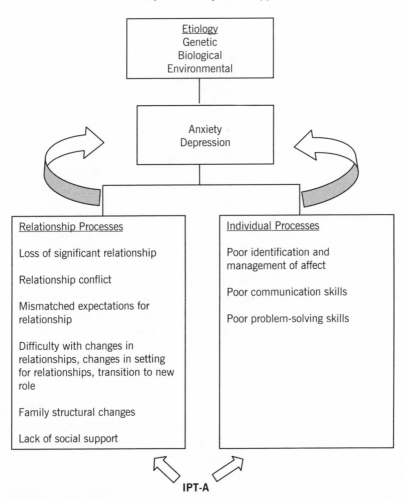

FIGURE 9.1. Transdiagnostic model of IPT-A for youth with depression and anxiety.

We are proposing that there are relationship processes that play a role in the development of anxiety and depression as well as individual processes, both of which are affected through treatment with IPT-A. The relationship processes, which correspond to the interpersonal problem areas, focus on interpersonal difficulties that can occur with either peers or family or both. They are not hypothesized necessarily to be a cause of the anxiety or depression but are interpersonal situations that have either triggered or maintained the anxiety or depression. As research has shown, adolescents with both depression and anxiety experience conflicts and social withdrawal within their relationships, and both depression and anxiety have been linked to the loss of a significant relationship (Starr & Davila, 2008). By conducting a thorough review of the important relationships in the adolescent's life, the IPT-A therapist helps the adolescent to identify and focus on the relationship that is most directly related to the maintenance of the current symptoms, which can easily include both anxious and depressive symptoms.

As previously mentioned, the problem area processes that are the focus in IPT-A include grief related to the loss through death of a significant person in one's life; conflict in relationships as a result of mismatched or unclear expectations for the parameters of the relationship; difficulties in making life transitions such as moving, changing schools, or parental divorce or remarriage that necessitate a change in one's role in relationships; and, last, the problem of social isolation and lack of social supports. As reflected by the inclusion of these problem areas in the various adaptations of IPT, these problem areas are relevant across development, culture, and diagnoses.

On an individual level, an adolescent has difficulty negotiating these peer and familial relationships because of a lack of effective affect management, communication, and problem-solving skills. Using the interpersonal inventory, the IPT-A therapist obtains examples of how the adolescent has attempted to address the problematic relationship, and these examples provide clues as to what skills need augmentation for the adolescent to be more successful in that relationship and in turn be less anxious and depressed. Teens with both depression and anxiety have difficulty managing their emotions, whether it be bottling feelings up inside until they explode in anger or expressing constant worries or negative affect within a relationship to the point of irritating or alienating the other person. IPT-A helps the adolescent to identify his or her emotions, link them to interpersonal events that may contribute to the feelings, and learn more effective ways to communicate feelings so the adolescent's needs can be met and the feelings can dissipate.

IPT-A focuses on teaching core communication skills, such as identifying the best time to have a conversation, postponing conversations if one is too emotionally upset, and communicating empathic statements that demonstrate the adolescent's ability to see the other person's perspective. These strategies help adolescents communicate thoughts and feelings with the other person in a way that is more likely to have a successful outcome, focusing on issues of timing, wording, perspective taking, and nonverbal messages. Last, adolescents are taught problem-solving skills to facilitate their ability to solve interpersonal problems. For adolescents with anxiety, the work may focus on how to communicate their concerns in a way that does not seem like excessive reassurance seeking, how to obtain information from others that may decrease their anxiety, as well as how to problem-solve situations to decrease avoidance due to anxiety. Using the techniques of role playing and "work at home" interpersonal experiments, the adolescents spend a significant part of the middle phase practicing these new communication and problem-solving skills both in session and outside of session, the latter being very similar to exposure exercises that are part of standard CBT treatments for anxiety. Parents and peers may be involved as needed to support the new interpersonal skills. In addition, they may be invited to participate to help change their interactions with the adolescent in order to decrease the adolescent's associated depressive and anxious feelings. The framework and techniques are applicable transdiagnostically, as the associated interpersonal difficulties for adolescents with these disorders occur regardless of the etiology of the disorders. If these techniques can ameliorate the difficulties, they can promote recovery.

Aspects of IPT-A That Would Require Modification

There are also several key elements of IPT-A that would need to be modified for a transdiagnostic approach. The psychoeducational component of IPT-A would be broadened to include discussions of anxiety, of what is known about the relationship between anxiety and interpersonal difficulties, and of available treatments and recovery information specifically for anxiety and/or comorbid depression and anxiety. The diagnoses would be discussed in regard to how our moods (anxious and depressed) can affect our relationships and vice versa and to how both depression and anxiety affect our ability to cope with life stressors. Similarly, the limited sick role would be modified to address the effects of anxiety on the adolescent's participation in his or her usual activities. The adolescent with anxiety would be similarly encouraged to push him- or herself to engage in normal activities with revised performance expectations and with encouragement that his or her performance will improve the more he or she engages in the activities and the more treatment assists in recovery. Although this may be more challenging for the adolescent with social anxiety, the parent would be similarly educated about the limited sick role, and both adolescent and parent would be helped to understand that avoidance only serves to maintain the anxiety and that exposure to small pieces of the usual activities will result in an eventual decrease in the concomitant anxiety.

Within the transdiagnostic approach, parent involvement can remain largely the same as in the original manual. The parent is involved in the initial phase to review diagnosis and available treatments, to discuss the current treatment approach, and to identify his or her role in treatment. More discussion may be needed to address the increased need to support the adolescent in the "work at home," including interpersonal experiments/exposures. In the middle phase, the parent would still be invited to participate in sessions as needed for work on communication and problem solving and also to assist as coach and support for the adolescent to engage in more of the exposure type of work-at-home exercises. The work at home would likely need to be modified to better address the difficulties of social anxiety. This might include more parental involvement in designing the work-at-home exposures so that parents can play more of a coaching role in their implementation. It might also include revising the experiments to address smaller components of the anxiety-related interpersonal situation so that the adolescent can master smaller pieces before moving on to the larger interpersonal issue. Last, based on our analyses of the effects of comorbid anxiety on treatment outcome, it might be beneficial to build in flexibility on the part of the clinician to extend the middle phase of treatment for adolescents with social anxiety to provide additional time to practice their interpersonal skills. We believe these additional sessions may improve the impact of IPT-A on adolescents with social anxiety.

Limitations of IPT-A as a Transdiagnostic Approach

Despite the elements of IPT-A that make it a potential transdiagnostic treatment for depression and anxiety, research on IPT-A as a transdiagnostic approach is in its infancy. We feel confident, given the findings mentioned herein, that IPT-A is a useful treatment approach for adolescents with comorbid depression and anxiety. IPT-A may also be effective for adolescents with GAD and panic disorder who do not have comorbid depression, although additional research is needed to examine this question. However, less evidence exists to support the treatment of other anxiety disorders, such as obsessive–compulsive disorder (OCD) or PTSD. In addition, findings from the IPT-A and IPT-AST research (Young et al., 2006b, 2012) suggest that social anxiety may fare best with an exposure component incorporated into treatment. Furthermore, given that IPT-A is a short-term treatment, it may be difficult to effectively target multiple diagnoses that require additional components without diffusing the effects of IPT-A, as has been found in other treatments that aimed to address comorbid conditions (e.g., Craske et al., 2007). To answer this question, future research should compare singular versus transdiagnostic approaches for depression and anxiety, something that is notably absent in this field (see Rohde, 2012).

Future Directions

This chapter has focused on IPT-A as a transdiagnostic approach for youth depression and anxiety. The usefulness of IPT-A as a transdiagnostic tool for other disorders is speculative. Given the efficacy of IPT in treating adult eating disorders and in preventing weight gain in overweight adolescent girls, there is potential for IPT-A to be used as a transdiagnostic treatment for disordered eating behaviors in youth. Such an approach would target the interpersonal problems that maintain disordered eating. Additional research is needed to examine the utility of IPT-A for youth with eating disorders. Beyond depressive disorders, certain anxiety disorders, and eating disorders, there is currently limited rationale for the use of IPT-A for other youth psychopathology.

At this stage, perhaps a more realistic and feasible approach is to incorporate an IPT-A-based module into existing treatments that do not already address interpersonal issues, assuming that interpersonal difficulties is one of the presenting problems. For example, in addition to treating OCD with exposure and response prevention, there may be significant problems with role disputes or role transitions that could be treated with an IPT-A module to help support the CBT work. Conflict between the adolescent and parents about how to manage the OCD might benefit from work on communication and problem solving. In addition, it may be necessary for parents to temporarily reassert control to implement the exposure exercises and manage the compulsions. Specific IPT techniques might help the adolescent and parents negotiate the adolescent's transition back to age-appropriate autonomy when the adolescent is ready and to help the adolescent communicate his or her feelings and concerns surrounding these transitions. Therefore, an additional area of inquiry would be to conduct research examining the efficacy of including IPT-A as a module or adjunctive treatment to another established approach to see whether this improves treatment outcomes. Other avenues of research include identifying which interpersonal factors are important across disorders and which may be disorder-specific, the impact of particular disorders on adolescents' significant relationships, and the role of these relationships in the recovery process. The results of such research would provide further information about the transdiagnostic utility of IPT-A, as well as the potential limitations of such an approach.

REFERENCES

Agras, W. S., Walsh, T., Fairburn, C. G., Wilson, G. T., & Kraemer, H. C. (2000). A multicenter comparison of cognitive-behavioral therapy and interpersonal psychotherapy for bulimia nervosa. *Archives of General Psychiatry, 57*, 459–466.

Barlow, D. H., Allen, L. B., & Choate, M. L. (2004). Toward a unified treatment for emotional disorders. *Behavior Therapy, 35*, 205–230.

Bleiberg, K. L., & Markowitz, J. C. (2005). A pilot study of interpersonal psychotherapy for posttraumatic stress disorder. *American Journal of Psychiatry, 162*, 181–183.

Bolton, P., Bass, J., Neugebauer, R., Verdeli, H., Clougherty, K. F., Wickramaratne, P., et al. (2003). Group interpersonal psychotherapy for depression in rural Uganda: A randomized controlled trial. *Journal of the American Medical Association, 289,* 3117–3124.

Borge, F., Hoffart, A., Sexton, H., Clark, D. M., Markowitz, J. C., & McManus, F. (2008). Residential cognitive therapy versus residential interpersonal therapy for social phobia: A randomized clinical trial. *Journal of Anxiety Disorders, 22,* 991–1010.

Borkovec, T. D., Newman, M. G., Pincus, A. L., & Lytle, R. (2002). A component analysis of cognitive-behavioral therapy for generalized anxiety disorder and the role of interpersonal problems. *Journal of Consulting and Clinical Psychology, 70,* 288–298.

Bosquet, M., & Egeland, B. (2006). The development and maintenance of anxiety symptoms from infancy through adolescence in a longitudinal sample. *Development and Psychopathology, 18,* 517–550.

Bowlby, J. (1977). The making and breaking of affectional bonds: II. Some principles of psychotherapy. *British Journal of Psychiatry, 130,* 421–431.

Campanini, R. F. B., Schoedl, A. F., Pupo, M. C., Costa, A. C. H., Krupnick, J. L., & Mello, M. F. (2010). Efficacy of interpersonal therapy-group format adapted to post-traumatic stress disorder: An open-label add-on trial. *Depression and Anxiety, 27,* 72–77.

Cassidy, J., Lichtenstein-Phelps, J., Sibrava, N. J., Thomas, C. L., Jr., & Borkovec, T. D. (2009). Generalized anxiety disorder: Connections with self-reported attachment. *Behavior Therapy, 40,* 23–38.

Chambless, D. L., Baker, M. J., Baucom, D. H., Beutler, L. E., Calhoun, K. S., Crits-Christoph, P., et al. (1998). Update on empirically validated therapies: II. *Clinical Psychologist, 51,* 3–16.

Chu, B. C., Colognori, D., Weissman, A. S., & Bannon, K. (2009). An initial description and pilot of group behavioral activation therapy for anxious and depressed youth. *Cognitive and Behavioral Practice, 16,* 408–419.

Chu, B. C., Merson, R. A., Zandberg, L. J., & Areizaga, M. (2012). Calibrating for comorbidity: Clinical decision-making in youth depression and anxiety. *Cognitive and Behavioral Practice, 19,* 5–16.

Craske, M. G., Farchione, T. J., Allen, L. B., Barrios, V., Stoyanova, M., & Rose, R. (2007). Cognitive behavioral therapy for panic disorder and comorbidity: More of the same or less of more? *Behaviour Research and Therapy, 45,* 1095–1109.

Cuijpers, P., Geraedts, A., van Oppen, P., Andersson, G., Markowitz, J. C., & van Straten, A. (2011). Interpersonal psychotherapy for depression: A meta-analysis. *American Journal of Psychiatry, 168,* 581–592.

Cuijpers, P., van Straten, A., Andersson, G., & van Oppen, P. (2008). Psychotherapy for depression in adults: A meta-analysis of comparative outcome studies. *Journal of Consulting and Clinical Psychology, 76,* 909–922.

Cyranowski, J. M., Frank, E., Shear, M. K., Swartz, H., Fagiolini, A., Scott, J., et al. (2005). Interpersonal psychotherapy for depression with panic spectrum symptoms: A pilot study. *Depression and Anxiety, 21,* 140–142.

Davila, J., Ramsay, M., Stroud, C. B., & Steinberg, S. J. (2005). Attachment as vulnerability to the development of psychopathology. In B. L. Hankin & J. R. Z. Abela (Eds.), *Development of psychopathology: A vulnerability–stress perspective* (pp. 215–242). Thousand Oaks, CA: Sage.

Dozois, D. J. A., Seeds, P. M., & Collins, K. A. (2009). Transdiagnostic approaches to the prevention of depression and anxiety. *Journal of Cognitive Psychotherapy, 23,* 44–59.

Ehrenreich, J. T., Goldstein, C. R., Wright, L. R., & Barlow, D. H. (2009). Development of a unified protocol for the treatment of emotional disorders in youth. *Child and Family Behavior Therapy, 31,* 20–37.

Elkin, I., Gibbons, R. D., Shea, M. T., Sotsky, S. M., Watkins, J. T., Pilkonis, P. A., et al. (1995). Initial severity and differential treatment outcome in the National Institute of Mental Health treatment of depression collaborative research program. *Journal of Consulting and Clinical Psychology, 63,* 841–847.

Elkin, I., Shea, M. T., Watkins, J. T., Imber, D. S., Sotsky, S. M., Collins, J. F., et al. (1989). National Institute of Mental Health treatment of depression collaborative research program. *Archives of General Psychiatry, 46,* 971–982.

Fairburn, C. G., Jones, R., Peveler, R. C., Carr, S. J., Solomon, R. A., O'Connor, M. E., et al. (1991). Three psychological treatments for bulimia nervosa: A comparative trial. *Archives of General Psychiatry, 48,* 463–469.

Fairburn, C. G., Jones, R., Peveler, R. C., Hope, R. A., & O'Connor, M. (1993). Psychotherapy and bulimia nervosa: Longer-term effects of interpersonal psychotherapy, behavior therapy, and cognitive behavior therapy. *Archives of General Psychiatry, 50,* 419–428.

Festa, C. C., & Ginsburg, G. S. (2011). Parental and peer predictors of social anxiety in youth. *Child Psychiatry and Human Development, 42,* 291–306.

Frank, E., Kupfer, D. J., Perel, J. M., Cornes, C., Jarrett, D. B., Mallinger, A. G., et al. (1990). Three-year outcomes for maintenance therapies in reccurent depression. *Archives of General Psychiatry, 47,* 1093–1099.

Frank, E., Kupfer, D. J., Thase, M. E., Mallinger, A. G., Swartz, H. A., Fagiolini, A. M., et al. (2005). Two-year outcomes for interpersonal and social rhythm therapy in individuals with bipolar I disorder. *Archives of General Psychiatry, 62,* 996–1004.

Frank, E., Kupfer, D. J., Buysse, D. J., Swartz, H. A., Pilkonis, P. A., Houck, P. R., et al. (2007). Randomized trial of weekly, twice-monthly, and monthly interpersonal psychotherapy as maintenance treatment for women with recurrent depression. *American Journal of Psychiatry, 164,* 761–767.

Garber, J., & Weersing, V. R. (2010). Comorbidity of anxiety and depression in youth: Implications for treatment and prevention. *Clinical Psychology: Science and Practice, 17,* 293–306.

Gazelle, H., & Ladd, G. W. (2003). Anxious solitude and peer exclusion: A diathesis–stress model of internalizing trajectories in childhood. *Child Development, 74,* 257–278.

Goodyer, I. M., & Altham, P. M. (1991). Lifetime exit events and recent social and family adversities in anxious and depressed school-age children and adolescents: I. *Journal of Affective Disorders, 21,* 219–228.

Hammen, C. (1991). *Depression runs in families: The social context of risk and resilience in children of depressed mothers.* New York: Springer-Verlag.

Kingery, J. N., Erdley, C. A., Marshall, K. C., Whitaker, K. G., & Reuter, T. R. (2010). Peer experiences of anxious and socially withdrawn youth: An integrative review of the developmental and clinical literature. *Clinical Child and Family Psychology Review, 13,* 91–128.

Klerman, G. L., DiMascio, A., Weissman, M., Prusoff, B., & Paykel, E. S. (1974). Treatment of depression by drugs and psychotherapy. *American Journal of Psychiatry, 131,* 186–191.

Krupnick, J. L., Green, B. L., Stockton, P., Miranda, J., Krause, E., & Mete, M. (2008). Group interpersonal psychotherapy for low-income women with posttraumatic stress disorder. *Psychotherapy Research, 18,* 497–507.

Lipsitz, J. D., Gur, M., Miller, N., Forand, N., Vermes, D., & Fyer, A. J. (2006). An open pilot study of interpersonal psychotherapy for panic disorder (IPT-PD). *Journal of Nervous and Mental Disease, 194,* 440–445.

Lipsitz, J. D., Gur, M., Vermes, D., Petkova, E., Cheng, J., Miller, N., et al. (2008). A randomized trial of interpersonal therapy versus supportive therapy for social anxiety disorder. *Depression and Anxiety, 25,* 542–553.

Lipsitz, J. D., Markowitz, J. C., Cherry, S., & Fyer, A. J. (1999). Open trial of interpersonal psychotherapy for the treatment of social phobia. *American Journal of Psychiatry, 156,* 1814–1816.

Luty, S. E., Carter, J. D., McKenzie, J. M., Rae, A. M., Frampton, C. M. A., Mulder, R. T., et al. (2007). Randomised controlled trial of interpersonal psychotherapy and cognitive-behavioural therapy for depression. *British Journal of Psychiatry, 190,* 496–502.

McLeod, B. D., Weisz, J. R., & Wood, J. J. (2007). Examining the association between parenting and childhood depression: A meta-analysis. *Clinical Psychology Review, 27,* 986–1003.

McLeod, B. D., Wood, J. J., & Weisz, J. R. (2007). Examining the association between parenting and childhood anxiety: A meta-analysis. *Clinical Psychology Review, 27,* 155–172.

Meyer, A. (1957). *Psychobiology: A science of man.* Springfield, IL: Charles C. Thomas.

Mufson, L., Dorta, K. P., Moreau, D., & Weissman, M. M. (2004). *Interpersonal psychotherapy for depressed adolescents* (2nd ed.). New York: Guilford Press.

Mufson, L., Dorta, K. P., Wickramaratne, P., Nomura, Y., Olfson, M., & Weissman, M. M. (2004). A randomized effectiveness trial of interpersonal psychotherapy for depressed adolescents. *Archives of General Psychiatry, 6,* 577–584.

Mufson, L., Weissman, M. M., Moreau, D., & Garfinkel, R. (1999). Efficacy of interpersonal psychotherapy for depressed adolescents. *Archives of General Psychiatry, 56,* 573–579.

Newman, M. G., & Erickson, T. M. (2010). Generalized anxiety disorder. In J. G. Beck (Ed.), *Interpersonal processes in the anxiety disorders: Implications for understanding psychopathology and treatment* (pp. 235–259). Washington, DC: American Psychological Association.

Rapee, R. M., & Szollos, A. A. (2002). Developmental antecedents of clinical anxiety in childhood. *Behaviour Change, 19,* 146–157.

Reynolds, C. F., III, Dew, M. A., Martire, L. M., Miller, M. D., Cyranowski, J. M., Lenze, E., et al. (2010). Treating depression to remission in older adults: A controlled evaluation of combined escitalopram with interpersonal psychotherapy versus escitalopram with depression care management. *International Journal of Geriatric Psychiatry, 25,* 1134–1141.

Reynolds, C. F., III, Frank, E., Perel, J. M., Imber, S. D., Cornes, C., Miller, M. D., et al. (1999). Nortriptyline and interpersonal psychotherapy as maintenance therapies for recurrent major depression: A randomized controlled trial in patients older than 59 years. *Journal of the American Medical Association, 281,* 39–45.

Roemer, L., Molina, S., & Borkovec, T. D. (1997). An investigation of worry content among generally anxious individuals. *Journal of Nervous and Mental Disease, 185,* 314–319.

Rohde, P. (2012). Applying transdiagnostic approaches to treatments with children and adolescents: Innovative models that are ready for more systematic evaluation. *Cognitive and Behavioral Practice, 19,* 83–86.

Rosselló, J., & Bernal, G. (1999). The efficacy of cognitive-behavioral and interpersonal treatments for depression in Puerto Rican adolescents. *Journal of Consulting and Clinical Psychology, 67,* 734–745.

Rosselló, J., Bernal, G., & Rivera-Medina, C. (2008). Individual and group CBT and IPT for Puerto Rican adolescents with depressive symptoms. *Cultural Diversity and Ethnic Minority Psychology, 14,* 234–245.

Rudolph, K. D., Hammen, C., Burge, D., Lindberg, N., Herzberg, D., & Daley, S. E. (2000). Toward an interpersonal life-stress model of depression: The developmental context of stress generation. *Development and Psychopathology, 12,* 215–234.

Sloane, R. B., Stapes, F. R., & Schneider, L. S. (1985). Interpersonal therapy versus nortriptyline for depression in the elderly. In G. D. Burrow, T. R. Norman, & L. Dennerstein (Eds.), *Clinical and pharmacological studies in psychiatric disorders* (pp. 344–346). London: Libbey.

Stangier, U., Schramm, E., Heidenreich, T., Berger, M., & Clark, D. M. (2011). Cognitive therapy vs. interpersonal psychotherapy in social anxiety disorder: A randomized controlled trial. *Archives of General Psychiatry, 68,* 692–700.

Starr, L. R., & Davila, J. (2008). Differentiating interpersonal correlates of depressive symptoms and social anxiety in adolescence: Implications for models of comorbidity. *Journal of Clinical Child and Adolescent Psychology, 37,* 337–349.

Stuart, S., Robertson, M., & O'Hara, M. W. (2006). The future of interpersonal psychotherapy. *Psychiatric Annals, 36,* 578–588.

Sullivan, H. S. (1953). *The interpersonal theory of psychiatry.* New York: Norton.

Talbot, N. L., Conwell, Y., O'Hara, M. W., Stuart, S., Ward, E. A., Gamble, S. A., et al. (2005). Interpersonal psychotherapy for depressed women with sexual abuse histories: A pilot study in a community mental health center. *Journal of Nervous and Mental Disease, 193,* 847–850.

Talbot, N. L., & Gamble, S. A. (2008). IPT for women with trauma histories in community mental health care. *Journal of Contemporary Psychotherapy, 38,* 35–44.

Tanofsky-Kraff, M., Wilfley, D. E., Young, J. F., Mufson, L., Yanovski, S. Z., Glasofer, D. R., et al. (2007). Preventing excessive weight gain in adolescents: Interpersonal psychotherapy for binge eating. *Obesity, 15,* 1345–1355.

Tanofsky-Kraff, M., Wilfley, D. E., Young, J. F., Mufson, L., Yanovski, S. Z., Glasofer, D. R., et al. (2010). A pilot study of interpersonal psychotherapy for preventing excess weight gain in adolescent girls at-risk for obesity. *International Journal of Eating Disorders, 43,* 701–706.

Verdeli, H., Clougherty, K., Bolton, P., Speelman, L., Ndogoni, L., Bass, J., et al.

(2003). Adapting group interpersonal psychotherapy for a developing country: Experience in rural Uganda. *World Psychiatry, 2,* 114–120.

Verdeli, H., Clougherty, K., Onyango, G., Lewandowski, E., Speelman, L., Betancourt, T., et al. (2008). Group interpersonal psychotherapy for depressed youth in IDP camps in northern Uganda: Adaptation and training. *Child and Adolescent Psychiatric Clinics of North America, 17,* 605–624.

Weersing, V. R., Gonzalez, A., Campo, J. V., & Lucas, A. N. (2008). Brief behavioral therapy for pediatric anxiety and depression: Piloting an integrated treatment approach. *Cognitive and Behavioral Practice, 15,* 126–139.

Weissman, M. M., Klerman, G. L., Paykel, E. S., Prusoff, B., & Hanson, B. (1974). Treatment effects on the social adjustment of depressed patients. *Archives of General Psychiatry, 30,* 771–778.

Weissman, M. M., Markowitz, J. C., & Klerman, G. L. (2000). *Comprehensive guide to interpersonal psychotherapy.* New York: Basic Books.

Weissman, M. M., Prusoff, B. A., DiMascio, A., Neu, C., Goklaney, M., & Klerman, G. L. (1979). The efficacy of drugs and psychotherapy in the treatment of acute depressive episodes. *American Journal of Psychiatry, 136,* 555–558.

Wilfley, D. E., Agras, W. S., Telch, C. F., Rossiter, E. M., Schneider, J. A. Cole, A. G., et al. (1993). Group cognitive-behavioral therapy and group interpersonal psychotherapy for the nonpurging bulimic individual: A controlled comparison. *Journal of Consulting and Clinical Psychology, 61,* 296–305.

Wilfley, D. E., Frank, M. A., Welch, R., Spurrell, E. B., & Rounsaville, B. J. (1998). Adapting interpersonal psychotherapy to a group format (IPT-G) for binge eating disorder: Toward a model for adapting empirically supported treatments. *Psychotherapy Research, 8,* 379–391.

Wilfley, D. E., Welch, R. R., Stein, R. I., Spurrell, E. B., Cohen, L. R., Saelens, B. E., et al. (2002). A randomized comparison of group cognitive-behavioral therapy and group interpersonal psychotherapy for the treatment of overweight individuals with binge-eating disorder. *Archives of General Psychiatry, 59,* 713–721.

Wilson, G. T., Wilfley, D. E., Agras, S., & Bryson, S. W. (2010). Psychological treatments of binge eating disorder. *Archives of General Psychiatry, 67,* 94–101.

Young, J. F., Makover, H. B., Cohen, J. R., Mufson, L., Gallop, R., & Benas, J. S. (2012). Interpersonal psychotherapy—adolescent skills training: Anxiety outcomes and impact of comorbidity. *Journal of Clinical Child and Adolescent Psychology, 41,* 640–653.

Young, J. F., & Mufson, L. (2003). *Manual for interpersonal psychotherapy—adolescent skills training (IPT-AST).* New York: Columbia University.

Young, J. F., Mufson, L., & Davies, M. (2006a). Efficacy of interpersonal psychotherapy—adolescent skills training: An indicated preventive intervention for depression. *Journal of Child Psychology and Psychiatry, 47,* 1254–1262.

Young, J. F., Mufson, L., & Davies, M. (2006b). Impact of comorbid anxiety in an effectiveness study of interpersonal psychotherapy for depressed adolescents. *Journal of the American Academy of Child and Adolescent Psychiatry, 45,* 904–912.

Young, J. F., Mufson, L., & Gallop, R. (2010). Preventing depression: A randomized trial of interpersonal psychotherapy—adolescent skills training. *Depression and Anxiety, 27,* 426–433.

CHAPTER 10

Dialectical Behavior Therapy for Emotion Dysregulation

Lorie A. Ritschel, Alec L. Miller, and Victoria Taylor

Dialectical behavior therapy (DBT; Linehan, 1993a, 1993b) is an evidence-based treatment originally developed for chronically suicidal adults with borderline personality disorder (BPD). BPD can be thought of as a disorder of emotional, behavioral, cognitive, intrapersonal, and interpersonal dysregulation (Linehan, 1993a); thus, the overarching goal of treatment is to intervene on this pervasive dysregulation and to help individuals with BPD modulate their emotions without engaging in ineffective compensatory or regulatory behaviors (e.g., suicidal or nonsuicidal self-injurious behaviors [NSSI]). According to DSM-5 (American Psychiatric Association, 2013), a diagnosis of BPD requires the presence of at least five out of a possible nine criteria, meaning that considerable variation in symptom presentation exists among individuals with BPD. Moreover, many individuals with BPD also meet criteria for comorbid Axis I disorders (Lieb, Zanarini, Schmahl, Linehan, & Bohus, 2004). In order to treat the myriad areas of dysregulation found among suicidal individuals diagnosed with BPD, Linehan designed DBT (1993a), a multimodal therapy that is both comprehensive and flexible.

DBT synthesizes four distinct theoretical foundations: dialectics, Zen philosophy, behaviorism, and the biosocial theory of emotion dysregulation. The term *dialectical* refers to the philosophy that there is no absolute truth; that is, seemingly opposite ideas (i.e., thesis and antithesis) can both be true at the same time, and their convergence produces a synthesis out of which a new dialectic may arise. As it applies to the practice of psychotherapy, a dialectical philosophy highlights the need for clients to work on simultaneously accepting and changing their thoughts, emotions, and behaviors. DBT therapists teach their patients to move away from black-and-white, "either–or" thinking and instead to view the world in accordance with the idea that there is no absolute truth. For example, a therapist might say, "I believe that you are doing the best you can; and, at the same time, you must do better at tolerating your distress if you want to reach your goals." By learning to reduce polarized thinking, clients achieve the ability to find a middle path, opening up novel pathways to problem solving and reducing cognitive rigidity.

At its core, DBT is a well-balanced blend of acceptance- and change-based strategies (Linehan, 1993a, 1993b). Acceptance-based interventions are primarily informed by the principles of Zen mindfulness practice and teach patients how to accept their reality without trying to change it (including their behaviors, emotions, and circumstances) through mindful and nonjudgmental participation. The change-based interventions used in DBT are largely predicated on the principles of behaviorism and include techniques such as exposure, contingency management, problem solving, and cognitive restructuring. For individuals with BPD, both strategies should be woven together in an iterative, balanced fashion, because individuals with BPD tend to find change without acceptance to be invalidating of their difficulties. At the same time, they are likely to find acceptance without change insufficient in helping them achieve the life they want (and invalidating in its own right).

Linehan's (1993a) biosocial theory posits that BPD emerges from the transaction between biological dysfunction in the individual's emotion regulation system and an invalidating environment. We describe these two elements in turn. Biological dysfunction comprises three components: high emotional sensitivity, pronounced emotional reactivity, and slow return to baseline (Linehan, 1993a). First, individuals with BPD tend to operate in a state of physiological hyperarousal (Ebner-Priemer et al., 2007; Kuo & Linehan, 2009), leaving them more vulnerable to emotional triggers and cues (both intra- and interpersonally). Second, individuals with BPD tend to be more reactive to emotional events than individuals without BPD (Bland, Williams, Scharer, & Manning, 2004; Ebner-Priemer et al., 2007). Given their higher level of emotional sensitivity, this reactivity can result in extreme emotional experiences, such as rage, panic, and profound dysphoria. Third, once dysregulated, individuals with BPD tend to take longer than individuals without BPD to return to emotional baseline (Kuo & Linehan, 2009; Yen, Zlotnick, & Costello, 2002). To draw an analogy, life for individuals with BPD is the emotional equivalent of going to the beach when you already have a sunburn (high baseline arousal), forgetting your sunscreen (greater reactivity to triggers), and having the kind of skin that takes a long time to get back to normal after a sunburn (slow return to baseline).

The second component of the biosocial theory is the invalidating environment. This term refers to any environment that negates, punishes, ignores, or corrects a person's emotions or behaviors *independent of the actual validity of the emotion or behavior*. In essence, an invalidating environment communicates that the individual's perceptions of and responses to the world simply do not make sense. Take the example of a child who is teased at school and reports to her parents that she feels sad when other kids make fun of her. Her parents respond by telling her it is stupid or wrong to feel sad about that and that instead she should be angry with the other kids and with her teachers for not protecting her from such bullying. What results is a mismatch between what the child is feeling and what she is told she *should* feel, which can lead to confusion about emotions and ambivalence about how to respond to a similar trigger (i.e., bullying) in the future. Alternatively, consider the teenager who struggles in his math class and has repeatedly asked his parents for help with homework or to get him a tutor. He comes home at the end of the week having failed a test for which he studied every day and is told that he should have "tried harder." As another example, when teens engage in NSSI, parents often remark that they are "just being manipulative" without recognizing that most teens engage in NSSI as a way to downregulate negative affect (Nock & Prinstein, 2004). These kinds of environments fail to teach the child to recognize, label, and respond to emotions appropriately, and they often inadvertently reinforce ineffective behavior on the part of the child. It is important to note that invalidating environments can include but are not limited to families, peers, school personnel, coaches, and mental health and medical providers (Miller, Rathus, & Linehan, 2007). In sum, the biosocial theory posits that the emotional and behavioral difficulties associated with BPD arise when a child who has difficulty regulating emotion is placed in an environment that pervasively and chronically communicates that the child's responses are inappropriate, faulty, inaccurate, or otherwise invalid (Koerner, Miller, & Wagner, 1998).

Empirical Support for the DBT Model

Standard DBT (i.e., Linehan, 1993a) is a principle-based treatment that includes weekly individual therapy, as-needed intersession telephone coaching, weekly skills-training groups, and weekly therapist consultation team meetings. DBT skills groups are manualized, didactic in nature, and focus on teaching four skill modules: Mindfulness, Interpersonal Effectiveness, Emotion Regulation, and Distress Tolerance. Based on their work with adolescents and their families, Miller, Rathus, and Linehan (2007) developed a fifth skill module titled "Walking the Middle Path," which we describe in greater detail later in this chapter. The Mindfulness module helps clients participate more fully in their lives by building nonjudgmental awareness of themselves and the world around them in the present moment. The Interpersonal Effectiveness module helps clients learn to effectively navigate relationships. The Emotion Regulation module helps clients learn to recognize their emotions and antecedent events, as well as how to cope in more adaptive and effective ways when emotions arise. The Distress Tolerance module helps clients learn to bear negative life events skillfully without engaging in behaviors that worsen the emotional or behavioral consequences of such events (e.g., NSSI, substance use). As we discuss in greater detail later in this chapter, the individual therapist helps the patient apply the skills learned in DBT group to the specific situations in her or his life in weekly sessions and coaching calls.

DBT has been adapted for use across a variety of age ranges, diagnostic categories, and treatment settings (Miller et al., 2007). The flexibility of the treatment and adaptability for such a wide variety of patients seems to be possible due to (1) the emphasis placed on balancing change and acceptance strategies and skills when treating multidiagnostic patients and (2) the focus on emotion dysregulation as the underlying cause of distress, rather than a focus on specific diagnostic categories. We first describe the empirical evidence of DBT; later in this chapter we discuss how the treatment has been adapted for use with patients with heterogeneous diagnoses.

DBT with Adults

There is ample evidence from numerous randomized controlled outpatient and inpatient trials that patients with chronic suicidality, NSSI, and those diagnosed with BPD benefit greatly from DBT (for a review, see Lynch, Trost, Salsman, & Linehan, 2007). The treatment has been shown to improve social and global adjustment while reducing attrition rates, decreasing inpatient psychiatric days and emergency room usage, and reducing the frequency and severity of suicide attempts, suicidal ideation, and NSSI (Bohus et al., 2003; Koons et al., 2001; Linehan et al., 1991, 2006; Lynch, Morse, Mendelson, & Robins, 2003; van den Bosch, Koeter, Stijnen, Verheul, & van den Brink, 2005; Verheul et al., 2003).

DBT research has been conducted in a variety of treatment settings, including outpatient (Linehan 1993a; Linehan et al., 1991, 2006; van den Bosch et al., 2005; Verheul et al., 2003), partial hospital (Ben-Porath, Wisniewski, & Warren, 2009; Gratz, Lacroce, & Gunderson, 2006), inpatient (Barley et al., 1993; Bohus et al., 2000, 2003; Koons et al., 2001; Linehan et al., 1999; Simpson et al., 1998) and forensic (Bradley & Follingstad, 2003; Berzins & Trestman 2004; Evershed et al., 2003) settings. Furthermore, DBT has been adapted for adults with a variety of presenting problems. Evidence published to date supports the use of DBT as a treatment for eating disorders (Hill, Craighead, & Safer, 2011; Safer, Telch, & Agras,

2001; Telch, Agras, & Linehan, 2001), treatment-resistant depression (Harley, Sprich, Safren, Jacobo, & Fava, 2008), and depression in older adults with mixed personality features (Lynch, 2000; Lynch et al., 2003). Other research has found that DBT is effective for BPD that is comorbid with substance abuse (Linehan et al., 1999, 2002; van den Bosch et al., 2005) and with eating disorders (Palmer et al., 2003).

DBT with Adolescents

Although many professionals are still reluctant to make a formal personality disorder diagnosis in adolescents, a substantial number of teenagers exhibit the chronic suicidality, NSSI, and emotion regulation difficulties that are the hallmark features of BPD in adults (Miller, Muehlenkamp, & Jacobson, 2008). Moreover, many of these adolescents receive multiple Axis I diagnoses, including mood, anxiety, substance use, and disruptive behavior disorders. Given these similarities in clinical presentation and the success of DBT with adults with BPD, Miller and colleagues (Miller, Rathus, Linehan, Wetzler, & Leigh, 1997; Miller et al., 2007; Rathus & Miller, 2002) adapted DBT for adolescents who have BPD features. According to a recent review (Groves, Backer, van den Bosch, & Miller, 2012), 12 published studies have examined the effectiveness of DBT with various adolescent populations using quasi-experimental designs. Two randomized controlled trials (RCTs) are in progress in Norway (Tørmoen et al., 2009) and New Zealand (Cooney, Davis, Thompson, & Stewart, 2008). In the last decade, various studies have evaluated DBT as a promising treatment for adolescents with various psychological disorders, including adolescents diagnosed with borderline personality features and who engage in suicidal behavior and/or NSSI (Fleischhaker, Munz, Böhme, Sixt, & Schulz, 2006; James, Taylor, Winmill, & Alfoadari, 2008; Rathus & Miller, 2002; Woodberry & Poponoe, 2008), as well as adolescents diagnosed with the following Axis I disorders: bipolar disorder (Goldstein, Axelson, Birmaher, & Brent, 2007); eating disorders (Safer, Lock, & Couturier, 2007; Salbach, Klinkowski, Pfeiffer, Lehmkuhl, & Korte, 2007; Salbach-Andrae, Bohnekamp, Pfeiffer, Lehmkuhl, & Miller, 2008); and oppositional defiant disorder (ODD) (Nelson-Gray et al., 2006). Finally, evidence suggests that DBT is promising for adolescents deemed by the courts to be juvenile offenders (Trupin, Stewart, Beach, & Boesky, 2002).

As is the case in the adult literature, DBT with adolescents has been adapted for use in a variety of settings, such as acute inpatient hospitals (Katz, Cox, Gunasekara, & Miller, 2004), long-term inpatient hospitals (McDonnell et al., 2010), residential treatment settings (Sunseri, 2004), forensic settings (Trupin et al., 2002), schools (Mason, Catucci, Lusk, & Johnson, 2009; Sally, Jackson, Carney, Kevelson, & Miller, 2002), and children's medical hospitals for youth with chronic medical conditions (Hashim, Vadnais, & Miller, in press). Thus, despite significant variability in populations, settings, structure, and format of treatment, these results suggest that DBT is a promising treatment for adolescents with a range of diagnostic and behavioral problems, including suicidal behaviors and NSSI and other problems associated with BPD, bipolar disorder, externalizing disorders, and eating disorders (Groves et al., 2012). While we await the results of RCTs applied to adolescents with varying disorders, our clinical wisdom, coupled with the results from the quasi-experimental and within-subjects treatment studies cited earlier, lend credibility to the notion that DBT is an appropriate model for transdiagnostic use with both adults and adolescents.

Why DBT Can Be Applied Transdiagnostically

Emotion dysregulation is widely considered to be the primary underlying feature of BPD in both adults and adolescents (Miller et al., 2007), as well as a key component of a variety of other psychological disorders (McRae & Gross, 2009). Difficulties in basic emotion regulation are often associated with a host of problematic behaviors (e.g., substance abuse, NSSI, suicide, binge eating; Selby, Anestis, Bender, & Joiner, 2009) and interpersonal difficulties (e.g., chaotic relationships, disorganized social networks; Clifton, Pilkonis, & McCarty, 2007), which are common transdiagnostic target behaviors. Moreover, difficulties with emotion regulation are posited to play a central role in both internalizing (Abela, Brozina, & Haigh, 2002; Lyubomirsky & Nolen-Hoeksema, 1995; McLaughlin, Hatzenbuehler, & Hilt, 2009; Zeman, Shipman, & Suveg, 2002) and externalizing (Kostiuk & Fouts, 2002; Leibenluft, Charney, & Pine, 2003) disorders in adolescents.

DBT provides a unifying theoretical model that explains disparate conditions via common mechanisms and provides principles and treatment strategies that are flexible enough to accommodate diverse problems. According to the biosocial theory that underpins DBT, the behavioral, cognitive, interpersonal, and intrapersonal dysregulation often seen in BPD stems from a core difficulty with emotion regulation; thus, the primary treatment target is to improve emotion regulatory capacities. Hence, although a patient may present with a heterogeneous and complicated diagnostic picture, DBT was designed to target the emotions and associated dysfunctional behaviors in a hierarchical, principle-based fashion (see Linehan, 1993a; Miller et al., 2007) rather than targeting the "disorder" or the "diagnosis" itself. For example, one adolescent with clinical depression may present with sadness, anhedonia, and social withdrawal, whereas another adolescent with depression may present with irritability, sleep disturbance, and suicidal ideation. Although both teens carry the same diagnosis, it is the specific behaviors and emotions that will be targeted within the DBT treatment model. Similarly, two patients may be assigned different diagnoses even if both engage in NSSI and make repeated suicide attempts. The DBT clinician places a higher priority on targeting these dysfunctional, problematic behaviors first before targeting the depression, social anxiety, or other diagnoses the youth may carry. If, of course, a patient presents with a pure and uncomplicated Axis I diagnosis for which a more straightforward treatment (e.g., CBT) exists, the clinician would be wise to target the presenting problem directly using streamlined interventions rather than implementing the hierarchical DBT approach to treatment we are describing. This recommendation is based in part on the comprehensive and time-intensive nature of DBT; that is, weekly individual and group therapy may not be warranted for a case of major depression that is likely to respond to a more streamlined empirically supported treatment (e.g., 12–16 sessions of individual CBT). Although some of the principles that underlie DBT may be applicable for straightforward Axis I disorders, and although emotion dysregulation may be a common treatment target even in uncomplicated cases, we advocate for treatment decisions based on a combination of empirical support and parsimony.

Transdiagnostic Theory Underlying DBT

The concept of a transdiagnostic treatment model can be applied both across and within patients. That is, a treatment can be considered transdiagnostic if it effectively treats a number of patients presenting for treatment with distinct diagnostic concerns (e.g., bipolar disorder, eating disorders, substance use disorders, BPD). Alternatively, a transdiagnostic treatment model can be used to treat one patient who presents with multiple diagnostic concerns (e.g., one patient who meets criteria for bipolar disorder, alcohol dependence, and BPD). DBT fits both of these types of models; the literature to date suggests that DBT is effective across various diagnoses (see previous discussion), as well as for patients who meet criteria for more than one diagnosis on Axes I and II (Groves et al., 2012; James et al., 2008). This flexibility can be explained in part by the fact that DBT is a principle-driven (rather than protocol-driven) approach to treatment. Whereas protocol-driven treatments typically are designed to address a specific diagnostic concern and generally unfold in a stepwise fashion (e.g., cognitive-behavior therapy [CBT]—Beck, Rush, Shaw, & Emery, 1979; panic control treatment—Barlow & Cerny, 1988), principle-driven treatments are designed to be flexibly implemented while adhering to therapeutic techniques unique to the model (e.g., acceptance and commitment therapy—Hayes, Strosahl, & Wilson, 1999; behavioral activation—Dimidjian et al., 2006). Like other principle-driven treatments, DBT was designed to target and treat emotional and behavioral dysregulation and their sequelae and thus can successfully be implemented across a range of diagnostic presentations. There are five basic elements of DBT that allow it to fit this definition of a transdiagnostic model, and we describe each one in turn.

1. *DBT targets emotion dysregulation in general rather than disorders specifically.* As discussed, a basic assumption of DBT is that individuals with BPD suffer from pervasive emotion regulation problems that have arisen through the transaction between difficulties in the endogenous emotion regulation system (e.g., hyperreactivity in the amygdala and decreased central serotonergic activity; New & Siever, 2002) and an invalidating environment (e.g., an environment that is a poor fit with this emotional vulnerability). This focus on emotion dysregulation in general allows the treatment to be crafted to fit the needs of patients with a range of diagnoses. Of course, an underlying problem with emotion regulation can produce a wide variety of symptoms and behavioral manifestations of distress and emotional responding; the DBT focus on both function and topography of behavior allows the therapist to move flexibly among these behavior targets as they are defined within the treatment hierarchy.

2. *Individual sessions are guided by a structured yet flexible target hierarchy.* Each individual DBT session follows a four-item target hierarchy that is designed to be both structured and flexible. In order to set the agenda for each session, patients receiving DBT are asked to complete diary cards each day that assess their urges and actions regarding target behaviors, the degree to which they experience various emotions, and skills used over the course of the week. Diary cards help the therapist and patient establish an agenda that is both consistent with the DBT target hierarchy and in line with helping the patient reach his or her goals. The principle behind the structure of this hierarchy is that anything that is likely to disrupt treatment must be addressed first and foremost. In particular, life-threatening behaviors (i.e., suicide attempts, urges, threats, or increased suicidal ideation) receive top priority in DBT for the simple reason that clients who kill themselves are no longer in treatment. In addition, patients who make suicide attempts or who struggle with high or increasing suicidal ideation are at risk for hospitalization, which also can disrupt treatment.[1] Self-harming behaviors (e.g., cutting, burning) are addressed next based on a similar rationale: NSSI is not only a significant

---

[1]To be clear, hospitalization can and should be used to ensure patient safety. That said, a primary goal of DBT is to reduce the duration and frequency of hospitalization and emergency room usage in the spirit of helping the patient create a life worth living. Data from a multitude of studies have demonstrated that DBT is indeed effective at achieving this goal.

risk for completed suicide (Nock, Joiner, Gordon, Lloyd-Richardson, & Prinstein, 2006) but is also antithetical to building a life worth living and often results in hospitalizations that disrupt treatment. After targeting life-threatening behaviors, the second agenda item on the treatment target hierarchy is referred to as therapy-interfering behaviors (TIB). These are any behaviors on the part of the patient, the family, *or the therapist* that increase the likelihood that therapy will end (either by the patient dropping out or the therapist "firing" the patient). Examples of patient TIB include nonattendance, lateness, incomplete homework, and too many or too few coaching calls. Examples of family TIB include not bringing teens to therapy, not attending skills-training groups, and maintaining a negative attitude toward DBT treatment or the DBT therapist. Examples of therapist TIB include pushing too hard for change without sufficient validation, acceptance of the patient's difficulties without helping him or her change, and not returning phone calls in a timely fashion.

The third agenda item on the treatment target hierarchy encompasses quality-of-life-interfering behaviors (QOL). This is the broadest of the agenda items and is structured collaboratively by the therapist and patient in order, from most to least life-impairing behaviors. QOL items include any other diagnosable psychiatric conditions (e.g., mood and anxiety disorders, substance-related disorders, etc.), medical conditions (e.g., diabetes), or conditions that potentially compromise a person's well-being, such as relationship, financial, employment, school, or housing issues. For example, a patient may present for treatment with panic attacks, depression, school difficulties, and a high-conflict relationship with a boyfriend. If the teen attends school that week and reports negligible panic attacks and depressed mood but substantial conflicts with her boyfriend, the QOL agenda would likely be set as follows: interpersonal conflicts with boyfriend, depression, panic attacks, and school.

The fourth agenda on the treatment target hierarchy is increasing behavioral skills. Hence, while the therapist and patient are attending to reducing treatment targets 1 (suicide, NSSI), 2 (TIB), and 3 (QOL), they are also trying to increase treatment target 4 (i.e., behavioral skills). The idea is to replace problematic and dysfunctional behaviors with prosocial and skillful behaviors. Although the DBT skills trainer is often responsible for providing the initial didactic training of these skills, the individual DBT therapist's role is to help the patient apply, strengthen, and generalize these skills to his or her daily life.

3. *DBT relies on effective case conceptualization.* DBT can be applied with a variety of patients and diagnoses because of its strong reliance on comprehensive and effective case conceptualization. With input from the consultation team, the therapist summarizes the patient's demographic information and history and then organizes his or her presenting

problems into primary and secondary treatment targets (see Figure 10.1 for a case conceptualization worksheet). As discussed previously, primary treatment targets include life-threatening, therapy-interfering, and quality-of-life-interfering behaviors. Linehan (1993a) identified numerous behavioral patterns that contribute to the maintenance of these primary target behaviors. These patterns are known as secondary treatment targets and include emotional vulnerability versus self-invalidation, active passivity versus apparent competence, and unrelenting crises versus inhibited grieving (for a discussion of these secondary targets, see Linehan, 1993a). For adolescent patients, Rathus and Miller (2000) identified another set of secondary targets that are used to characterize the patient and her or his interactions with her or his primary environment (i.e., families, school personnel, therapists). These targets include excessive leniency versus authoritarian control, normalizing pathological behavior versus pathologizing normative behaviors, and forcing autonomy versus fostering dependence (see Miller et al., 2007). Finally, the therapist evaluates and summarizes the patient's skill strengths and deficits according to the DBT skill modules.

This type of conceptualization allows for the inclusion of *all* of the patient's difficulties and strengths, both intra- and interpersonally, as well as across diagnostic categories. Moreover, environmental factors (e.g., different rules implemented by different caretakers) that may be reinforcing unskillful behaviors are incorporated, allowing the therapist to take a broad view of the patient's life outside of the therapy setting. Case conceptualizations can and should change over time; we advise therapists to complete a case conceptualization form early in treatment (around session 4), to present this case conceptualization to the consultation team for feedback and discussion, and to periodically update the form. In addition to the immediate treatment utility that DBT case conceptualizations provide, they also yield meaningful data on the changes occurring over the course of treatment. Such rich data can be shared with patients and their families and are a particularly useful tool for therapists preparing for treatment termination when patients have met their treatment goals.

4. *DBT includes four stages of treatment and provides a comprehensive framework.* The overarching course of DBT treatment is structured in four stages preceded by a pretreatment stage, all of which have associ-ated treatment goals (see Linehan, 1993a, for a discussion of these treatment stages). At initial presentation, patients are considered to be in the pretreatment stage, during which the therapist helps the patient operationalize problems, identify goals, and make a commitment to working on those goals and to DBT treatment. In Stage 1, the predominant problem is severe behavioral dyscontrol, and the associated treatment goal is behavioral control. Adolescent patients are typically asked (depending on

Patient's Name: _____

Date treatment began: _____

Date of this case conceptualization: _____

This is the _____ case conceptualization I have completed for this patient.

Dates of previous completed conceptualizations:

    Baseline/beginning of treatment: _____

    During treatment: _____

Demographic Information and History: _____

_____

_____

_____

_____

_____

Primary Treatment Targets

Life-threatening: _____

_____

TIB (patient and therapist): _____

_____

QOL (most to least severe): _____

_____

Secondary Treatment Targets

Emotional vulnerability: _____

_____

Self-invalidation: _____

_____

Active-passivity: _____

_____

Apparent competence: _____

_____

Unrelenting crisis: _____

_____

Inhibited grieving: _____

_____

(continued)

FIGURE 10.1. DBT case conceptualization worksheet.

Adolescent/Family Secondary Targets

Excessive leniency: _____

_____

Authoritarian control: _____

_____

Normalizing pathology: _____

_____

Pathologizing the norm: _____

_____

Forcing autonomy: _____

_____

Fostering dependence: _____

Assessment of Patient Skills

Mindfulness: _____

_____

Emotion regulation: _____

_____

Distress tolerance: _____

_____

Interpersonal effectiveness: _____

_____

Assessment of Family Middle Path Skills

Behaviorism: _____

_____

Validation: _____

_____

Dialectics: _____

_____

FIGURE 10.1. *(continued)*

the specific treatment program) to commit to a minimum of 6 months of treatment,[2] during which the primary focus is to reduce problematic behaviors (e.g., suicide attempts, NSSI, substance use, depression, school difficulties, interpersonal conflicts). As behavioral control is achieved and the patient stabilizes, she or he moves into Stage 2, in which the predominant problem is quiet desperation, and the associated treatment goal is emotional experiencing. For patients who have endured traumatic life events, including severe social alienation, neglect, and abuse, their trauma histories are addressed in Stage 2 via prolonged exposure therapy (Harned & Linehan, 2008). When a patient reaches Stage 3, the focus is on ordinary problems in living, with the goal of learning to experience typical happiness and unhappiness. Possible interventions useful to address Stage 3 targets include, but are not limited to, problem solving, standard CBT, and family therapy. Finally, the predominant problem in Stage 4 is a feeling of incompleteness, and the associated treatment goal is to develop meaning and a sense of joy and freedom. It is important to note that there is no time requirement with any of these stages; that is, one patient may accomplish his or her Stage 1 goals in 3 months, whereas another patient may remain in Stage 1 for 6 months. In addition, these stages are not mutually exclusive; a patient who has progressed to Stage 2 may revert to Stage 1 treatment targets following a major life stressor or resurgence of behavioral dyscontrol.[3]

5. *Different skills for different people or for the same person at different times.* Finally, DBT teaches skills that can be flexibly implemented according to the patient's needs. Although many Stage 1 patients need skills from all of the modules taught in the skills-training group, some patients may place greater emphasis on certain skills than others. For example, a teen who is engaging in frequent NSSI may spend more time practicing distress tolerance skills, whereas a teen who has discontinued self-harm but who continues to experience significant social phobia may spend more time practicing the emotion regulation skill of opposite action. Importantly, patients and therapists work together collaboratively to ensure that (1) patients acquire the full array of DBT skills and (2) those skills are strengthened and generalized as needed for that particular individual.

DBT's Transdiagnostic Strategies and Techniques

There are five functions of comprehensive DBT treatment, all of which apply to any adolescent patient experiencing emotional, behavioral, or

[2]Adults are asked to commit to 1 year.

[3]It is important to note that no empirical studies have addressed the use of DBT beyond Stage 2.

interpersonal dysregulation. The first function is *to enhance the patient's overall capabilities*, with a special emphasis on emotion regulation. The second is *to improve motivational factors*. Therapists assess factors that interfere with behavioral change and, based on this assessment, choose from a variety of interventions (e.g., skills coaching, cognitive restructuring, exposure, modification of behavioral contingencies). The third is *to ensure generalization to the adolescent's natural environment*. By remaining accessible between sessions for telephone consultation, therapists encourage adolescents to call for skills coaching during real-life situations and stressors.[4] The fourth function is *to enhance therapist capabilities and his or her motivation to treat effectively*. The DBT consultation team provides a supportive network of therapists who offer "therapy for the therapist." The functions of the team are to provide validation, to troubleshoot problems, to generate empathy toward the patient and his or her family, and to assist in case conceptualization. Perhaps most essential in working with youth with complex problems and their families, the consultation team also assesses and treats therapist burnout. Finally, the fifth function of DBT is *to structure the environment so that treatment can be implemented effectively by the patient*. By holding family sessions on an as-needed basis and by requiring family members to accompany patients to skills-training groups, DBT ensures that adolescents are working toward change within their family systems so that negative behaviors are not reinforced.

A closer examination of the structure of skills training and individual DBT further highlights the transdiagnostic nature of DBT treatment strategies. Each of the five modules that are taught in group skills training were designed to target a specific area of dysregulation: the Mindfulness module targets identity dysregulation (e.g., poor self-awareness, poor attentional control); Distress Tolerance targets behavioral dysregulation; Emotion Regulation targets emotion dysregulation; Interpersonal Effectiveness targets interpersonal and relational dysregulation; and Walking the Middle Path targets cognitive and familial dysregulation.

First, skills trainers teach mindfulness skills in an effort to address adolescents' confusion about self and to improve attentional capacity. As teens' ability to engage in abstract and hypothetical reasoning emerges, adolescents become more self-aware and self-reflective (Wagner, Rathus, & Miller, 2006). Coupled with the normative adolescent task of identity development, these new cognitive abilities leave some adolescents feeling overwhelmed. The practice of mindfulness in DBT is a behavioral application of an eastern meditative practice that directs one's attention to what is occurring in the present moment while maintaining a

---

[4]Some adolescent DBT programs also encourage family members who are simultaneously participating in skills training to contact the skills trainers for coaching related to challenging issues they are having with their adolescents (Miller et al., 2007).

compassionate, nonjudgmental stance. Research has suggested the utility of combining mindfulness therapy with CBT for relapse prevention and symptom reduction in a variety of disorders, including depression (Segal, Williams, & Teasdale, 2002), generalized anxiety disorder (Rapgay, Bystritsky, Dafter, & Spearman, 2011), and substance abuse (Breslin, Zack, & McMain, 2002). DBT presents "wise mind" as a balance between emotion and reason in which one can use intuition to engage in the moment and to act only after considering one's thoughts and emotions. DBT provides adolescents with three mindfulness skills to achieve wise mind (*observe, describe,* and *participate*) and three skills for remaining mindful (*don't judge, stay focused,* and *do what works*). By learning to observe and describe without judging, adolescents gain knowledge about their thoughts, feelings, physiological reactions, and urges. Mindfulness can thus enhance self-knowledge and self-awareness so that adolescents can make decisions with both emotional and rational input (Wagner et al., 2006).

Mindfulness underscores all of the DBT skills and modalities of treatment; in fact, mindfulness skills are taught between each of the other skill modules (see Figure 10.2). Adolescents and their family members learn mindfulness formally in skills-training groups, practice it in individual psychotherapy, and use it as needed during telephone consultations and when practicing skills between sessions. Mindfulness is of greatest import for patients who become emotionally dysregulated and then engage in

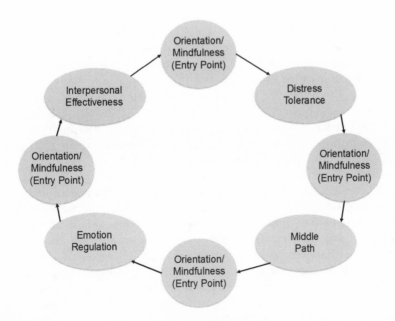

FIGURE 10.2. Entry points and order of skills-training modules in DBT-A groups.

impulsive behaviors. By improving an adolescent's ability to observe and identify their negative affective states, to notice their urges, and to listen to "wise mind" prior to acting, mindfulness can help effectively reduce emotional outbursts, suicide attempts, NSSI, and any other problematic behavior engendered by negative emotions.

The Distress Tolerance module addresses impulsive and reactive behaviors. Skills trainers teach adolescents how to radically accept situations they cannot change, to make "pros" and "cons" lists to help them skillfully evaluate whether to engage in effective or ineffective behaviors, and to use crisis survival skills such as distraction and self-soothing to stop them from making problematic situations worse. Crisis survival skills can be used for patients at risk for suicide, NSSI, running away, using drugs, school refusal, blurting out in class, fighting, binging/restricting food, or engaging in other problematic behaviors. Doodling, playing a video game, listening to music, eating a favorite food, and applying lotion to one's body are all examples of distress tolerance skills. By providing alternative "replacement" behaviors to their heretofore problematic urges/behaviors, DBT therapists use tenets of classical and operant conditioning to teach adolescents to pair new, nonharmful behaviors with feeling better and to reward teens for skillful behavior.

The Emotion Regulation module teaches adolescents how to engage in more positive events and how to reduce vulnerability to negative emotions. Skills trainers teach adolescents to identify and "ride out" uncomfortable emotions so as to expose adolescents to the inevitability and finite nature of such emotions, as well as to teach them that emotions communicate important information to themselves and others. Adolescents learn to differentiate between primary and secondary emotions, to identify unjustified emotions, and to act opposite to their emotional urges as a way to change unhelpful or unjustified emotions. They learn how to increase positive emotions by engaging in pleasant activities and building mastery. They also learn to reduce their vulnerability to emotions by improving sleep hygiene and eating habits, reducing drug and alcohol use, taking prescribed medications regularly, getting regular exercise, and treating physical illnesses.

The Interpersonal Effectiveness module teaches adolescents how to communicate effectively and how to prioritize their interpersonal goals and objectives (i.e., improve and maintain existing relationships, meet a specific goal, or keep their self-respect). Adolescents are taught about the various barriers to being interpersonally effective, such as worry thoughts, indecision, and the power of the environment (e.g., parents, teachers, the legal system). They learn how to negotiate effectively, how to say no to unreasonable or unjustified requests in a skillful manner, and how to modify their nonverbal communication style to be more interpersonally effective. Importantly, patients are taught that even the most skillful people do not always get what they want and that they may need to modify their goals accordingly.

The Walking the Middle Path module was developed to address certain skill deficits that commonly appeared among emotionally dysregulated families. Specifically, Miller and colleagues (2007) noticed that some caregivers and teens had the capacity for skillful behavior outside of their families but that they became invalidating and nondialectical in thought and action in emotional situations that involved other family members. Moreover, they tended to apply ineffective punishments and missed opportunities to effectively reinforce desired behaviors when emotions flared up. In an effort to target these family difficulties, Miller and colleagues designed the Middle Path module, which incorporates three additional skill sets for multifamily skills-training groups: validation, behavioral principles, and dialectical thinking and acting. Validation teaches patients and families how to engage in perspective taking and how to skillfully articulate another person's viewpoint without necessarily agreeing with it. Behaviorism teaches families how to apply the principles of positive and negative reinforcement, shaping, extinction, and effective punishment in the family environment. Finally, dialectics helps adolescents and their parents understand how to think and act dialectically in order to navigate the tensions that arise between teens and parents (described earlier in this chapter) in an effort to help them find a "middle path" and avert extreme thinking and behavioral patterns. Although some families may struggle more with one of these areas than another, the skills are intended to be broadly applicable across dyads within families, as well as families as a whole.

Transdiagnostic Mechanisms Targeted by the DBT Model

As we have discussed throughout this chapter, DBT targets behaviors and mechanisms found across a spectrum of emotional disorders, including emotion dysregulation, confusion about self (i.e., poor self-awareness and attentional control), impulsivity, and interpersonal conflict. Emotion dysregulation is often described as being at the core of most psychological difficulties (see Gross, 2007), although it varies in its topography across disorders. DBT also targets behavioral dysregulation, including impulsive behaviors such as suicide attempts and NSSI. In addition to BPD (Miller et al., 2008), suicidal behaviors among adolescents also are associated with bipolar disorder (Goldstein et al., 2007), depression (Shaffer et al., 1996), anxiety (Lewinsohn, Rohde, & Seeley, 1996), posttraumatic stress disorder (PTSD) (Giaconia et al., 1995), and disruptive behavior disorders, including conduct disorder (Lewinsohn, Klein, & Seeley, 1995; Marttunen, Aro, Henriksson, & Lonnqvist, 1991). Moreover, several researchers have found that aggression with impulsivity is linked to suicidal behaviors among youth (Brent et al., 1994; Grosz et al., 1994; Pfeffer, Newcorn, Kaplan, Mizruchi, & Plutchik, 1988). Other research has shown that adolescents who attempt or commit suicide frequently use or abuse substances; thus, substance use is a primary risk factor for adolescent suicide (for a review, see Miller et al., 2007).

Clinical Vignette

"Stacy," a 16-year-old Caucasian female, presented for therapy in the DBT program after being discharged from a residential treatment facility that focused on remediating substance dependence. At intake, she endorsed symptoms consistent with diagnoses of major depression, generalized anxiety disorder, substance abuse, eating disorder not otherwise specified, and BPD. She also endorsed a history of sexual trauma and several associated symptoms of PTSD, though her symptoms were insufficient to warrant an independent diagnosis. Stacy's parents noted that she had displayed symptoms of depression and anxiety dating back to early childhood. She began cutting herself and experiencing suicidal ideation around age 11. She noted that self-harm, restricted eating, and substance use all functioned to regulate negative emotions and that she tended to "rotate" among these emotion regulation strategies. She had been hospitalized six times prior to starting DBT: twice for suicide attempts and four times for severe NSSI. In addition to her mood difficulties, Stacy and her parents reported that Stacy had been involved in several chaotic romantic relationships and that arguments with her current boyfriend were frequent triggers for Stacy's cutting. Stacy's parents reported that Stacy had reached her developmental milestones appropriately but that she had been difficult to soothe as a baby. They noted high emotionality in Stacy throughout early childhood and adolescence, stating that perceived slights from friends were often enough to prompt alternating sadness and anger for several days and that she often wound up "cutting off" her friendships in the wake of minor altercations. They also reported that Stacy had consistently been a high academic achiever and that she was extremely self-critical and perfectionistic.

Stacy committed to 6 months of individual therapy and group skills training. Her therapist devised a case conceptualization (see Figure 10.3) of Stacy that was reviewed by the consultation team and revised every 3 months throughout treatment. Although Stacy initially expressed some reluctance to engage in therapy, she indicated that she liked the structure of both the skills-training group and individual therapy. In particular, she made good use of her diary card to track problem behaviors and began to see the links between substance use, fights with her boyfriend, mood dysregulation, poor self-management (especially with regard to sleep),

Patient's Name: _Stacy_

Date treatment began: _7/1/2011_

Date of this case conceptualization: _8/1/2011_

This is the _1st_ case conceptualization I have completed for this patient.

Dates of previous completed conceptualizations:

    Baseline/beginning of treatment: _____

    During treatment: _N/A_

Demographic Information and History: _16yo Caucasian female, presents for_ _treatment following 2 months in residential substance abuse treatment_ _facility. History significant for 6 inpatient hospitalizations (2 suicide_ _attempts, 4 NSSI by cutting, burning). Sexual trauma at age 13. Mood_ _lability is present; pt reports significant symptoms of depression and_ _anxiety as well as restricted eating periodically. She denies history of_ _mania or psychotic symptoms. Meets criteria at intake for MDD, GAD,_ _EDNOS, and BPD._

Primary Treatment Targets

Life-threatening: _Elevated suicidal ideation, repeated suicide attempts,_ _NSSI occurring 5–10 times a week._

TIB (patient and therapist): _Initial refusal to complete diary card, some_ _verbally aggressive in-session behaviors, followed by high shame and_ _dissociation, which disrupts session._

QOL (most to least severe): _Depression, anxiety, some continued substance_ _use (marijuana), chaotic relationship with boyfriend, extreme anger_ _displays at home (e.g., breaks objects, screams at parents), unprotected/_ _high-risk sexual intercourse with relatively unknown partners._

Secondary Treatment Targets

Emotional vulnerability: _There have been glimpses of this in two sessions,_ _but thus far pt has generally presented with more self-invalidation_ _than emotional vulnerability. She is clearly reluctant to cry in session_ _and has difficulty making eye contact. At times asks to end sessions_ _early._

Self-invalidation: _Often describes self as "weak" following ineffective_ _behaviors, even with an understandable/difficult/justified trigger;_

(continued)

FIGURE 10.3. Sample initial case conceptualization in DBT: Defining treatment targets.

frequently articulates that she "should" be able to deal with her problems without outside help; highly self-critical for perceived imperfections (academic, familial, body image).

Active-passivity: Particularly problematic with regard to boyfriend; also displayed in terms of improving relationship with parents ("they make the rules, there's nothing I can do about it").

Apparent competence: In first four sessions, has articulated at some point in each session that she's "fine" and doesn't need help.

Unrelenting crisis: Frantic calls from parents each week to date describing a "meltdown" at home; pt reports that abusive nature of relationship with b.f. is escalating into physical violence; pt seeking drugs in known dangerous area of town; states that she is often "a mess" for 2–3 days following negative interactions with parents or b.f.

Inhibited grieving: Manifests in session as tendency to change topic when discussing painful emotional situations; is often reluctant to put difficult items from the week on therapy agenda.

Adolescent/Family Secondary Targets

Excessive leniency: Is given fairly substantial allowance, free use of family car, and generally does not have a curfew, even during school week. Pt does not set many rules for self.

Authoritarian control: Parents periodically get "fed up" and make long and stringent lists of rules that would be difficult for any teen to follow.

Normalizing pathology: Pt and parents minimize marijuana use, even in the home. Pt minimizes NSSI and eating-disordered behavior, saying "all my friends do it too."

Pathologizing the norm: Parents consider body piercing (ears, nose) equivalent to NSSI and describe pt's style of dress as "how crazy people look" (pt tends to wear jeans with holes in them and t-shirts with provocative political slogans or shirts with obscenities).

Forcing autonomy: Pt largely expected to manage own schedule without consistent rules or guidance for how to do so.

Fostering dependence: Pt has few chores around house and has difficulty taking care of herself when parents are away (e.g., does not know how to cook for herself, wash clothes).

FIGURE 10.3. (continued)

and eventual ineffective emotion regulation strategies (e.g., cutting, food restriction). Stacy's suicidal ideation decreased quickly, and she made no more suicide attempts during treatment, although she continued to struggle with other primary treatment targets during her first 6 months in treatment. She eventually discontinued all self-harming behaviors, as well as food restriction, although she elected to continue smoking marijuana periodically. A visual representation of changes in these symptoms over the first 6 months of treatment is presented in Figure 10.4. In terms of TIB, Stacy and her therapist most frequently discussed the fact that Stacy was hesitant to make coaching calls, particularly during weeks when she engaged in NSSI.

As the year progressed, Stacy and her therapist spent the majority of their time dealing with QOL targets. In particular, they spent a considerable amount of time discussing Stacy's relationship with her boyfriend, who had become increasingly verbally and emotionally abusive over the course of the year. This agenda item provided the therapist ample opportunity to address secondary treatment targets, as presented in Figure 10.3. In addition, Stacy and her parents worked on the adolescent and family dilemmas presented in the Middle Path module. Her parents became aware of their tendency to alternate between excessive leniency (e.g., allowing Stacy to stay at a friend's house all week with no curfews, overlooking drug use in the home) and authoritarian control. For example, when they got fed up with Stacy's behavior, they made long lists of house rules that included daily drug testing, no social outings, and daily food allowances that were strictly monitored. Over time, Stacy and her parents worked to find a middle path to dealing with their similarities and differences, and they benefitted tremendously from learning to

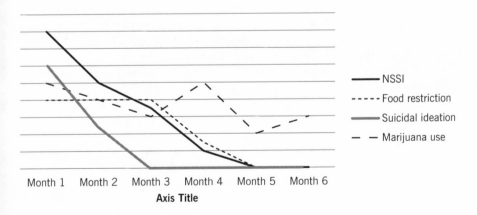

FIGURE 10.4. Example graph of symptom changes over the first 6 months of treatment.

validate each other's experiences. Stacy's parents worked toward developing a reasonable set of house rules, as well as appropriate rewards and consequences. They learned to implement skills both inter- and intrapersonally and maintained a "DBT culture" within their home.

After 1 year of therapy, Stacy had met her Stage 1 treatment targets. She elected to stay in individual therapy for an additional year to work on Stage 2 and 3 goals; during this time she also joined the DBT graduate group. In these contexts, she and her therapist were able to discuss her sexual trauma and eventually to work on developing healthier relationships and better self-esteem and to reduce her tendency to self-invalidate. The remaining portion of her therapy was devoted to ordinary problems in living; in particular, she and her therapist spent time applying DBT skills to the college application process, using the pros and cons list and wise mind skills to select a university that would be the best fit for Stacy.

Limits of the DBT Approach

DBT for adolescents and families is a comprehensive, wraparound treatment model that requires resources for specially trained individual therapists who are consistently available for telephone consultation, group leaders who are also available for telephone consultation for parents, a weekly 2-hour multifamily skills group, a weekly DBT consultation team, and often a weekly 90-minute DBT graduate group for adolescents who have completed the skills training group. Thus, full-package DBT is an intensive treatment for youth with multiple problems and their family members. Given the intensive nature of DBT with adolescents, this treatment is not relevant for those disorders for which simpler treatment options are just as (if not more) effective, such as noncomorbid anxiety disorders and unipolar depression. For those diagnostic categories in which CBT alone is effective (e.g., major depression), investing in DBT would be useful only for those individual patients who are not experiencing symptom relief due to other complex needs and who are beginning to present with more complex emotional and behavioral dysregulation. In addition to the substantial commitment required of families who participate in DBT, the treatment can also be difficult to implement, depending on the structure of the system within which it is being offered. For example, therapists must be trained in DBT and available to co-lead groups, to conduct individual therapy, and to take coaching calls. Systems must be willing to provide time for consultation teams and as-needed supervision to protect against therapist burnout.

There are several patient populations for whom DBT could be effective but whom it could be challenging to accommodate, such as cases in which the family component is difficult or impossible to incorporate. In such cases, the DBT treatment model may need to be modified. Nelson-Gray and colleagues (2006) implemented a DBT treatment program for a group of 32 adolescents with ODD whose family members were unable to attend treatment. The authors modified the treatment so that adolescents attended a weekly adolescent-only skills-training group without individual therapy, multifamily skills training, or telephone consultation. In addition to the financial incentives that were provided to improve homework compliance, the manual was modified to make the material more age-appropriate. The authors reported posttreatment decreases in symptoms of ODD and externalizing behavior problems. Thus, Nelson-Gray and colleagues demonstrated that adolescent DBT can be implemented effectively using adolescent-only groups when necessary.

Similarly, the DBT treatment manual for adolescents and families has been modified to accommodate difficulties specific to adolescents with eating disorders (Salbach et al., 2007) and bipolar disorder (Goldstein et al., 2007). Specifically, these authors added a psychoeducation component for these disorders; they also modified some of the skills in order to better target the specific needs of these populations. For example, when treating patients with eating disorders, modifying DBT to focus on issues of weight and eating is called for, as this patient population faces risks that are not addressed in the standard model.

Trupin and colleagues (2002) provide another example of modifying the adolescent DBT manual to treat a particular population. In this case, the authors conducted a controlled trial comparing a treatment unit receiving DBT, a general population unit receiving DBT, and a general population unit receiving treatment as usual (TAU) among females in a juvenile correctional facility. The authors added behavioral targets specific to unit problematic behaviors and offense-related behaviors. The goal of this treatment protocol was to move members from severe behavioral dyscontrol to behavioral control. Although the study had some methodological difficulties that precluded direct comparisons across conditions, the behavior problems on the DBT treatment unit decreased significantly. Importantly, the staff's punitive actions toward adolescents on the unit were significantly lower in the DBT condition.

Future Directions

DBT is a promising treatment for youth with multiple problems. Numerous quasi-experimental studies and open trials have found DBT to be effective in reducing severe behavioral and emotional dysregulation. Several RCTs are under way to confirm whether DBT is effective for suicidal adolescents with multiple diagnoses, including BPD. Because DBT is a comprehensive, principle-based treatment that flexibly targets numerous problems based on a treatment target hierarchy, DBT therapists are accustomed to treating clients who present with a range of diagnoses and problem behaviors. As a result, based on the aforementioned research and our own clinical experience, we believe DBT to be an ideal treatment for transdiagnostic applications. Future researchers evaluating DBT should consider conducting component analyses and briefer applications of this treatment for youth in other settings, including schools and medical inpatient units.

REFERENCES

Abela, J. R. Z., Brozina, K., & Haigh, E. P. (2002). An examination of the response styles theory of depression in third- and seventh-grade children: A short-term longitudinal study. *Journal of Abnormal Child Psychology, 30*, 515–527.

American Psychiatric Association. (2013). *Diagnostic and statistical manual of mental disorders* (5th ed.). Arlington, VA: Author.

Barley, W. D., Buie, S. E., Peterson, E. W., Hollingsworth, A. S., Griva, M., Hickerson, S. C., et al. (1993). Development of an inpatient cognitive-behavioral treatment program for borderline personality disorder. *Journal of Personality Disorders, 7*, 232–240.

Barlow, D. H., & Cerny, J. A. (1988). *Psychological treatment of panic.* New York: Guilford Press.

Beck, A. T., Rush, A. J., Shaw, B. F., & Emery, G. (1979). *Cognitive therapy of depression.* New York: Guilford Press.

Ben-Porath, D. D., Wisniewski, L., & Warren, M. (2009). Differential treatment response for eating disordered patients with and without a comorbid borderline personality diagnosis using a dialectical behavior therapy-informed approach. *Eating Disorders, 17*, 225–241.

Berzins, L. G., & Trestman, R. L. (2004). The development and implementation of dialectical behavior therapy in forensic settings. *International Journal of Forensic Mental Health, 3*, 93–103.

Bland, A. R., Williams, C. A., Scharer, K., & Manning, S. (2004). Emotion processing in borderline personality disorder. *Issues in Mental Health Nursing, 25*, 655–672.

Bohus, M., Haaf, B., Simms, T., Limberger, M. F., Schmahl, C., Unckel, C., et al. (2003). Effectiveness of inpatient dialectical behavioral therapy for borderline personality disorder: A controlled trial. *Behavior Research and Therapy, 42*, 487–499.

Bohus, M., Haaf, B., Stiglmayr, C., Pohl, U., Bohme, R., & Linehan, M. (2000). Evaluation of inpatient dialectical–behavioral therapy for borderline personality disorder: A prospective study. *Behavior Research and Therapy, 38*, 875–887.

Bradley, R. G., & Follingstad, D. R. (2003). Group therapy for incarcerated women who experienced interpersonal violence: A pilot study. *Journal of Traumatic Stress, 16*, 337–340.

Brent, D. A., Johnson, B. A., Perper, J., Connolly, J., Bridge, J., Bartle, S., et al.

(1994). Personality disorder, personality traits, impulsive violence, and completed suicide in adolescents. *Journal of the American Academy of Child Adolescent Psychiatry, 33*(8), 1080–1086.

Breslin, F. C., Zack, M., & McMain, S. (2002). An information-processing analysis of mindfulness: Implications for relapse prevention in the treatment of substance abuse. *Clinical Psychology: Science and Practice, 9*, 275–293.

Clifton, A., Pilkonis, P. A., & McCarty, C. (2007). Social networks in borderline personality disorder. *Journal of Personality Disorders, 21*, 434–442.

Cooney, E., Davis, K., Thompson, P., & Stewart, J. (2008). Pilot study of dialectical behavior therapy for suicidal adolescents. Retrieved September 9, 2011, from *www.tepou.co.nz/knowledge-exchange/research/view/listing/112.*

Dimidjian, S., Hollon, S. D., Dobson, K. S., Schmaling, K. B., Kohlenberg, R. J., Addis, M. E., et al. (2006). Randomized trial of behavioral activation, cognitive therapy, and antidepressant medication in the acute treatment of adults with major depression. *Journal of Consulting and Clinical Psychology, 74*, 658–670.

Ebner-Priemer, U. W., Welch, S. S., Grossman, P., Reisch, T., Linehan, M. M., & Bohus, M. (2007). Psychophysiological ambulatory assessment of affective dysregulation in borderline personality disorder. *Psychiatry Research, 150*, 265–275.

Evershed, S., Tennant, A., Boomer, D., Rees, A., Barkham, M., & Watsons, A. (2003). Practice-based outcomes of dialectical behavior therapy (DBT) targeting anger and violence, with male forensic patients: A pragmatic and non-contemporaneous comparison. *Criminal Behavior and Mental Health, 13*, 198–213.

Fleischhaker, C., Munz, M., Böhme, R., Sixt, B., & Schulz, E. (2006). Dialectical behavior therapy for adolescents (DBT-A): A pilot study on the therapy of suicidal, parasuicidal, and self-injurious behavior in female patients with a borderline disorder. *Zeitschrift für Kinder- und Jugendpsychiatrie und Psychotherapie, 34*, 15–25.

Giaconia, R. M., Reinherz, H. Z., Silverman, A. B., Pakiz, B., Frost, A. K., & Cohen, E. (1995). Traumas and posttraumatic stress disorder in a community population of older adolescents. *Journal of the American Academy of Child and Adolescent Psychiatry, 34*, 1369–1380.

Goldstein, T. R., Axelson, D. A., Birmaher, B., & Brent, D. A. (2007). Dialectical behavior therapy for adolescents with bipolar disorder: A 1-year open trial. *Journal of American Academic Child and Adolescent Psychiatry, 46*, 820–839.

Gratz, K. L., Lacroce, D. M., & Gunderson, J. G. (2006). Measuring changes in symptoms relevant to borderline personality disorder following short-term treatment across partial hospital and intensive outpatient levels of care. *Journal of Psychiatric Practice, 12*, 153–159.

Gross, J. J. (Ed.). (2007). *Handbook of emotion regulation.* New York: Guilford Press.

Grosz, D. E., Lipschitz, D. S., Eldar, S., Finkelstein, G., Blackwood, N., Gerbino-Rosen, G., et al. (1994). Correlates of violence risk in hospitalized adolescents. *Comprehensive Psychiatry, 35*, 296–300.

Groves, S., Backer, H. S., van den Bosch, W., & Miller, A. (2012). Dialectical behavior therapy with adolescents: A review. *Child and Adolescent Mental Health, 17*, 65–75.

Harley, R., Sprich, S., Safren, S., Jacobo, M., & Fava, M. (2008). Adaptation of dialectical behavior therapy skills training group for treatment-resistant depression. *Journal of Nervous Mental Disease, 196*, 136–143.

Harned, M. S., & Linehan, M. M. (2008). Integrating dialectical behavior therapy and prolonged exposure to treat co-occurring borderline personality disorder and PTSD: Two case studies. *Cognitive and Behavioral Practice, 15*, 263–276

Hashim, B. L., Vadnais, M., & Miller, A. L. (in press). Improving adherence in adolescent chronic kidney disease: A DBT feasibility trial. *Clinical Practice in Pediatric Psychology.*

Hayes, S. C., Strosahl, K., & Wilson, K. G. (1999). *Acceptance and commitment therapy: An experiential approach to behavior change.* New York: Guilford Press.

Hill, D. M., Craighead, L. W., & Safer, D. L. (2011). Appetite-focused dialectical behavior therapy for the treatment of binge eating with purging: A preliminary trial. *International Journal of Eating Disorders, 44*, 249–261.

James, A. C., Taylor, A., Winmill, L., & Alfoadari, K. (2008). A preliminary community study of dialectical behaviour therapy (DBT) with adolescent females demonstrating persistent, deliberate self-harm (DSH). *Child and Adolescent Mental Health, 13*, 148–152.

Katz, L. Y., Cox, B. J., Gunasekara, S., & Miller, A. L. (2004). Feasibility of dialectical behavior therapy for suicidal adolescent inpatients. *Journal of the American Academy of Child and Adolescent Psychiatry, 43*, 276–282.

Koerner, K., Miller, A. L., & Wagner, A. W. (1998). Dialectical behavior therapy: Part I. Principle-based intervention for patients with multiple problems. *Journal of Practical Psychiatry and Behavioral Health, 4*, 28–36.

Koons, C. R., Robins, C. J., Tweed, J. L., Lynch, T.R., Gonzalez, A.M., Morse, J. Q., et al. (2001). Efficacy of dialectical behavior therapy in women veterans with borderline personality disorder. *Behavioral Therapy, 32*, 371–390.

Kostiuk, L. M., & Fouts, G. T. (2002). Understanding of emotions and emotion regulation in adolescent females with conduct problems: A qualitative analysis. *Qualitative Report, 7*. Retrieved July 21, 2011, from *www.nova.edu/ssss/qr/qr7-1/kostiuk.html.*

Kuo, J. R., & Linehan, M. M. (2009). Disentangling emotion processes in borderline personality disorder: Physiological and self-reported assessment of biological vulnerability, baseline intensity, and reactivity to emotionally evocative stimuli. *Journal of Abnormal Psychology, 118*, 531–544.

Leibenluft, E., Charney, D. F., & Pine, D. (2003), Researching the pathophysiology of pediatric bipolar disorder. *Biological Psychiatry, 53*, 1009–1020.

Lewinsohn, P. M., Klein, D. N., & Seeley, J. R. (1995). Bipolar disorders in a community sample of older adolescents: Prevalence, phenomenology, comorbidity, and course. *Journal of the American Academy of Child and Adolescent Psychiatry, 34*, 454–463.

Lewinsohn, P. M., Rohde, P., & Seeley, J. R. (1996). Adolescent suicidal ideation and attempts: Prevalence, risk factors, and clinical implications. *Clinical Psychology: Science and Practice, 3*, 25–46.

Lieb, K., Zanarini, M. C., Schmahl, C., Linehan, M. M., & Bohus, M. (2004). Borderline personality disorder. *Lancet, 364*, 453–461.

Linehan, M. M. (1993a). *Cognitive-behavioral treatment of borderline personality disorder.* New York: Guilford Press.

Linehan, M. M. (1993b). *Skills training manual for treating borderline personality disorder.* New York: Guilford Press.

Linehan, M. M., Armstrong, H. E., Suarez, A., Allmon, D., & Heard, H. L. (1991). Cognitive- behavioral treatment of chronically parasuicidal borderline patients. *Archives of General Psychiatry, 48,* 1060–1064.

Linehan, M. M., Comtois, K. A., Murray, A. M., Brown, M. Z., Gallop, R. J., Heard, H. L., et al. (2006). Two-year randomized controlled trial and follow-up of dialectical behavior therapy vs. therapy by experts for suicidal behaviors and borderline personality disorder. *Archives of General Psychiatry, 64,* 727–766.

Linehan, M. M., Dimeff, L. A., Reynolds, S. K., Comtois, K. A., Welch, S. S., Heagerty, P., et al. (2002). Dialectical behavior therapy versus comprehensive validation therapy plus 12-step for the treatment of opioid dependent women meeting criteria for borderline personally disorder. *Drug and Alcohol Dependence, 67,* 13–26.

Linehan, M. M., Heard, H. L., & Armstrong, H. E. (1993). Naturalistic follow-up of a behavioral treatment for chronically parasuicidal borderline patients. *Archives of General Psychiatry, 50,* 971–974.

Linehan, M. M., Schmidt, H., III, Dimeff, L. A., Craft, J. C., Kanter, J., & Comtois, K. A. (1999). Dialectical behavior therapy for patients with borderline personality disorder and drug dependence. *American Journal on Addictions, 8,* 279–292.

Lynch, T. R. (2000). Treatment of depression with personality disorder comorbidity using dialectical behavior therapy. *Cognitive and Behavioral Practice, 7,* 468–477.

Lynch, T. R., Morse, J. Q., Mendelson, T., & Robins, C. J. (2003). Dialectical behavior therapy for depressed older adults: A randomized pilot study. *American Journal of Geriatric Psychiatry, 11,* 33–45.

Lynch, T. R., Trost, W. T., Salsman, N., & Linehan, M. M. (2007). Dialectical behavior therapy for borderline personality disorder. *Annual Review of Clinical Psychology, 3,* 181–205.

Lyubomirsky, S., & Nolen-Hoeksema, S. (1995). Effects of self-focused rumination on negative thinking and interpersonal problem-solving. *Journal of Personality and Social Psychology, 69,* 176–190.

Marttunen, M. J., Aro, H. M., Henriksson, M. M., & Lonnqvist, J. K. (1991). Antisocial behavior in adolescent suicide. *Acta Psychiatrica Scandinavica, 89,* 167–173.

Mason, P., Catucci, D., Lusk, V., & Johnson, M. (2009, November). *An initial program evaluation of modified dialectical behavioral therapy adolescent skills training in a school setting.* Poster presented at the 14th annual conference of the International Society for the Improvement and Teaching of Dialectical Behavioral Therapy, New York.

McDonnell, M. G., Tarantino, J., Dubose, A. P., Matestic, P., Steinmetz, K., Galbreath, H., et al. (2010). A pilot evaluation of dialectical behavioral therapy in adolescent long-term inpatient care. *Child and Adolescent Mental Health, 15,* 193–196.

McLaughlin, K. A., Hatzenbuehler, M. L., & Hilt, L. M. (2009). Emotion dysregulation as a mechanism linking peer victimization to internalizing symptoms in adolescents. *Journal of Consulting and Clinical Psychology, 77,* 894–904.

McRae, K., & Gross, J. J. (2009). Emotion regulation. In D. Sander & K Scherer (Eds.), *Oxford companion to the affective sciences* (pp. 337–339). New York: Oxford University Press.

Miller, A. L., Muehlenkamp, J. J., & Jacobson, C. M. (2008). Fact or fiction: Diagnosing borderline personality disorder in adolescents. *Clinical Psychology Review, 28,* 969–981.

Miller, A. L., Rathus, J. H., & Linehan, M. M. (2007). *Dialectical behavior therapy with suicidal adolescents.* New York: Guilford Press.

Miller, A. L., Rathus, J. H., Linehan, M. M., Wetzler, S., & Leigh, E. (1997). Dialectical behavior therapy adapted for suicidal adolescents. *Journal of Practical Psychiatry and Behavioral Health, 3,* 78–86.

Miller, A. L., Wagner, E. E., & Rathus, J. H. (2004). Dialectical behavior therapy for suicidal multi-problem adolescents. In H. Steiner (Ed.), *Handbook of mental health interventions in children and adolescents: An integrated developmental approach* (pp. 659–684). San Francisco: Jossey-Bass.

National Institute of Mental Health. (2011). Borderline personality disorder. Retrieved August 29, 2011, from *www.nimh.nih.gov/health/publications/borderline-personality-disorder/index.shtml.*

Nelson-Gray, R. O., Keane, S. P., Hurst, R. M., Mitchell, J. T., Warburton, J. B., Chok, J. T., et al. (2006). A modified DBT skills training program for oppositional defiant adolescents: Promising preliminary findings. *Behaviuor Research and Therapy, 44,* 1811–1820.

New, A. S., & Siever, L. J. (2002). The neurobiology and genetics of borderline personality disorder. *Psychiatric Annals, 32,* 329–336.

Nock, M. K., Joiner, T. E., Gordon, K. H., Lloyd-Richardson, E., & Prinstein, M. J. (2006). Non- suicidal self-injury among adolescents: Diagnostic correlates and relation to suicide attempts. *Psychiatry Research, 144,* 65–72.

Nock, M. K., & Prinstein, M. J. (2004). A functional approach to the assessment of self-mutilative behavior in adolescents. *Journal of Consulting and Clinical Psychology, 72,* 885–890.

Palmer, R. L., Birchall, H., Damani, S., Gatward, N., McGrain, L., & Parker, L. (2003). A dialectical behavior therapy program for people with an eating disorder and borderline personality disorder: Description and outcome. *International Journal of Eating Disorders, 33,* 281–286.

Pfeffer, C. R., Newcorn, J. H., Kaplan, G., Mizruchi, M. S., & Plutchik, R. (1988). Suicidal behavior in adolescent psychiatric inpatients. *Journal of the American Academy of Child Psychiatry, 27,* 357–361.

Rapgay, L., Bystritsky, A., Dafter, R., & Spearman, M. (2011). New strategies for combining mindfulness with integrative cognitive behavioral therapy for the treatment of generalized anxiety disorder. *Journal of Rational-Emotive Cognitive-Behavior Therapy, 29,* 92–119.

Rathus, J. H., & Miller, A. L. (2000). Introduction to special section on dialectical behavior therapy. *Cognitive and Behavioral Practice, 7,* 420–425.

Rathus, J. H., & Miller, A. L. (2002). Dialectical behavior therapy adapted for suicidal adolescents. *Suicide and Life-Threatening Behavior, 32,* 146–157.

Safer, D. L., Lock, J., & Couturier, J. L. (2007). Dialectical behavior therapy modified for adolescent binge eating disorder: A case report. *Cognitive and Behavioral Practice, 14,* 157–167.

Safer, D. L., Telch, C. F., & Agras, W. S. (2001). Dialectical behavior therapy adapted for bulimia: A case report. *International Journal of Eating Disorders, 30,* 101–106.

Salbach, H., Klinkowski, N., Pfeiffer, U., Lehmkuhl, U., & Korte, A. (2007). Dialectical behavior therapy for adolescent patients with anorexia and bulimia nervosa (DBT-AN/BN): A pilot study. *Practice of Child Psychology and Child Psychiatry, 56,* 91–108.

Salbach-Andrae, H., Bohnekamp, I., Pfeiffer, E., Lehmkuhl, U., & Miller, A. L. (2008). Dialectical behavior therapy of anorexia and bulimia nervosa among adolescents: A case series. *Cognitive and Behavioral Practice, 15,* 415–425.

Sally, M., Jackson, L., Carney, J., Kevelson, J., & Miller, A. L. (2002, November). *Implementing DBT skills training groups in an underperforming high school.* Poster presented at the 7th annual conference of the International Society for the Improvement and Teaching of Dialectical Behavioral Therapy, Reno, Nevada.

Selby, E. A., Anestis, M. D., Bender, T. W., & Joiner, T. E. (2009). An exploration of the emotional cascade model in borderline personality disorder. *Journal of Abnormal Psychology, 118,* 375–387.

Segal, Z. V., Williams, J. M. G., & Teasdale, J. D. (2002). *Mindfulness-based cognitive therapy for depression: A new approach to preventing relapse.* New York: Guilford Press.

Shaffer, D., Gould, M. S., Fisher, P., Trautman, P., Moreau, D., Kleinman, M., et al. (1996). Psychiatric diagnosis in child and adolescent suicide. *Archives of General Psychiatry, 53,* 339–348.

Simpson, E. B., Pistorello, J., Begin, A., Costello, E., Levinson, J., Mulberry, S., et al. (1998). Focus on women: Use of dialectical behavior therapy in a partial hospital program for women with borderline personality disorder. *Psychiatric Services, 49,* 669–673.

Sunseri, P. A. (2004). Preliminary outcomes on the use of dialectical behavior therapy to reduce hospitalization among adolescents in residential care. *Residential Treatment for Children and Youth, 21,* 59–76.

Telch, C. F., Agras, W. S., & Linehan, M. M. (2001). Dialectical behavior therapy for binge eating disorder. *Journal of Consulting and Clinical Psychology, 69,* 1061–1065.

Tørmoen, A. J., Mehlum, L., Haga, E., Grøholt, B., Larsson, B., & Miller, A. (2009, November). *Dialectical behavior therapy with suicidal and self-harming adolescents: Preliminary results of a pilot study.* Poster presented at the 14th annual conference of the International Society for the Improvement and Teaching of Dialectical Behavioral Therapy, New York.

Trupin, E. W., Stewart, D. G., Beach, B., & Boesky, L. (2002). Effectiveness of dialectical behaviour therapy program for incarcerated female juvenile offenders. *Child and Adolescent Mental Health, 7,* 121–127.

van den Bosch, L. M., Koeter, M. W., Stijnen, T., Verheul, R., & van den Brink, W. (2005). Sustained efficacy of dialectical behavior therapy for borderline personality disorder. *Behavior Research and Therapy, 43,* 1231–1241.

Verheul, R., van den Bosch, L. M., Koeter, M. W., De Ridder, M. A., Stijnen, T., & van den Brink, W. (2003). Dialectical behavior therapy for women with borderline personality disorder: 12-month, randomized clinical trial in the Netherlands. *British Journal of Psychiatry, 182,* 135–140.

Wagner, E., Rathus, J. H., & Miller, A. L. (2006). Mindfulness in dialectical behavior therapy (DBT) for adolescents. In R. A. Baer (Ed.), *Mindfulness-based treatment approaches: Clinician's guide to evidence base and applications.* Amsterdam: Elsevier Academic Press.

Woodberry, K. A., & Popenoe, E. J. (2008). Implementing dialectical behavior therapy with adolescents and their families in a community outpatient clinic. *Cognitive and Behavioral Practice, 15,* 277–286.

Yen, S., Zlotnick, C., & Costello, E. (2002). Affect regulation in women with borderline personality disorder traits. *Nervous and Mental Disease, 190,* 693–696.

Zeman, J., Shipman, K., & Suveg, C. (2002). Anger and sadness regulation: Predictions to internalizing and externalizing symptoms in children. *Journal of Clinical Child and Adolescent Psychology, 31,* 393–398.

CHAPTER 11

Acceptance and Commitment Therapy

Lisa W. Coyne, Kirstin B. Birtwell, Louise McHugh, and Kelly G. Wilson

Third-wave cognitive and behavior therapies (Hayes, Villatte, Levin, & Hildebrandt, 2011) involve a transdiagnostic approach concerned not with the elimination of symptoms but rather with building broad, flexible behavioral repertoires (Ruiz, 2010). Acceptance and commitment therapy (ACT; Hayes, Strosahl, & Wilson, 1999, 2012) is a prominent example of a transdiagnostic therapeutic approach. Rather than focusing on symptom reduction, ACT encourages acceptance of aversive private experiences so that one can pursue meaningful and valued activities. ACT has received substantial empirical support across numerous disorder categories (Ruiz, 2010; Öst, 2008).

ACT is grounded in basic behavioral science, more specifically, behavior analysis (e.g., Cooper, Heron, & Heward, 2007) and relational frame theory (RFT; Hayes, Barnes-Holmes, & Roche, 2001). This grounding not only ensures that ACT is coherent and evidence based but also allows for the continued refinement of therapy at the process level, thus facilitating its ongoing evolution and development. In this chapter, we describe ACT and its evidence base with adults and youth, its underlying philosophy and theoretical model, its conceptualization of experiential avoidance as a transdiagnostic process characterizing psychopathology, and its application as a transdiagnostic therapy.

ACT Efficacy across Disorders

The ACT approach to psychological dysfunction has been shown to be effective across a wide range of clinical and subclinical presentations.

233

Effect sizes have been found to be medium to large and have further improved at follow-up (Ruiz, 2010). In fact, the Substance Abuse and Mental Health Services Administration (SAMHSA) of the U.S. government has recently listed ACT as an empirically supported method as part of its National Registry of Evidence-Based Programs and Practices (U.S. Department of Health & Human Services, 2011). ACT is also considered an empirically validated treatment by the American Psychological Association and is recognized as having moderate to strong research support for chronic pain, obsessive–compulsive disorder (OCD), mixed anxiety-depression, and psychosis (*www.div12.org/PsychologicalTreatments/treatments.html*).

In addition to the areas cited, ACT trials with adult samples using single-case, open-trial, and randomized-trial methodology have demonstrated positive outcomes for individuals with the following presentations: personality disorders (e.g., borderline personality disorder), substance abuse, smoking cessation, diabetes management, epilepsy, cancer, and weight loss (for comprehensive reviews, see Hayes, Luoma, Bond, Masuda, & Lillis, 2006; Ruiz, 2010). At present, more than 50 randomized clinical trials (RCTs) of ACT have been published, are in press, or are in preparation (see Table 11.1). Although promising results have surfaced thus far, replication and further research in new domains are needed—especially with youth.

Despite the breadth and depth of empirical investigation with adults, studies exploring ACT-based treatment adaptations for children, adolescents, and families have been limited in both quantity and scope (e.g., small sample size, single-case or uncontrolled studies, lack of interstudy consistency). Nonetheless, researchers are analyzing ACT-based protocols for children and adolescents suffering from various mental health disorders, chronic pain, eating disorders, and sickle cell disease. In addition, two published studies have evaluated ACT for parent populations, and several other trials are under way.

Though the field is only in its infancy, child- and adolescent-targeted ACT trials have demonstrated largely favorable outcomes for a range of mental health challenges. For example, Hayes, Boyd, and Sewell (2011) recently published results from an RCT with depressed adolescents, comparing ACT with a treatment-as-usual (TAU) condition. Participants in the ACT condition reported significantly lower depression levels than those in the TAU group and evidenced further improvement from post-treatment to 3-month follow-up. In addition, Morris and Greco (2002) implemented an ACT-based protocol with socially anxious youngsters and reported a reduction of social anxiety and increased school attendance. In nonclinical populations, ACT resulted in less experiential avoidance, more social confidence, parent-reported shorter "episodes of anxiety," and return to school for an 18-year-old developmentally delayed female

TABLE 11.1. Articles Concerning Randomized Clinical Trials of ACT

Study	Problem/diagnosis	N	Main findings
Zettle & Hayes (1986)	Depression	18	ACT is more effective than CT.
Zettle & Rains (1989)	Depression	31	ACT is as effective as CT and CT + distancing.
Bond & Bunce (2000)	Worksite stress and anxiety	90	ACT is more effective than behavioral approach and both are better than wait-list control.
Bach & Hayes (2002)	Psychotic inpatients	80	ACT reduces rehospitalization over a 4-month follow-up as compared with TAU.
Zettle (2003)	Math anxiety	24	ACT is comparable to systematic desensitization in reducing math anxiety, but systematic desensitization reduces trait anxiety more than ACT.
Dahl, Wilson, & Nilsson (2004)	Stress and pain symptoms	19	ACT is more effective than TAU.
Gifford et al. (2004)	Smoking cessation	76	Quit rates are similar at posttreatment but 1-year follow-up shows that the ACT group maintains gains while the NRT quit rates decline.
Hayes, Bissett, et al. (2004)	Stigmatizing attitudes and burnout in substance abuse counselors	93	ACT is more effective than control.
Hayes, Wilson, et al. (2004)	Polysubstance abuse	114; methadone maintenance (n = 38), addition of ACT (n = 42), or intensive twelve-step facilitation (ITSF; n = 44)	No differences at posttreatment, but ACT is more effective at 6-month follow-up.

(continued)

235

TABLE 11.1. *(continued)*

Study	Problem/diagnosis	N	Main findings
Gaudiano & Herbert (2006)	Inpatients with psychotic symptoms	40	ACT is more effective than TAU.
Gratz & Gunderson (2006)	Borderline personality disorder	22	ACT/DBT combo is more effective than TAU.
Lundgren, Dahl, Melin, & Kees (2006)	Drug refractory epilepsy	27	ACT reduces seizures significantly more than supportive therapy.
Woods, Wetterneck, & Flessner (2006)	Trichotillomania	25	ACT plus habit reversal is more effective than wait-list control.
Forman, Herbert, Moitra, Yeomans, & Geller (2007)	Anxiety and depression	101	Participants improve similarly with ACT and CT.
Gregg, Callaghan, Hayes, & Glenn-Lawson (2007)	Diabetes	81	ACT + patient education is more effective than patient education.
Lappalainen et al. (2007)	Outpatient	14	ACT is more effective than CBT at posttreatment and 6-month follow-up.
Masuda et al. (2007)	Psychological disorder stigma	96	ACT reduces mental health stigma significantly, but education reduces stigma among participants who are relatively flexible and nonavoidant to begin with.
Páez, Luciano, & Gutiérrez (2007)	Women diagnosed and treated for breast cancer	12	ACT is more effective than CBT at 1-year follow-up.
Vowles et al. (2007)	Chronic pain	74	Acceptance group improves more than pain control and practice conditions.
Lundgren, Dahl, Yardi, & Melin (2008)	Epilepsy patients with drug-refractory seizures	18	ACT reduces seizures more than yoga, but both improve QOL.

Study	Population	N	Findings
Luoma et al. (2007)	Drug counselors	30	ACT-based supervision group following training in group drug counseling increase group drug counseling adoption in drug and alcohol counselors.
Roemer, Orsillo, & Salters-Pedneault (2008)	Generalized anxiety disorder	31	ACT-based protocol (ABBT) produces positive outcomes maintained at 3- and 9-month follow-up.
Varra, Hayes, Roget, & Fisher (2008)	Clinicians	59	ACT is more effective than psychoeducation alone ($d = .85$).
Wicksell, Ahlqvist, Bring, Melin, & Olsson (2008)	Chronic pain and whiplash associated disorders (WAD)	21	ACT is more effective than TAU.
Lillis, Hayes, Bunting, & Masuda (2009)	Obesity	84	ACT reduces stigma, increases QOL, and reduces weight.
Peterson & Zettle (2009)	Comorbid depression and alcohol	24	ACT and TAU produce similar outcomes, but ACT uses less time.
Tapper et al. (2009)	Obesity	62	ACT group has drop in BMI (compared with wait-list controls).
Wicksell, Melin, Lekander, & Olsson (2009)	Pediatric pain	32	ACT performs significantly better than multidisciplinary treatment plus amitriptyline (MDT).
Flaxman & Bond (2010)	Worksite stress	107	ACT and SIT (stress inoculation training) are equally effective; ACT is mediated by psychological flexibility; SIT is not successfully mediated by cognitive change.
Flaxman & Bond (2010)	Worksite stress	311	ACT is better than wait-list control.
Fledderus, Bohlmeijer, Smit, & Westerhof (2010)	Mild to moderate psychological distress	93	ACT shows good outcomes compared with wait-list control.

(continued)

TABLE 11.1. *(continued)*

Study	Problem/diagnosis	N	Main findings
Hinton & Gaynor (2010)	Psychological distress, dysphoria, and low self-esteem	22	Group receiving ACT component (cognitive defusion) demonstrates better outcomes than wait-list controls.
Johnston, Foster, Shennan, Starkey, & Johnson (2010)	Chronic pain	14	ACT is helpful for chronic pain.
Juarascio, Forman, & Herbert (2010)	Comorbid eating pathology	55	ACT produces greater reductions in eating pathology and greater increases in global functioning than CT.
Smout et al. (2010)	Methamphetamine use disorders	104	ACT is no more effective than CBT in retaining or treating methamphetamine users.
Twohig et al. (2010)	Obsessive–compulsive disorder	79	ACT has good outcomes in comparison with progressive relaxation training.
Bohlmeijer, Fledderus, Rokx, & Pieterse (2011)	Mild to moderate depressive symptomotology	93	Significant reduction in depressive symptomatology (Cohen's $d = .60$) for ACT group compared with wait-list control.
Brinkborg, Michanek, Hesser, & Berglund (2011)	Stress and burnout in social workers	106	ACT is more effective than wait-list control.
Brown et al. (2011)	Test anxiety	16	Similar outcomes are seen on self-reports (ACT vs. CT), but ACT participants do objectively better on test scores in school.
Butryn, Forman, Hoffman, Shaw, & Juarascio (2011)	Promoting physical activity	54	ACT participants increase their physical activity level more than psychoeducation participants.

Study	Population	N	Outcomes
Fledderus, Bohlmeijer, Pieterse, & Schreurs (2011)	Depression	376	ACT group has reductions in depression, anxiety, fatigue, and experiential avoidance and improvements in positive mental health and mindfulness; sustained at follow-up.
Hayes, Boyd, & Sewell (2011)	Adolescent depression	30	Good outcomes (~60% in ACT show clinically significant change; d = .38 at posttreatment and 1.45 at follow-up).
Muto, Hayes, & Jeffcoat (2011)	Japanese college students living abroad	70	Better general mental health at posttreatment and follow-up. Moderately and above depressed, stressed, and severely anxious students show improvement compared with those not receiving the book. Outcomes are mediated and moderated by psychological flexibility.
Weineland, Arvidsson, Kakoulidis, & Dahl (2012)	Bariatric surgery patients	39	ACT is more effective than TAU.
Wetherell et al. (2011)	Chronic pain	114	ACT is comparable to CBT.
Pearson, Follette, & Hayes (2012)	Body dissatisfaction and disordered eating attitudes	73	ACT helps with body dissatisfaction and disordered eating attitudes.
Gifford et al. (2011)	Smoking cessation	303	ACT has good outcomes in comparison with FAP + Zyban and Zyban.
Westin et al. (2011)	Tinnitus distress	64	ACT does better than tinnitus retraining therapy in reducing the interference and distress from tinnitus.
Luoma, Kohlenberg, Hayes, & Fletcher (2012)	Substance use disorder	133	ACT intervention results in smaller immediate gains in shame, but larger reductions at 4-month follow-up.

(Brown & Hooper, 2009). In two studies using a group intervention, ACT was also shown to reduce anxiety associated with chess performance in a nonclinical population of adolescents (Ruiz & Luciano, 2006) and to improve objectively measured chess performance (Ruiz & Luciano, 2012), compared with a wait-list control. ACT also appears useful with parent distress (Blackledge & Hayes, 2006) and impaired parenting (Coyne & Wilson, 2004).

ACT has been successful with children and adolescents experiencing behavioral health conditions, including chronic pain (Wicksell, Dahl, Magnusson, & Olsson, 2005; Wicksell, Melin, Lekander, & Olsson, 2009; Wicksell, Melin, & Olsson, 2007), eating disorders (Heffner, Sperry, & Eifert, 2002; Merwin, Timko, Zucker, Martin, & Moskovich, 2010), and sickle cell disease (Masuda, Cohen, Wicksell, Kemani, & Johnson, 2011). In one well-designed small RCT with 32 adolescents described as severely disabled by chronic pain, Wicksell and colleagues (2009) compared the efficacy of ACT with that of a multidisciplinary treatment (MDT) based on a biobehavioral model of pain. MDT consisted of treatment by a psychiatrist, a child psychologist, a physiotherapist, and a pain physician as needed by individual patients, as well as amitriptyline use. ACT participants reported significantly improved functional ability (i.e., global functioning despite the presence of pain), fear of reinjury, pain interference, and quality of life compared with the MDT group, and these gains were maintained over time. Although preliminary findings regarding ACT efficacy with youth must be interpreted cautiously, they represent a compelling rationale for further study. ACT has a strong theoretical basis, and research suggests that it may be used flexibly (and transdiagnostically) in diverse children, adolescents, and families.

ACT as a Transdiagnostic Approach to Psychopathology

Ideally, transdiagnostic approaches to treatment may be used flexibly across a variety of client presentations, populations, and contexts. A truly advantageous transdiagnostic approach must be informed by weaknesses in our current diagnostic system (discussed elsewhere in this book) and must hold onto current models of diagnostic categories lightly. Additionally, it should identify a common psychological process that spans various types and levels of psychological dysfunction. Moreover, its goal would be to identify a mechanism (or mechanisms) of dysfunction that are amenable to change, rather than stable traits or individual-difference factors. Finally, that identified process should be shown to be the "active ingredient" in clinical change when measured and tracked in the context of treatment studies. Given its theoretical and empirical background, ACT clearly fits this description.

Theoretical Background of ACT: Functional Contextual Behaviorism

ACT assumes that psychological events are ongoing and best viewed within a situational and historical context. To this end, ACT has been called a "functional contextual" approach to human behavior. ACT assumes that behaviors can have different functions for any one individual in different settings, that different behaviors can belong to similar functional domains, and that behavioral change is optimally achieved through manipulation of contextual factors. ACT also relies on the premise that contextual events regulate and organize behaviors (including cognitions) and link them with one another (Hayes et al., 2006).

Given its underlying philosophy of science, ACT seeks to influence behavior through the contextual variables that maintain it. In contrast, when speaking in diagnostic terms, we speak in terms of associated symptoms that exist outside of context. The process of "diagnosing" refers to detecting a constellation of linked symptoms that are part of some presumably meaningful category of illness. In ACT, what is more important than "diagnosis" is a functional analytical approach to behavior, couched in a thorough understanding of contemporary basic research on verbal behavior (Hayes et al., 2001), and inclusive of private events as well as the context in which they occur. The assessment procedure and goals thus differ markedly from traditional diagnostic methods. More specifically, an ACT therapist would be interested in behaviors that don't "work" in the way the client wants them to, even though the client still engages in them in a rigid, narrow way.

ACT and RFT and Basic Research

Whereas several transdiagnostic approaches described in this book draw on basic emotion science and its related fields (neurobiology, cognitive affective neuroscience, etc.), ACT draws from learning theory, specifically contemporary behavioral research that examines the development of language processes. Perhaps the most important feature of ACT is that it is founded on aspects of RFT (Hayes et al., 2001), a modern behavior analytical approach to language and cognition.

According to RFT, language and cognition can be understood in terms of the learned capacity to relate stimuli under arbitrary contextual control, referred to as relational framing (see Hayes et al., 2001). To understand the meaning of "contextual control," consider this example. A mother tells a child that "Shrek is taller than Donkey," and when she asks who is shorter, he answers, "Donkey." His reply is based on the contextual cue "taller." He has previously learned to "relationally frame" stimuli in accordance with the relation of comparison in the presence of this cue, and thus, when he hears it, he frames Shrek and Donkey in this way and "derives" that Donkey is shorter.

RFT argues that humans learn to relationally frame based on exposure to contingencies of reinforcement in the socioverbal community. The earliest and arguably most fundamental example of relational framing that children learn (at around the age of 18 months) is the relation of coordination (sameness) between words and their referents (e.g., the spoken word "tree" is the same as an actual tree; see Lipkens, Hayes, & Hayes, 1993). With continued exposure to the socioverbal environment, they gradually learn a variety of alternative frames, such as bigger–smaller (comparison), different from (distinction), and "a type of" (hierarchical; e.g., a dachshund is a type of dog). These frames are often arbitrary; for example, children learn through social conventions that a dime is worth more than a nickel, even though it is physically smaller. Eventually children's framing generalizes so that the contextual cues alone control the response pattern (see Barnes-Holmes, Barnes-Holmes, Smeets, Strand, & Friman, 2004 for an empirical example of training the relational frame of comparison; and see Hayes et al., 2001, for a more comprehensive list and description of characteristics of particular families of relational frames). RFT researchers have provided an increasing quantity of empirical evidence showing the diversity of patterns of framing as well as how they can be established and influenced (e.g., Dymond & Barnes, 1997; Roche & Barnes, 1996; Steele & Hayes, 1991).

According to RFT (Hayes et al., 2001), the way in which we verbally relate stimuli may be at the source of psychological suffering. RFT suggests that we learn to relate (relationally frame) things in our environment and that this relational activity can change the psychological functions of those things. This so-called "transformation of function" (TOF) can be highly useful in many contexts. For example, a child may learn to hit a baseball or softball by receiving step-by-step instructions from an adult on how to swing a bat. In this case, the child (via relational learning) may associate the notion of a bat as a wooden object used in baseball with the idea of a bat as a way in which to hit a home run (i.e., the bat comes to have positive psychological properties, such as positive emotion, fond memories, or eager anticipation and hope). Or perhaps the baseball bat can also come to remind the child of the loving relationship that he or she has with the parent (of that moment in time). In either case, the bat comes to have particular psychological functions for the child, derived through relational framing in this particular context.

TOF can also be problematic in some contexts. For example, the same child might be unsuccessful at hitting the ball, and consequently may define him- or herself as a physically awkward or nonathletic individual. Because the bat in this context may come to have unpleasant psychological properties, the child may avoid Little League altogether, thus precluding many of the pleasant experiences this might have afforded him or her. It may be painful or embarrassing not to be able to hit a ball well, but those added self-evaluations of "I'm physically awkward" or "I'm not athletic" and their subsequent avoidance are what ACT would term *suffering*.

An ACT model of psychopathology assumes that humans encounter pain, stress, and loss and that these experiences are part of life. However, *suffering* arises through the interaction of language processes with direct contingencies that create an unhelpful persistence and singular focus on managing or minimizing pain that precludes engagement in behavior toward valued domains. This end result is called *psychological inflexibility* and is thought to arise from weak, ineffective contextual control over associative learning processes. This process illustrates two elements that ACT posits are central to the development and maintenance of psychological problems. The first is *cognitive fusion*, which in technical terms refers to "excessive or improper regulation of behavior by verbal processes"— specifically, derived relational networks (Hayes, Strosahl, & Wilson, 1999, p. 304; Hayes et al., 2006). In more general terms, this refers to the tendency to experience one's own thoughts and beliefs as literal or true. An individual is unable to consider actual environmental contingencies when they are fused with his or her own cognitive content, and consequently he or she is less likely to respond in effective, adaptive ways. Because verbal or cognitive elements are treated as real, an individual may become engaged in a pervasive pattern of avoidance of such elements.

The attempt to change, minimize, or otherwise control unwanted psychological experiences is termed *experiential avoidance*, and it is the second element targeted by ACT (Hayes, Wilson, Strosahl, Gifford, & Follette, 1996). This avoidance, in limited doses or used in the short term without excessive personal costs, is not a problem per se. However, when individuals demonstrate excessive reliance on managing cognitive or verbal experiences, it is thought to contribute to the development of maladaptive behavioral repertoires. Exclusive reliance on experiential avoidance draws attention inward, toward the goals of managing unmanageable psychological events, and thus precluding attention to other, more meaningful pursuits.

What is Experiential Avoidance?

ACT would define experiential avoidance as a functional class of behavior that includes both antecedent and consequent emotion regulatory strategies that target suppression of unwanted or unpleasant private events. Experiential avoidance in and of itself is not a terrible thing and can actually be quite useful in the short term. For example, a child might look away from the doctor and the needle when getting a shot and thus might feel less afraid (Coyne, McHugh, & Martinez, 2011). However, sole or excessive reliance on experiential avoidance is where the real problem lies. Emotions, whether positive or negative, intense or less so, are viewed as normal parts of human experience. Experiential avoidance, then, can be defined functionally as "an inability to persist in goal-directed behavior in the presence of difficult thoughts and emotions" (Boulanger, Hayes, & Pistorello, 2010). Simply put, it is not our emotions that are the problem; it's what we do with them and about them when they occur—or, more specifically, what we do to prevent them from occurring and to escape them when they do occur.

If an individual is engaged in experiential avoidance (i.e., attempts to stop thinking about/feeling/experiencing unpleasant private events), his or her attention is narrowly focused on those events rather than on external contingencies. In this way, individuals are not in contact with the world, and, more important, they cannot access external reinforcers of adaptive behavior. In general, there is always an array of stimuli, internal and external, that influences individuals' behavior. However, an individual engaged in experiential avoidance focuses narrowly on only a subset of available stimuli, and thus the psychological functions of other available stimuli go unnoticed and consequently cannot influence behavior. This may be problematic in several ways, including in a therapy setting.

Consider the example of a child with social phobia engaged in exposure exercises, such as speaking in the front of a classroom. If the child is unwilling to engage in exposure, despite the urging of her therapist, she may engage in cognitive strategies that she feels may protect her from her anxiety during that experience. She may try to distract herself, or tell herself to "hang on until it's over," or tell herself "you shouldn't feel this anxious," rather than flexibly letting her awareness contain the exposure. This process appears to explain why anxiety does not extinguish in some individuals, despite their exposure to feared activities (Clark, 2001). From an ACT perspective, these behaviors constitute rigid, difficult-to-extinguish functional avoidance strategies.

These cognitive avoidance strategies create a secondary problem: The youngster just described may begin to evaluate her own success (or lack thereof) in managing her emotions. Now, in addition to her anxiety, her cognitive avoidance strategies may have inadvertently created *new* content she wishes to avoid (i.e., suffering): such thoughts as "There's something wrong with me because I can't manage my anxiety" and "I'm a failure at speaking to my class." In addition, although engagement in cognitive avoidance may reduce her anxiety in the short term, it may also preclude her from experiencing other aspects of the situation—for example, that perhaps her classmates are enjoying her talk, or that she has made a good joke, or that her teacher is smiling in approval. Thus, even though she has engaged in exposure, her cognitive avoidance has prevented the

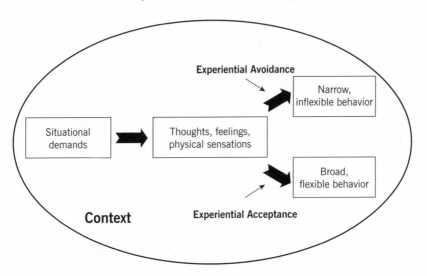

FIGURE 11.1. Conceptual model of experiential avoidance.

possibility of her public speaking behavior coming under the control of other available discriminative stimuli. Consequently, she is likely to continue to engage in narrow and inflexible safety-seeking strategies, including more cognitive avoidance (see Figure 11.1 for an illustration).

Experiential Avoidance as a Transdiagnostic Process in Psychopathology

There is growing evidence that in adult populations, experiential avoidance plays a role in the development and maintenance of psychopathology, as well as in treatment outcome (for reviews, see Boulanger, 2010; Chowla & Ostafin, 2007; Hayes et al., 2006). A recent meta-analysis demonstrated that experiential avoidance accounted for 16–28% of variance in psychological difficulties and had a moderately strong relationship (average $r = .5$) with varying forms of psychopathology, including depression, anxiety, and psychological distress in clinical and nonclinical populations and across diagnostic categories (Hayes et al., 2006). There is also evidence that experiential avoidance moderates response to experimentally induced stressors, including panic (Karekla, Forsyth, & Kelly, 2004), anxiety, and stress (Feldner, Zvolensky, Eifert, & Spira, 2003), and that it mediates treatment outcome in interventions for diabetes (Gregg, Callaghan, Hayes, & Glenn-Lawson, 2007), epilepsy (Lundgren, Dahl, & Hayes. 2008), stress (Bond & Bunce, 2000), smoking (Gifford et al., 2004), and weight control (Lillis, Hayes, Bunting, & Masuda, 2009).

In youth populations, experiential avoidance has been implicated in adolescent well-being and prosocial tendencies (Ciarrochi, Kashdan, Leeson, Heaven, & Jordan, 2011), emotional and behavioral difficulties (Greco, Lambert, & Baer, 2008), and chronic pain (McCracken, Gauntlett-Gilbert, & Eccleston, 2010). Experiential avoidance also appears important in samples of youth who experience specific psychosocial stressors. In a sample of 85 gay, lesbian, and bisexual teens, experiential avoidance and self-critical thoughts together mediated the relationship between verbal bullying and depression, which suggests that avoidant coping used to deal with verbal abuse may confer greater risk of depression (Armelie, Delahanty, & Bloarts, 2010). Finally, experiential avoidance has been implicated in parenting stress and psychological functioning (Blackledge & Hayes, 2006; Cheron, Ehrenreich, & Pincus, 2009; Coyne & Silvia, 2007; Coyne & Thompson, 2011), parenting behaviors (Berlin, Sato, Jastrowski, Woods, & Davies, 2006; Coyne & Burke-Currie, 2011; Murrell, Wilson, LaBorde, Drake, & Rogers, 2009; Shea & Coyne, 2011), the quality of parent–child relationships (Shea & Coyne, 2011), and child emotional and behavioral functioning across developmental periods from birth (Greco et al., 2005) to early adulthood (Berlin et al., 2006; for a review, see Coyne, McHugh, & Martinez, 2011). Studies targeting experiential avoidance in parents have demonstrated decreases in parent distress in parents of autistic children (Blackledge & Hayes, 2006).

How Does ACT Target Cognitive Fusion and Experiential Avoidance?

ACT targets experiential avoidance and cognitive fusion by attempting to undermine the negative effects of language while capitalizing on the positive effects. RFT and ACT suggest that clients' verbal structures are circulating the message that "undesirable thought content is a barrier to effective living." Two strategies are traditionally used to change this system: (1) changing the situation so as to change the content; (2) changing the content directly by avoiding it, disputing it, arguing with it, challenging it, justifying it, rationalizing it, denying it, ignoring it, tolerating it, and so forth. Despite implicit and explicit societal rules that specify otherwise, trying to successfully implement these functional avoidance strategies is futile and counterproductive.

Children and teens exposed to ACT treatment are brought through a series of experiential activities (exercises and metaphors) used to allow them to see for themselves how change attempts described previously are "unworkable" and to see that there is another option, which involves halting counterproductive avoidance strategies and instead focusing on pursuing their values. Put simply, clients stop trying to remove aversive experiences from their lives and start working for appetitives, or pleasant

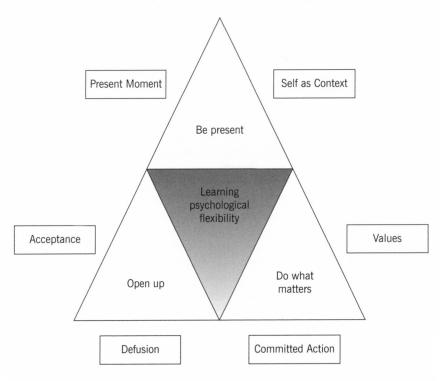

FIGURE 11.2. Core ACT processes expressed as a triflex. From Harris (2009, p. 13). Copyright 2009 by Russ Harris. Adapted with permission from New Harbinger Publications.

stimuli. Hence, after using experiential exercises to undermine the negative influence of language, ACT also facilitates values-directed behavior in children's everyday lives, even in the face of discomfort and distress. This is often referred to as *psychological flexibility*, which is defined as engaging in effective, flexible behavior even in the presence of unwanted or unpleasant thoughts, emotions, and physiological responses, and it is the goal of ACT treatment. To describe it in its simplest terms, psychological flexibility is "the ability to open up, be present, and do what matters," illustrated in Figure 11.2 as a "triflex" (Harris, 2009, p. 12).

ACT Therapy Components and Applications

ACT is made up of six components that can be divided into two broad groups: acceptance and mindfulness processes (acceptance, defusion) and commitment and behavior change processes (values, committed action), with the components present-moment awareness and self as context overlapping in each group.

The first component of ACT is *cognitive defusion*, which targets cognitive fusion, and can be conceptualized as deliteralization of thoughts. In other words, it refers to the process through which an individual comes to understand that his or her thoughts are merely verbal events rather than actual events. For example, rather than a thought being perceived as a literal truth and serving as antecedents to avoidance, an individual might say, "I am having the thought that . . . ." The second component is *acceptance*. Acceptance is an alternative to experiential avoidance and comprises awareness and compassionate acceptance of unpleasant material without any attempts to alter or avoid it. In the case of chronic physical pain, an ACT therapist might draw a client's attention to it or ask him or her to deliberately notice its quality, rather than distracting him- or herself from it. *Present-moment awareness*, the third ACT component, is defined as ongoing, nonevaluative awareness of psychological and environmental events as they occur on a moment-to-moment basis (this is also called *mindfulness*). The goal of present-moment awareness is to be in direct, continuous contact with the world.

Self as context is the fourth component of ACT and refers to the awareness that the self is experienced as a constant, unchanging perspective from which one can observe thoughts, emotions, and external experiences as they come and go. The fifth component, *values*, refers to the individual's domains of importance. They are not goals that can be attained but rather are guiding principles that are thought to motivate sustained and complex chains of behavior (Wilson & Murrell, 2004). Because behaviors are enacted in the service of values, these behaviors themselves may come to have some of the rewarding psychological properties of the valued domain. Sixth, ACT is also very explicit in its goal of fostering *committed action* in the service of one's valued goals. When individuals engage in committed action in the service of their values, they are typically brought into contact with previously avoided psychological experiences. To make a commitment to continued engagement in these behaviors implies willingness to have those experiences and to persist in one's behaviors, even in the face of psychological discomfort. This is a cornerstone of the ACT model of psychological flexibility—to continue to pursue valued ends in the face of discomfort or stress.

The following case example illustrates the adaptation of ACT for a middle-school-age child with significant comorbidity and functional impairment. For children and teens, ACT is often used with other traditional behavioral interventions, such as contingency management, parent management training, and skills building. Therefore, the intervention described next highlights how ACT may be integrated with these techniques.

Case Example: ACT for School Refusal

Identifying Features of Client

Joseph, a 12-year-old, typically developing, slightly obese Caucasian male, was initially referred by his mother, Ms. N., to a university psychological treatment center in the rural Southeast to address problems of chronic school refusal, anxiety, depression, noncompliance, and disruptive behavior both at home and in school. At the time of his assessment in April, Joseph had missed 69 days of school. He was failing, despite having gotten all A's and B's in the first 9 weeks of the school year, due to poor attendance and refusal to complete schoolwork at home. This followed a year in which he had been home-schooled due to his school avoidance. Joseph described numerous anxiety and somatic symptoms while in school, and he reported experiencing continued verbal and physical bullying, as well as unsympathetic teachers. While at home, Joseph mostly slept or watched TV, growing argumentative and violent when his mother encouraged him to go back to school. The school had informed Joseph's parents that they were to be fined and potentially jailed for educational neglect. Consequently, Mr. and Mrs. N. hoped that intervention would help Joseph return to school.

Past Treatment History

Ms. N. reported that Joseph had an extensive history of psychiatric treatment beginning 3 years before, subsequent to the death of his grandfather, to whom he was very close. Joseph received both inpatient and outpatient services at various points. He stated that he was hospitalized for "anxiety" because he got "real bad sick" when away from his parents. A series of pharmacological treatments had been tried, and currently Joseph was taking 1000 mg of Depakote for "mood swings," in addition to 15 mg of Paxil for "agitation and worry."

Assessment from an ACT Perspective

An ACT case conceptualization begins with a functional assessment to ascertain client behaviors that are unhelpful and reflective of experiential avoidance. With children, this includes assessment of the child's behavior, the family's response, and the nature of past treatment. In all three domains, Joseph's excessive anxiety and worry was seen as the cause of school refusal. Joseph avoided situations that elicited his anxiety—specifically school, but also any situations involving separation from his family. Therefore, Joseph's behavior constituted a functional avoidance strategy.

A variety of contingencies, both verbally mediated and immediately experienced, supported Joseph's experiential avoidance. Considered from an ecological perspective, these contingencies existed in Joseph's immediate environment (his family), as well as at school, in the treatment community, and in the broader culture.

1. Joseph perceived his anxiety as "unbearable," and he engaged in situational avoidance to prevent its occurrence, as well as to escape (e.g., promising to attend school in response to his mother's demands to go and then failing to follow through; leaving school as soon as he was dropped off; engaging in fights at school that resulted in his being sent home; spending time in the nurse's office; "falling asleep" at his desk).

2. Joseph's mother accommodated his anxiety by making, and then failing to enforce, demands to attend school. She allowed him to stay home if he was "too upset."

3. Medical and mental health professionals supported Joseph's and his family's view that in order for him to return to school, his anxiety should be eliminated. They identified the anxiety-related cognition and emotion as "the problem" and, in an effort to eliminate anxiety, provided treatments aimed at altering the intensity and frequency of "the problem."

4. The culture teaches us that negative affect and cognition, unless relatively short in duration, are abnormal and problematic. For example, when Joseph showed anxiety in school, he was bullied by peers, who called him derogatory names.

5. To the extent that anxiety avoidance tactics and unilateral acts by the client (staying home from school) reduce anxiety, these "solutions" will be immediately reinforced by these reductions. Thus Joseph's multitude of anxiety avoidance strategies constitutes a narrow, inflexible behavioral repertoire that ultimately results in more sustained and intense anxiety over time. Moreover, the failure of these strategies to remove anxiety may have also contributed to Joseph's depression and externalizing behaviors.

ACT as a Solution

From an ACT perspective, excessive attempts to control anxiety, rather than the anxiety itself, are seen as pathogenic. Therefore, we aim our efforts at disrupting the socioverbal context that establishes and maintains functional avoidance strategies. The first phase of the treatment of this young man involved a fairly straightforward reorganization of contingencies having to do with school attendance. The second phase of treatment is more specific to ACT and addressed the contingencies relevant to the establishment and maintenance of experiential avoidance. This latter set of contingencies are the focus of most of the following discussion.

During the course of treatment, the family met with therapist once per week for sessions lasting between 1 and 2 hours, for approximately 8 months (April to December). Both Joseph and his mother attended the majority of sessions, although each also attended separately, as needed.

Phase 1: Organization of Contingencies Regarding School Attendance

At the outset of treatment, the therapist instructed Joseph's mother to stop trying to get him to attend school. It was clear that her attempts to argue, cajole, threaten, and beg Joseph to attend school were unproductive with respect to school attendance and also highly disruptive of the family's home life. If he refused to go to school, Joseph was to restrict his activity to resting or at most reading, but he ought not to engage in any activity that might be too stimulating, including watching television, going outside, or playing any games. Above all, Joseph's parents were admonished not to attempt in any way to argue, convince, or coerce Joseph into attending school. Joseph's therapist also put in place a reward system through which he could earn the privilege of participating in activities such as bowling or riding his go-cart, provided he attend a certain number of days of school during the week. This part of the intervention is a straightforward application of the principle of relativity of reinforcement (e.g., Timberlake & Allison, 1974): the therapist greatly decreased the availability of reinforcement at home and increased it contingent on school attendance.

In addition to this contingency-management component of treatment, Joseph, his mother, and the therapist began a conversation that focused on the following question: "In a world where you could take a direction in life that you really care about, what direction might you take?" The balance of this discussion of intervention focuses on the ACT components of the treatment and about what got in the way of Joseph moving in that valued direction.

Phase 2: Targeting Experiential Avoidance

Treatment of experiential avoidance begins by aggregating a functional class of avoidant behaviors and helping the client to make psychological contact with those behaviors and their results. The parents of this young man were quite sympathetic to the obvious distress that he was experiencing at school. The case conceptualization presented to them by other professionals was generally consistent with a lay view of anxiety problems. That is, Joseph behaved badly because he was feeling overwhelming anxiety and worry when he went to school. He felt that in order for him to attend school, anxiety and worry would need to be reduced. Thus the therapist began treatment by carefully going over all of the ways that the family and Joseph had tried to eliminate or at least reduce anxiety. This intervention, called *creative hopelessness*, strives to undermine the client's desire to control private events. The intervention has a variety of functions. First, if attempts at control are truly pathogenic, we need to extinguish these responses. However, the client has actually been engaged in wholly sensible responses: in virtually every domain of life, attempts to remove oneself from pain are adaptive. Unfortunately, when such strategies are used to eliminate unwanted private events such as thoughts, emotions, or physical sensations, the result is their paradoxical amplification. In creative hopelessness interventions, ACT therapists pit entirely sensible avoidance strategies, again and again, against the client's experience of the unworkability of those strategies to manage private events. One aim of this intervention is to make a direct connection between a functional class of control strategies and their directly experienced, devastating consequences. Specifically, this includes the failure of these strategies to manage the anxiety in the long term.

Phase 3: Acceptance and Mindfulness Processes

In ACT, individuals are taught mindfulness and acceptance in an experiential way, such that they may simply notice and detach from their thoughts and appreciate the present moment without evaluation or response. Here is an example, adapted from Coyne, Burke, and Freeman (2008), of how present-moment awareness was described to Joseph:

> THERAPIST: I'd like to show you a way to be what we call "mindful," and to really notice what's going on around you. Would that be OK? (*Joseph nods.*) We're going to practice being explorers. Do you know what explorers do?
>
> JOSEPH: They travel really far, even if they don't know the way. They discover stuff.
>
> THERAPIST: How do you think they do that?
>
> JOSEPH: I'm not sure. Maybe they start off on a journey?
>
> THERAPIST: That's exactly right. Explorers get curious about stuff, and they set out to find out. They might be scared, or not know the right direction, but they do their best and start off anyway. But here's the trick—they are curious about what will happen, but they watch what happens without trying make stuff happen.
>
> JOSEPH: I'm not sure I understand.
>
> THERAPIST: Think of it this way. If you were at a restaurant and saw another kid eating a hot fudge sundae, what do you think about?
>
> JOSEPH: How yummy it might be! And I want to eat it!
>
> THERAPIST: Yup. And you probably imagine what the cold, vanilla ice cream will taste like, and wonder whether it's sweet, or maybe a

little melty because of the hot fudge, and if the brownie is chewy, and has chips in it. But you wouldn't go over to that kid and take his ice cream sundae, right? Well, that's like what an explorer does—noticing stuff, and being curious about it, without trying to change it. That's what we call being mindful. Can we try to practice that right now?

JOSEPH: All right.

THERAPIST: OK. Close your eyes . . . get comfy in your chair . . . notice how your body feels . . . where it touches the chair, where your feet touch the floor . . . notice all the sounds you hear . . . see how many different ones you can notice . . . see if you can notice how warm or cool the room is . . . see if you can feel the chair beneath you, holding you up . . . see if you can notice your breathing, gently, in and out . . . notice that the air is cool when you breathe it in, and warmer as you breathe it out. Now notice what you are thinking . . . if you are seeing pictures in your head, see if you can print them on the screen on your cellphone, like little texts or photos . . . imagine that each thought or picture in your head is on your phone . . . and just look at it until it passes and a new text or picture pops in . . . .

Defusion. In order to target Joseph's cognitive fusion with the idea that going to school was impossible, the next phase of treatment involved *defusion*, which refers to exposure to unwanted private events such that they cease to be experienced as literal *truths*. The therapist introduced this concept to Joseph and his mother in the following way. To begin, he asked Joseph to imagine that he wanted very badly to leave the therapy room.

THERAPIST: If you wanted to leave this room, you could assume that the door was locked or assume that the door was unlocked. Right?

JOSEPH: Sure.

THERAPIST: What if you assumed that the door was unlocked . . . what would you do?

JOSEPH: I'd leave.

THERAPIST: Right. You'd get up, walk over to the door, and turn the knob. What if you assumed the door was locked?

JOSEPH: I don't know . . . wait until someone unlocked it I guess.

THERAPIST: OK. Could you assume that the door was unlocked, even if you believed that it was locked. That is, could you have the thought "the door is locked" while getting up and walking over to the door and turning the knob.

JOSEPH: Yes.

THERAPIST: OK. We are going to play a little game. In this game, I am going to ask you to assume that something is possible, even though your mind may say that it is not. Are you willing to play?

JOSEPH: I guess so.

Acceptance. Acceptance, like present-moment awareness, is a component of mindfulness. It involves giving oneself permission to experience the whole of one's experiences in a compassionate, nondefensive way. Acceptance can be particularly useful for parents who have difficulty tolerating their child's behavior or strong negative emotion. Here is an example, adapted from Coyne and Murrell (2009), of how an acceptance exercise was used with Joseph's mother:

THERAPIST: There's a Buddhist saying that, paraphrased, is something like, Don't speak unless you can improve on the silence. When Joseph is fearful and arguing with you about going to school, you have a choice about what you can do. You can engage him, and from what you tell me, the situation quickly escalates. But what if there's another way?

MRS. N.: I'm not sure what that would be.

THERAPIST: We call it "acceptance," or nonjudgmental awareness of whatever you are feeling—all of your thoughts and feelings in response to Joseph, as well as all the thoughts and feelings that he expresses. Are you willing to try it here, right now, for a few minutes?

MRS. N.: Um, sure. I'm just not sure how to do it.

THERAPIST: That's OK. Let me try to show you, and let's see what happens. (*Client nods.*) Please close your eyes, and take a few moments to simply notice your breath. (*Client does so.*) I want you to imagine Joseph standing in front of you when he is anxious. Imagine the look on his face, his eyes, how he is breathing, if he is flushed, his posture, how quickly he moves, how he sounds when he speaks. Practice simply seeing him, how anxious he is. Don't try to change or solve anything, or help, or soothe him. There is no need. Simply be. Appreciate all the feelings he is showing you in this moment. Imagine that he sees you noticing him. Take a few moments to simply experience being with him.

Self-as-Context. A simple way to understand the "self-as-context" component of ACT is as perspective taking. It involves meta-awareness of one's experiences, or the ability to experience a stable, safe, and whole sense of self that holds thoughts, emotions, and physical sensations briefly as they pass. Self-as-context awareness involves the ability to distinguish a few simple relational frames: I–you; here–there; and now–then (McHugh, Barnes-Holmes, & Barnes-Holmes, 2004). Here is an example of how the therapist introduced self-as-context to Joseph through an experiential exercise called "the Treehouse" (Coyne & Murrell, 2009):

> "When you are angry, close your eyes, and imagine you are in a tree-house. Outside the window of your treehouse is the sky, and it is stormy. Your feelings and thoughts about school and being away from home are the stormclouds—you can watch them safely from inside your treehouse. You are high up in the tree, so you are close to them, but you are far enough away to be safe in the treehouse. Watch what they do outside the window. What do they look like? Are they moving slowly or quickly? Is there lightning? Thunder? Rain? Let me know how they move, and when they come and go."

Phase 4: Behavior Change Processes

Valuing. If symptom removal is not the work of therapy, what then? In order to identify treatment targets in ACT, one needs to establish the client's sense of direction. As with any behavioral intervention, clinicians need to assess for reinforcers that are sufficiently potent to motivate therapeutic activity. Identifying reinforcers that are available in the individual's day-to-day environment and that are the naturally occurring consequences of the desired behavior is optimal, as behavior brought under the control of such consequences has the greatest potential to be maintained posttreatment. In ACT, therapists conduct a values assessment because many of the strongest reinforcers available for people lie well outside the realm of primary reinforcers (e.g., going to heaven, being thought a good parent, being a pillar of the community, making a scientific contribution). Therapists thus assess for values in areas such as education, family, and social relations, among others. ACT therapists often ask children to generate lists of behaviors that are consistent with their values, as well as those that are inconsistent. Joseph had a great fondness for a certain university in the South, as do many young people from that area. When asked if he would like to attend that university when he finished school, he agreed that he would definitely like that. In order to attend a university, Joseph knew he had to do well in school. Therefore, he identified his value as "being an extraordinary student."

Committed Action. What ensued was a conversation about what would need to happen in order for Joseph to attend that university. Joseph stated that he would have to go to school. The therapist asked Joseph: "If therapy could be about you being an extraordinary student, would that be something you would be willing to work for?" The therapist then went on to ask him to imagine that this was possible and then instructed Joseph to ask himself a few questions: "If this could really work—you could become an extraordinary student—would it be worth feeling anxious, if that were the cost?" "What if you had to feel even more anxious than you ever felt, but in the end, you got to be an extraordinary student?"

To begin to more clearly delineate behaviors that would assist Joseph in becoming an extraordinary student, the clinician worked with him on discriminating those behaviors that "worked" and those that didn't. For example, he identified going to school, paying attention in class, staying in his seat, raising his hand if he had a question, and staying out of fights when he was mad as behaviors that "worked." Things that didn't work included arguing with his mother, staying home and sleeping all day, and telling the nurse he was sick so that he could go home.

Thus Joseph agreed to a treatment contract that involved working on becoming an extraordinary student as a project. Joseph was told that being an extraordinary student is like a team sport. His therapist asked him to imagine what would happen if he played on a football team (he loved football) in which the other team had eleven players, but his team had fifty players. Joseph could see the advantage of having a large team, and it was clear that his family and teachers at school would be important members of the team. Joseph and his therapist developed a recruiting strategy that had the following elements.

1. Approaching the person he wanted to recruit.
2. Stating his intention for the school year (being an extraordinary student).
3. Acknowledging the person's skepticism if he or she had known him the previous year. This usually took the form of: "I know this sounds kind of impossible, and I don't expect you to believe me just yet, but I intend to be an extraordinary student this year."
4. Repairing damaged relationships where necessary. This step typically involved saying something like: "I realize that I behaved very badly in your class last year. I know that my behavior was disrespectful. I know that I made it impossible for you to teach me anything."
5. Finally, Joseph asked the teacher to be on his team. This usually took the following form: "I know that to do this, I will need a lot of help. I am building a team to help me be an extraordinary student. Would you please be on my team and help me to be an extraordinary student this year?"

It is worth noting that this commitment exercise involved massive exposure to avoided psychological and environmental content. In order to do the exercises, Joseph had to go to school. He had to interact with teachers. Who likes to admit when they have been wrong? To enhance the probability of this work being done, the therapist conducted defusion and exposure work on past academic failures, because any attempt on Joseph's part to do better in school would almost certainly occasion memories of past school failures. Consequently, Joseph needed to develop greater flexibility in his reactions to his thoughts about failure. In addition, the therapist told Joseph that if he did this task, his experience in school might be completely transformed. The therapist asked him to imagine a world in which enemies became friends, in which mistakes that he made could help him to move ahead, and in which things that once seemed impossible became possible. To his delight, Joseph's recruiting efforts were met with no less than astonishment by his teachers. He did not receive a single negative response to his recruiting efforts.

Conclusions

The theories, mechanisms, and implementation of ACT have been shown to be efficacious across a wide range of adult populations. Though the child/adolescent ACT literature is only in its early stages, the overall effects are promising. In order to move forward, future work is needed, especially prospective studies of experiential avoidance and cognitive fusion as common or transdiagnostic risk factors in younger samples of children. Furthermore, the process of experiential avoidance should be more broadly measured, using observational tools, other report measures, and lab-based analogue indices. Finally, intervention studies should compare ACT or ACT-based interventions with traditional evidence-based strategies to determine whether ACT approaches parallel or improve on them. Perhaps most important, experiential avoidance should be assessed as a mediator or moderator of treatment outcome in clinical trials with children, adolescents, and parents. In sum, ACT may be a relatively ideal transdiagnostic model, given its clear linkage between treatment components, theory, and empirical data. Furthermore, the goals of ACT are not only malleable to various clinical presentations, but they are also accessible to youth at different developmental levels. Thus ACT demonstrates significant transdiagnostic potential for children, adolescents, and families.

REFERENCES

Armelie, A. P., Delahanty, P. L., & Boarts, J. M. (2010, July). *The impact of verbal abuse on depression symptoms in lesbian, gay, and bisexual youth: The roles of self-criticism and psychological inflexibility.* Poster presented at the annual meeting of the Association for Contextual and Behavioral Science, Reno, NV.

Bach, P., & Hayes, S. C. (2002). The use of acceptance and commitment therapy to prevent the rehospitalization of psychotic patients: A randomized controlled trial. *Journal of Consulting and Clinical Psychology, 70*(5), 1129–1139.

Barnes-Holmes, Y., Barnes-Holmes, D., Smeets, P. M., Strand, P., & Friman, P. (2004). Establishing relational responding in accordance with more-than and less-than as generalized operant behavior in young children. *International Journal of Psychology and Psychological Therapy, 4,* 531–558.

Berlin, K., Sato, A., Jastrowski, K., Woods, D., & Davies, W. H. (2006, November). Effects of experiential avoidance on parenting practices and adolescent outcomes. In K. S. Berlin & A. R. Murrell (Chairs), *Extending acceptance and mindfulness research to parents, families, and adolescents: Process, empirical findings, clinical implications, and future directions.* Symposium conducted at the annual meeting of the Association for Behavioral and Cognitive Therapies, Chicago.

Blackledge, J. T., & Hayes, S. C. (2006). Using acceptance and commitment training in the support for parents of children diagnosed with autism. *Child and Family Behavior Therapy, 28,* 1–18.

Bohlmeijer, E. T., Fledderus, M., Rokx, T. A. J. J., & Pieterse, M. E. (2011). Efficacy of an early intervention based on acceptance and commitment therapy for adults with depressive symptomatology: Evaluation in a randomized controlled trial. *Behaviour Research and Therapy, 49,* 62–67.

Bond, F. W., & Bunce, D. (2000). Mediators of change in emotion-focused and problem-focused worksite stress management interventions. *Journal of Occupational Health Psychology, 5,* 156–163.

Boulanger, J. L., Hayes, S. C., & Pistorello, J. (2010). Experiential avoidance as a functional contextual concept. In A. M. Kring & D. M. Sloan (Eds.), *Emotion regulation and psychopathology: A transdiagnostic approach to etiology and treatment* (pp. 107–134). New York: Guilford Press.

Brinkborg, H., Michanek, J., Hesser, H., & Berglund, G. (2011). Acceptance and commitment therapy for the treatment of stress among social workers: A randomized controlled trial. *Behaviour Research and Therapy, 49,* 389–398.

Brown, L. A., Forman, E. M., Herbert, J. D., Hoffman, K. L., Yuen, E. K., & Goetter, E. M. (2011). A randomized controlled trial of acceptance-based behavior therapy and cognitive therapy for test anxiety: A pilot study. *Behavior Modification, 35,* 31–53.

Brown, F., & Hooper, S. (2009). Acceptance and commitment therapy (ACT) with a learning disabled young person experiencing anxious and obsessive thoughts. *Journal of Intellectual Disabilities, 13,* 195–201.

Butryn, M. L., Forman, E., Hoffman, K., Shaw, J., & Juarascio, A. (2011). A pilot study of acceptance and commitment therapy for promotion of physical activity. *Journal of Physical Activity and Health, 8*(4), 516–522.

Cheron, D. M., Ehrenreich, J. T., & Pincus, D. B. (2009). Assessment of parental experiential avoidance in a clinical sample of children with anxiety disorders. *Child Psychiatry and Human Development, 40,* 383–403.

Chowla, N., & Ostafin, B. (2007). Experiential avoidance as a functional dimensional approach to psychopathology: An empirical review. *Journal of Clinical Psychology, 63,* 871–890.

Ciarrochi, J., Kashdan, T., Leeson, P., Heaven, P. C. L., & Jordon, C. (2011). On being aware and accepting: A one-year longitudinal study into adolescent well-being. *Journal of Adolescence, 34,* 695–703.

Clark, D. M. (2001). A cognitive perspective on social phobia. In W. R. Crozier & L. E. Alden (Eds.), *International handbook of social anxiety: Concepts, research and interventions related to the self and shyness* (pp. 405–430). Chichester, UK: Wiley.

Cooper, J. O., Heron, T. E., & Heward, W. L. (1987). *Applied behavior analysis* (2nd ed.). Upper Saddle River, NJ: Pearson.

Coyne, L. W., Burke, A. M., & Freeman, J. B. (2008). Cognitive-behavioral treatment. In M. Herson & A. M. Gross (Eds.), *Handbook of clinical psychology: Vol. 2. Children and adolescents* (pp. 694–727). Hoboken, NJ: Wiley.

Coyne, L. W., & Burke-Currie, A. (2011). *Mothers' attitudes towards children's emotions and emotional and behavioral regulation strategies.* Manuscript in preparation.

Coyne, L. W., McHugh, L., & Martinez, E. R. (2011). Acceptance and commitment therapy (ACT): Advances and applications with children, adolescents, and families. *Child and Adolescent Psychiatric Clinics of North America, 20,* 379–399.

Coyne, L. W., & Murrell, A. R. (2009). *The joy of parenting: An acceptance and commitment therapy guide to effective parenting in the early years.* Oakland, CA: New Harbinger.

Coyne, L. W., & Silvia, K. A. (2007, July). *Does mindfulness influence parent–child interactions?: Preliminary findings from an experimental study.* Poster presented at the World Congress of Behavioural and Cognitive Therapies, Barcelona, Spain.

Coyne, L., & Thompson, A. (2011). Maternal depression, locus of control, and emotion regulatory strategy as predictors of preschoolers' internalizing problems. *Journal of Child and Family Studies, 20,* 873–883.

Coyne, L. W., & Wilson, K. G. (2004). The role of cognitive fusion in impaired parenting: An RFT analysis. *International Journal of Psychology and Psychological Therapy, 4,* 469–486.

Dahl, J., Wilson, K. G., & Nilsson, A. (2004). Acceptance and commitment therapy and the treatment of persons at risk for long-term disability resulting from stress and pain symptoms: A preliminary randomized trial. *Behavior Therapy, 35,* 785–802.

Dymond, S., & Barnes, D. (1997). Behavior-analytic approaches to self-awareness. *Psychological Record, 47,* 181–200.

Feldner, M. T., Zvolensky, M. J., Eifert, G. H., & Spira, A. P. (2003). Emotional avoidance: An experimental test of individual differences and response suppression using biological challenge. *Behaviour Research and Therapy, 41,* 403–411.

Flaxman, P. E., & Bond, F. W. (2010). A randomized worksite comparison of acceptance and commitment therapy and stress inoculation training. *Behavior Research and Therapy, 48,* 816–820.

Fledderus, M., Bohlmeijer, E. T., Pieterse, M. E., & Schreurs, K. M. G. (2012). Acceptance and commitment therapy as guided self-help for psychological distress and positive mental health: A randomized controlled trial. *Psychological Medicine, 42*(3), 485–495.

Fledderus, M., Bohlmeijer, E. T., Smit, F., & Westerhof, G. B. (2010). Mental health promotion as a new goal in public mental health care: A randomized controlled trial of an intervention enhancing psychological flexibility. *American Journal of Public Health, 100*(12), 2372–2378.

Forman, E. M., Herbert, J. D., Moitra, E., Yeomans, P. D., & Geller, P. A. (2007). A randomized controlled effectiveness trial of acceptance and commitment therapy and cognitive therapy for anxiety and depression. *Behavior Modification, 31*(6), 772–799.

Gaudiano, B. A., & Herbert, J. D. (2006). Acute treatment of inpatients with psychotic symptoms using acceptance and commitment therapy: Pilot results. *Behaviour Research and Therapy, 44*(3), 415–437.

Gifford, E. V., Kohlenberg, B. S., Hayes, S. C., Antonuccio, D. O., Piasecki, M. M., Rasmussen-Hall, M. L., et al. (2004). Applying a functional acceptance based model to smoking cessation: An initial trial of acceptance and commitment therapy. *Behavior Therapy, 35*, 689–705.

Gifford, E. V., Kohlenberg, B. S., Hayes, S. C., Pierson, H. M., Piasecki, M. P., Antonuccio, D. O., et al. (2011). Does acceptance and relationship focused behavior therapy contribute to bupropion outcomes?: A randomized controlled trial of functional analytic psychotherapy and acceptance and commitment therapy for smoking cessation. *Behavior Therapy, 42*, 700–715.

Gratz, K. L., & Gunderson, J. G. (2006). Preliminary data on an acceptance-based emotion regulation group intervention for deliberate self-harm among women with borderline personality disorder. *Behavior Therapy, 37*(1), 25–35.

Greco, L. A., Heffner, M., Poe, S., Ritchie, S., Polak, M., & Lynch, S. K., (2005). Maternal adjustment following preterm birth: Contributions of experiential avoidance. *Behavior Therapy, 36*, 177–184.

Greco, L. A., Lambert, W., & Baer, R. A. (2008). Psychological inflexibility in childhood and adolescence: Development and evaluation of the Avoidance and Fusion Questionnaire for Youth. *Psychological Assessment, 20*, 93–102.

Gregg, J. A., Callaghan, G. M., Hayes, S. C., & Glenn-Lawson, J. L. (2007). Improving diabetes self-management through acceptance, mindfulness, and values: A randomized controlled trial. *Journal of Consulting and Clinical Psychology, 75*, 336–343.

Harris, R. (2009). *ACT made simple: An easy-to-read primer on acceptance and commitment therapy.* Oakland, CA: New Harbinger.

Hayes, S. C., Barnes-Holmes, D., & Roche, B. (2001). *Relational frame theory: A post-Skinnerian account of human language and cognition.* New York: Kluwer Academic.

Hayes, S. C., Bissett, R., Roget, N., Padilla, M., Kohlenberg, B. S., Fisher, G., et al. (2004). The impact of acceptance and commitment training and multicultural training on the stigmatizing attitudes and professional burnout of substance abuse counselors. *Behavior Therapy, 35*, 821–835.

Hayes, L., Boyd, C. P., & Sewell, J. (2011). Acceptance and commitment therapy for the treatment of adolescent depression: A pilot study in a psychiatric outpatient setting. *Mindfulness, 2*(2), 86–94.

Hayes, S., Luoma, J., Bond, F., Masuda, A., & Lillis, J. (2006). Acceptance and commitment therapy: Model, processes and outcomes. *Behaviour Research and Therapy, 44*, 1–25.

Hayes, S. C., Strosahl, K. D., & Wilson, K. G. (1999). *Acceptance and commitment therapy: An experiential approach to behavior change*. New York: Guilford Press.

Hayes, S. C., Strosahl, K. D., & Wilson, K. G. (2012). *Acceptance and commitment therapy: The process and practice of mindful change* (2nd ed.). New York: Guilford Press.

Hayes, S. C., Villatte, M., Levin, M., & Hildebrandt, M. (2011). Open, aware, and active: Contextual approaches as an emerging trend in the behavioral and cognitive therapies. *Annual Review of Clinical Psychology, 7*, 141–168.

Hayes, S. C., Wilson, K. G., Gifford, E. V., Bissett, R., Piasecki, M., Batten, S. V., et al. (2004). A preliminary trial of twelve-step facilitation and acceptance and commitment therapy with polysubstance-abusing methadone-maintained opiate addicts. *Behavior Therapy, 35*(4), 667–688.

Hayes, S. C., Wilson, K. G., Strosahl, K. D., Gifford, E. V., & Follette, V. M. (1996). Experiential avoidance and behavioral disorders: A functional dimensional approach to diagnosis and treatment. *Journal of Consulting and Clinical Psychology, 64*, 1152–1168.

Heffner, M., Sperry, J., & Eifert, G. H. (2002). Acceptance and commitment therapy in the treatment of an adolescent female with anorexia nervosa: A case example. *Cognitive and Behavioral Practice, 9*, 232–236.

Hinton, M. J., & Gaynor, S. T. (2010). Cognitive defusion for psychological distress, dysphoria, and low self-esteem: A randomized technique evaluation trial of vocalizing strategies. *International Journal of Behavioral Consultation and Therapy, 6*, 164–185.

Juarascio, A. S., Forman, E. M., & Herbert, J. D. (2010). Acceptance and commitment therapy versus cognitive therapy for the treatment of comorbid eating pathology. *Behavior Modification, 34*, 175–190.

Karekla, M., Forsyth, J. P., & Kelly, M. M. (2004). Emotional avoidance and panicogenic responding to a biological challenge procedure. *Behavior Therapy, 35*, 725–746.

Lappalainen, R., Lehtonen, T., Skarp, E., Taubert, E., Ojanen, M., & Hayes, S. C. (2007). The impact of CBT and ACT models using psychology trainee therapists: A preliminary controlled effectiveness trial. *Behavior Modification, 31*(4), 488–511.

Lillis, J., Hayes, S. C., Bunting, K., & Masuda, A. (2009). Teaching acceptance and mindfulness to improve the lives of the obese: A preliminary test of a theoretical model. *Annals of Behavioral Medicine, 37*, 58–69.

Lipkens, G., Hayes, S. C., & Hayes, L. J. (1993). Longitudinal study of derived stimulus relations in an infant. *Journal of Experimental Child Psychology, 56*, 201–239.

Lundgren, T., Dahl, J., & Hayes, S. C. (2008). Evaluation of mediators of change in the treatment of epilepsy with acceptance and commitment therapy. *Journal of Behavior Medicine, 31*, 225–235.

Lundgren, T., Dahl, J., Melin, L., & Kies, B. (2006). Evaluation of acceptance and commitment therapy for drug refractory epilepsy: A randomized controlled trial in South Africa—a pilot study. *Epilepsia, 47*(12), 2173–2179.

Lundgren, T., Dahl, J., Yardi, N., & Melin, J. (2008). Acceptance and commitment therapy and yoga for drug refractory epilepsy: A randomized controlled trial. *Epilepsy and Behavior, 13*, 102–108.

Luoma, J. B., Hayes, S. C., Twohig, M. P., Roget, N., Fisher, G., Padilla, M., et al. (2007). Augmenting continuing education with psychologically focused group consultation: Effects on adoption of group drug counseling. *Psychotherapy: Theory, Research, Practice, Training, 44*(4), 463–469.

Luoma, J. B., Kohlenberg, B. S., Hayes, S. C., & Fletcher, L. (2012). Slow and steady wins the race: A randomized clinical trial of acceptance and commitment therapy targeting shame in substance use disorders. *Journal of Consulting and Clinical Psychology, 80*, 43–51.

Masuda, A., Cohen, L. L., Wicksell, R. K., Kemani, M. K., & Johnson, A. (2011). A case study: Acceptance and commitment therapy for pediatric sickle cell disease. *Journal of Pediatric Psychology, 36*, 398–408.

Masuda, A., Hayes, S. C., Fletcher, L. B., Seignourel, P. J., Bunting, K., Herbst, S. A., et al. (2007). The impact of acceptance and commitment therapy versus education on stigma toward people with psychological disorders. *Behaviour Research and Therapy, 45*(11), 2764–2772.

McCracken, L. M., Gauntlett-Gilbert, J., & Eccleston, C. (2010). Acceptance of pain in adolescents with chronic pain: Validation of an adapted assessment instrument and preliminary correlation analyses. *European Journal of Pain, 14*, 316–320.

McHugh, L., Barnes-Holmes, D., & Barnes-Holmes, Y. (2004). A relational frame account of the development of complex cognitive phenomena: Perspective-taking, false belief understanding, and deception. *International Journal of Psychology and Psychological Therapy, 4*, 303–324.

Merwin, R. M., Timko, A. C., Zucker, N. L., Martin, L., & Moskovich, A. A. (2010, July). *ACT-based family intervention for adolescents with anorexia nervosa.* Paper presented at the annual meeting of the Association for Behavioral and Contextual Science, Reno, NV.

Morris, T. L., & Greco, L. A. (2002). Incorporating parents and peers in the assessment and treatment of childhood anxiety. In L. VandeCreek & T. L. Jackson (Eds.), *Innovations in clinical practice: A source book* (Vol. 20, pp. 75–85). Sarasota, FL: Professional Resource Press/Professional Resource Exchange.

Murrell, A. R., Wilson, K. G., LaBorde, C. T., Drake, C. E., & Rogers, L. J. (2009). Relational responding in parents. *Behavior Analyst Today, 9*, 196–214.

Muto, T., Hayes, S. C., & Jeffcoat, T. (2011). The effectiveness of acceptance and commitment therapy bibliotherapy for enhancing the psychological health of Japanese college students living abroad. *Behavior Therapy, 42*, 323–335.

Öst, L. (2008). Efficacy of the third wave of behavioral therapies: A systematic review and meta-analysis. *Behaviour Research and Therapy, 46*, 296–321.

Páez, M., Luciano, M. C., & Gutiérrez, O. (2007). Tratamiento psicológico para el afrontamiento del cáncer de mama: Estudio comparativo entre estrategias de aceptación y de control cognitivo [Psychological treatment for breast cancer: Comparison between acceptance based and cognitive control based strategies]. *Psicooncología, 4*, 75–95.

Pearson, A. N., Follette, V. M., & Hayes, S. C. (2012). A pilot study of acceptance and commitment therapy as a workshop intervention for body dissatisfaction and disordered eating attitudes. *Cognitive and Behavioral Practice, 19,* 181–197.

Petersen, C. L., & Zettle, R. D. (2009). Treating inpatients with comorbid depression and alcohol use disorders: A comparison of acceptance and commitment therapy and treatment as usual. *Psychological Record, 59,* 521–536.

Roche, B., & Barnes, D. (1996). Arbitrarily applicable relational responding and human sexual categorization: A critical test of the derived difference relation. *Psychological Record, 46,* 451–475.

Roemer, L., Orsillo, S. M., & Salters-Pedneault, K. (2008). Efficacy of an acceptance-based behavior therapy for generalized anxiety disorder: Evaluation in a randomized controlled trial. *Journal of Consulting and Clinical Psychology, 76*(6), 1083–1089.

Ruiz, F. J. (2010). A review of acceptance and commitment therapy (ACT) empirical evidence: Correlational, experimental psychopathology, component and outcome studies. *International Journal of Psychology and Psychological Therapy, 10,* 125–162.

Ruiz, F. J., & Luciano, C. (2006, May). Improving chess performance with ACT. In J. T. Blackledge (Chair), *Applications of acceptance and commitment therapy with children and adolescents.* Symposium conducted at the annual meeting of the Association for Behavior Analysis, Atlanta, GA.

Ruiz, F. J., & Luciano, C. (2012). Improving international-level chess players' performance with an acceptance-based protocol. *Psychological Record, 62,* 447–461.

Shea, S., & Coyne, L. W. (2011). Maternal dysphoric mood, stress, and parenting practices in mothers of Head Start preschoolers: The role of experiential avoidance. *Journal of Child and Family Behavior Therapy, 33,* 231–247.

Smout, M. F., Longo, M., Harrison, S., Minniti, R., Wickes, W., & White, J. M. (2010). Psychosocial treatment for methamphetamine use disorders: A preliminary randomized controlled trial of cognitive behavior therapy and acceptance and commitment therapy. *Substance Abuse, 31,* 98–107.

Steele, D., & Hayes, S. (1991). Stimulus equivalence and arbitrarily applicable relational responding. *Journal of the Experimental Analysis of Behavior, 56,* 519–555.

Timberlake, W., & Allison, J. (1974). Response deprivation: An empirical approach to instrumental performance. *Psychological Review, 81,* 146–164.

Twohig, M. P., Hayes, S. C., Plumb, J. C., Pruitt, L. D., Collins, A. B., Hazlett-Stevens, H., et al. (2010). A randomized clinical trial of acceptance and commitment therapy vs. progressive relaxation training for obsessive compulsive disorder. *Journal of Consulting and Clinical Psychology, 78,* 705–716.

U.S. Department of Health and Human Services, Substance Abuse and Mental Health Services Administration, National Registry of Evidence-Based Programs and Practices (NREPP). (2011). Acceptance and commitment therapy (ACT). Retrieved from *http://174.140.153.167/viewintervention.aspx?id=191.*

Varra, A. A., Hayes, S. C., Roget, N., & Fisher, G. (2008). A randomized control trial examining the effect of acceptance and commitment training on clinician willingness to use evidence-based pharmacotherapy. *Journal of Consulting and Clinical Psychology, 76,* 449–458.

Vowles, K. E., McNeil, D. W., Gross, R. T., McDaniel, M., Mouse, A., Bates, M., et al. (2007). Effects of pain acceptance and pain control strategies on physical impairment in individuals with chronic low back pain. *Behavior Therapy, 38,* 412–425.

Weineland, S., Arvidsson, D., Kakoulidis, T. P., & Dahl, J. (2012). Acceptance and commitment therapy for bariatric surgery patients: A pilot RCT. *Obesity Research and Clinical Practice, 6,* 21–30.

Westin, V., Schulin, M., Hesser, H., Karlsson, M., Noe, R., Olofsson, U., et al. (2011). Acceptance and commitment therapy versus tinnitus retraining therapy in the treatment of tinnitus: A randomised controlled trial. *Behaviour Research and Therapy, 49,* 737–747.

Wetherell, J., Afari, N., Rutledge, T., Sorrell, J. T., Stoddard, J. A., Petkus, A. J., et al. (2011). A randomized, controlled trial of acceptance and commitment therapy and cognitive-behavioral therapy for chronic pain. *Pain, 152,* 2098–2107.

Wicksell, R. K., Ahlqvist, J., Bring, A., Melin, L., & Olsson, G. L. (2008). Can exposure and acceptance strategies improve functioning and life satisfaction in people with chronic pain and whiplash-associated disorders (WAD)?: A randomized controlled trial. *Cognitive Behaviour Therapy, 37*(3), 1–14.

Wicksell, R. K., Dahl, J., Magnusson, B., & Olsson, G. L. (2005). Using acceptance and commitment therapy in the rehabilitation of an adolescent female with chronic pain: A case example. *Cognitive and Behavioral Practice, 12,* 415–423.

Wicksell, R. K., Melin, L., Lekander, M., & Olsson, G. L. (2009). Evaluating the effectiveness of exposure and acceptance strategies to improve functioning and quality of life in longstanding pediatric pain: A randomized controlled trial. *Pain, 141,* 248–257.

Wicksell, R., Melin, L., & Olsson, G. (2007). Exposure and acceptance in the rehabilitation of adolescents with idiopathic chronic pain: A pilot study. *European Journal of Pain, 11,* 267–274.

Wilson, K. G., & Murrell, A. (2004). Values work in acceptance and commitment therapy: Setting a course for behavioral treatment. In S. Hayes, V. M. Follette, & M. M. Linehan (Eds.), *Mindfulness and acceptance: Expanding the cognitive-behavioural tradition* (pp. 120–151). New York: Guilford Press.

Woods, D. W., Wetterneck, C. T., & Flessner, C. A. (2006). A controlled evaluation of acceptance and commitment therapy plus habit reversal for trichotillomania. *Behaviour Research and Therapy, 44,* 639–656.

Zettle, R. D. (2003). Acceptance and commitment therapy vs. systematic desensitization in treatment of mathematics anxiety. *Psychological Record, 53*(2), 197–215.

Zettle, R. D., & Hayes, S. C. (1986). Dysfunctional control by client verbal behavior: The context of reason giving. *Analysis of Verbal Behavior, 4,* 30–38.

Zettle, R. D., & Rains, J. C. (1989). Group cognitive and contextual therapies in treatment of depression. *Journal of Clinical Psychology, 45,* 438–445.

PART IV

Transdiagnostic Treatment Approaches

CHAPTER 12

The Unified Protocols for the Treatment of Emotional Disorders in Children and Adolescents

Jill Ehrenreich-May, Alexander H. Queen, Emily L. Bilek, Cara S. Remmes, and Kristen K. Marciel

This chapter discusses the rationale, development, and preliminary efficacy of two emotion-focused, transdiagnostic cognitive-behavioral (CBT) treatments for emotional disorders in youth, using anxiety and depressive disorders as primary targets for change in initial research. The first of these treatments is the Unified Protocol for the Treatment of Emotional Disorders in Adolescents (UP-A; Ehrenreich et al., 2008), an individual treatment for adolescents ages 12–17 years with a principal diagnosis of any anxiety disorder, any depressive disorder, or any combination of these. The second treatment is the Unified Protocol for Children: Emotion Detectives (UP-C:ED; Ehrenreich-May & Bilek, 2009), a group-based program for children ages 7–12 years and a downward extension of the UP-A. The chapter begins with a brief discussion of anxiety and depression in youth, as well as benefits of a non-disorder-specific approach when considering the commonalities and overlap between such emotional disorders in childhood and adolescence.

Youth Anxiety and Depression:
Phenomenology and Treatment Response

Anxiety disorders are among the most common psychological disorders in children and adolescents, with 12-month prevalence estimates of 10–21% in the general population (Beesdo, Knappe, & Pine, 2009; Costello, Mustillo, Erkanli, Keeler, & Angold, 2003; Pine, 1994). Unipolar depressive disorders (i.e., major depressive disorder [MDD], dysthymic disorder [DD]) are also common, particularly in adolescence, when prevalence rates rise to 4–7% (Costello et al., 2002), comparable to depressive disorder rates in adulthood (Narrow, Rae, Robins, & Regier, 2002). The prevalence of depressive episodes is even higher, with approximately 28% of individuals experiencing a depressive episode before age 18 (Lewinsohn, Rohde, & Seeley, 1998). Both youth anxiety and depression are chronic conditions (Birmaher, Mustillo, Erkanli, Keeler, & Angold, 1996; Keller, Lavori, Mueller, & Endicott, 1992) associated with negative effects on social and academic functioning (Brunstein-Klomek, Marrocco, Kleinman, Schonfeld, & Gould, 2007; Messer & Beidel, 1994; Sheeber, Davis, Leve, Hops, & Tildesley, 2007), as well as increased risk of negative outcomes in adulthood, including poor occupational functioning, substance abuse, and suicide (Geller, Zimerman, Williams, Bolhofner, & Craney, 2001; Weissman et al., 1999).

In addition to their unique prevalence rates and impairments, a high degree of diagnostic comorbidity also exists between youth anxiety and depressive disorders. A meta-analysis by Brady and Kendall (1992) revealed that across multiple settings (e.g., community settings, inpatient facilities, pediatric clinics), 15.9–61.9% of children and adolescents met diagnostic criteria for at least one anxiety disorder and a concurrent depressive disorder. Rates of anxiety and depression comorbidity are higher among older children and adolescents (Ollendick, Shortt, & Sander, 2005; Strauss, Last, Hersen, & Kazdin, 1988), as well as treatment-seeking youth (Brady & Kendall, 1992). In addition to diagnostic comorbidity, anxiety and depressive symptoms show a moderately strong correlation ($r = .34$), even after controlling for overlapping items on self-report anxiety and depression measures (Stark & Laurent, 2001). Beyond their high co-occurrence, youth anxiety and depression share a number of common biological and environmental risk factors, including behaviorally inhibited temperament (Caspi et al., 1996; Gladstone, Parker, Mitchell, Wilhelm, & Malhi, 2005; Pérez-Edgar & Fox, 2005), negative early life experiences (Chorpita & Barlow, 1998), and deficits in emotion regulation (Hannesdottir & Ollendick, 2007; Kovacs, Joormann, & Gotlib, 2008; Southam-Gerow & Kendall, 2000; Suveg & Zeman, 2004).

Despite this high degree of comorbidity and common risk factors, many youth with anxiety disorders and comorbid depression have been excluded from treatment trials for youth anxiety (e.g., the Child/Adolescent Multimodal Study [CAMS]; Kendall et al., 2010; Walkup et al., 2008). This historical exclusion of youth with comorbid disorders in clinical trials is troubling, given consistent evidence that children and adolescents with comorbid anxiety and depression present with greater baseline diagnostic severity, more severe anxiety and depression symptomatology, and poorer family and peer relationships than youth with either disorder alone (Masi, Favilla, Mucci, & Millepiedi, 2000; O'Neil, Podell, Benjamin, & Kendall, 2010; Starr & Davila, 2008; Strauss et al., 1988). In regard to outcomes, youth with comorbid depressive disorders tend to be poorer responders to anxiety-focused treatment than youth with anxiety disorders alone (Berman, Weems, Silverman, & Kurtines, 2000; Crawley, Beidas, Benjamin, Martin, & Kendall, 2008; Suveg, Sood, Comer, & Kendall, 2009). On a symptom level, higher self-reported and parent-reported youth depressive symptoms at baseline predicted poorer treatment response at posttreatment and 12-month follow-up in both child and family CBT, compared with youth with lower depressive symptoms (O'Neil & Kendall, 2012). In addition, some studies have found that a comorbid anxiety disorder predicts poorer treatment response to CBT for depression in youth (Curry et al., 2006), although others have found the opposite effect (Brent et al., 1998; Rohde, Clark, Lewinsohn, Seeley, & Kaufman, 2001).

Given the generally poorer treatment response of individuals with comorbid conditions to disorder-specific CBT, the use of a transdiagnostic approach that targets the common processes of internalizing disorders may improve outcomes for those traditionally unresponsive to CBT, as well as those presenting with a more disorder-specific problem focus. In addition, a transdiagnostic treatment for emotional disorders may appeal to community clinicians, given the lesser burden of learning a singular protocol as opposed to having to learn multiple disorder-specific manuals (McHugh & Barlow, 2010). In the following sections, we first present a theoretical rationale for the UP-A and UP-C:ED, based primarily on findings within emotion science, cognition, and behavior modification. We then present information regarding the treatment structure and content for these two transdiagnostic protocols. Last, we present preliminary findings from each trial that offer empirical evidence to support the use of these transdiagnostic approaches.

Theoretical Basis for the Unified Protocols for Emotional Disorders

The UP-A and UP-C:ED have a strong theoretical basis in emotion regulation (ER) research, cognitive science, and literature on behavioral modification. Research within emotion science indicates that anxiety and depression share a number of underlying affective and ER characteristics.

For instance, high negative affect (NA) has been shown to be a risk factor for the development of both anxiety and depressive disorders (Brown, Chorpita, & Barlow, 1998; Chorpita, Daleiden, Moffitt, Yim, & Umemoto, 2000; Lonigan & Phillips, 2001). Anxiety and depression are also associated with increased usage of maladaptive ER strategies, including emotional avoidance and suppression of negative emotions (Campbell-Sills, Barlow, Brown, & Hofmann, 2006; Tull & Roemer, 2007). In addition to suppression of negative emotion, individuals with depression demonstrate an attenuated response to pleasant emotions (Allen, Trinder, & Brennan, 1999; Sloan, Strauss, Quirk, & Sajatovic, 1997; Sloan, Strauss, & Wisner, 2001). Although some of these emotion regulation processes have been understudied in child and adolescent populations, youth anxiety and depression have been shown to be related to poorer emotional awareness (Penza-Clyve & Zeman, 2002), as well as to high inhibition of worry, sadness, and anger (Chaplin, 2006; Zeman, Shipman, & Suveg, 2002).

The theoretical model underlying the UP-A and UP-C:ED is Gross and Thompson's (2007) modal model of emotions and ER. According to this model, emotions consist of experiential, physiological, and behavioral reactions to external and internal stimuli, and ER refers to the use of cognitive and behavioral processes to modulate the intensity, duration, or expression of emotions. This model enumerates five core ER strategies that run parallel to the generation of emotions: (1) *situation selection*, which involves approaching situations believed to generate pleasurable emotions and avoiding situations believed to produce uncomfortable emotions (e.g., avoidance of threat, social withdrawal); (2) *situation modification*, or modifying the situation to reduce the emotional intensity generated (e.g., use of safety objects, excessive reassurance seeking); (3) *attentional deployment*, which involves directing attention toward or away from pleasurable or uncomfortable emotions (e.g., worry, rumination); (4) *cognitive change*, which refers to the use of reframing techniques to increase or decrease the emotional significance of the situation; and (5) *response modulation*, or directly altering one's emotional experience through physiological or behavioral manners (Gross & Thompson, 2007). Importantly, this model is non-emotion-specific and can be generalized to cognitive and behavioral responses to a broad range of negative emotions (e.g., anger, sadness, worry, fear, guilt, disgust) and, of greater relevance to depression (e.g., Sloan et al., 2001), responses to positive emotions (e.g., pleasure, joy, excitement). Given that this model is not anxiety-specific or depression-specific but rather can be applied to how individuals with anxiety, depression, or their combination experience and respond to a broad array of emotions, it is an ideal model for an emotion-focused, transdiagnostic treatment for emotional disorders.

Using the modal model as a theoretical guide, the UP-A and UP-C:ED incorporate ER skills within traditional CBT for youth anxiety and depression. This is accomplished by targeting three core components relevant to emotional responding: (1) modifying cognitive appraisals of emotions and emotion-provoking stimuli; (2) promoting action tendencies that are incongruent with maladaptive emotion-driven behaviors (EDBs); and (3) preventing emotional avoidance (Campbell-Sills & Barlow, 2007). Thus, although components of standard CBT for youth anxiety and depression (e.g., psychoeducation, cognitive reappraisal, exposure, behavioral activation, problem solving) are utilized within these protocols, these skills are refocused to target the ways in which youth experience, evaluate, and respond to emotions more broadly. As a result, this approach is theorized to positively affect ER more broadly than anxiety-disorder-specific or depressive-disorder-specific manuals. For example, CBT for youth anxiety has been shown to improve regulation of worry, but not anger or sadness (Suveg et al., 2009).

The UP-A: Treatment Structure, Content, and Case Study

The UP-A (Ehrenreich et al., 2008) is an emotion-focused, transdiagnostic CBT for adolescents (ages 12–17) with a principal anxiety disorder diagnosis, principal depressive disorder diagnosis, or coprincipal anxiety and depressive disorder diagnoses. Although not the focus of initial investigation, the UP-A may theoretically be useful for adolescents with comorbid, noninternalizing diagnoses (e.g., attention-deficit/hyperactivity disorder [ADHD]) or other co-occurring issues with ER (e.g., nonsuicidal self-injury, other mood regulation difficulties), as long as anxiety or depressive symptoms may be considered primary concerns at present. The UP-A is a downward extension and adaptation of the unified protocol (UP; Barlow, Allen, & Choate, 2004), a transdiagnostic treatment for adults with anxiety and depressive disorders that shares the same theoretical basis and focus on the broad context of emotional experiences as the UP-A. However, although the adult and adolescent protocols share the same theoretical approach, as well as numerous treatment components, the UP-A contains a number of developmental adaptations, including using worksheets to concretize material, relating didactic content to topics relevant to adolescents (i.e., peer relationships, academic worries), greater focus on building treatment motivation, and involving parents in treatment.

UP-A Structure

The UP-A follows a modular treatment structure in which treatment can be delivered flexibly based on client needs and is designed to be delivered within 8–21 weekly sessions. The UP-A is divided into five main treatment modules and three optional modules. Although all modules are delivered in sequential order, the number of sessions devoted to a particular module is allowed to vary, dependent on client needs or characteristics. In this regard, the UP-A is particularly client-driven and encourages the clinician to make use of its overarching principles flexibly to meet particular client needs. For instance, a clinician may devote more sessions to enhancing the skill of cognitive reappraisal for an adolescent with high metacognitive skills. In contrast, for an adolescent with low metacognitive skills, less time may be devoted to cognitive reappraisal, whereas behavioral strategies (e.g., behavioral activation) may be given more clinical focus. Although the number of modules may vary, Table 12.1 illustrates the recommended number of sessions and the skills taught within each module. In addition, Table 12.1 notes the corresponding process within Gross and Thompson's (2007) model of ER that is targeted within each module.

UP-A Content

The UP-A contains five required modules. In the first module, adolescent clients and their parents are introduced to treatment. The initial session focuses on establishing rapport with the adolescent. In addition, treatment goals and benefits of change are reviewed to build motivation. In subsequent sessions during the first module, the function and parts of emotions (thoughts, physical sensations, and emotion-driven behaviors) are reviewed. A core theme introduced in this module is that emotions

TABLE 12.1. UP-A: Required Treatment Modules

Module	Recommended number of sessions	Content	Corresponding emotion regulation process in Gross and Thompson's (2007) modal model
1	One to three	Emotion education, emotional awareness	
2	One to three	Generalized emotion exposures, nonjudgmental awareness	Attentional deployment
3	One to three	Cognitive reappraisal, problem solving	Cognitive change
4	Four or more	Interoceptive and in vivo exposures, behavioral activation	Situation selection, situation modification, and response modulation
5	One to two	Skill consolidation, relapse prevention	

are "normal, natural, and necessary." Emotional awareness is embedded within a functional assessment of emotions, including helping adolescent patients learn to identify the antecedents, behaviors, and consequences associated with various emotional experiences (e.g., fear when speaking in front of the class, sadness resulting from a romantic breakup). This assessment is used to guide case conceptualization, as well as working with the adolescent to develop an emotion and avoidance hierarchy (EAH). The EAH is developed to rank various situations, as well as the emotions elicited in these situations, based on which are most commonly avoided by the adolescent, as well as which evoke the greatest distress for the patient.

In addition, the role of the adolescent's parent or parents in treatment is discussed. The importance of parental involvement is first examined, including how educating the parent(s) about skills the adolescent is learning in treatment will better allow them to be an effective support system for him or her. Except in rare exceptions (e.g., interfering levels of parental psychopathology or extreme parent–child conflict), adolescents are not given the option of no parental involvement. However, different methods by which to include parents are discussed. Most typically, parents are brought back to the clinic room in the last 5–10 minutes to discuss the treatment content from that session, with the adolescent present. However, other options for including parents (e.g., check-in with parent without the adolescent present, individual sessions with parent plus check-in) are discussed with the adolescent, to ascertain what will be the most comfortable.

The second module of treatment includes generalized emotion exposures, generated through traditional mood-induction paradigms (i.e., watching a sad or happy movie clip or musical piece). During these generalized emotion exposures, clients are encouraged to "fully feel" their emotions and avoid attempts to alter or suppress their emotional experience. In addition, mindfulness-based strategies (Kabat-Zinn, 1994) are incorporated into treatment and framed through "nonjudgmental awareness" of emotional experiences, in which adolescents are encouraged to attend to their emotions but refrain from judgment. Given that emotional suppression is associated with increased sympathetic arousal and anxiety symptomatology (Campbell-Sills et al., 2006; Tull & Roemer, 2007), the goal of this module is to begin a process of emotional experiencing and acceptance, even of uncomfortable emotions (i.e., fear, sadness, anger). It is recommended that adolescents progress from these more generalized emotion exposures to more personalized experiences with opposite behavioral action as treatment progresses.

The third module of treatment focuses on reappraisal of emotions and emotion-evoking situations, which corresponds to the first core component: modifying cognitive appraisals. Cognitive reappraisal is introduced to the adolescent as "detective thinking," in which clients first learn to recognize cognitive errors ("thinking traps") and then apply strategies to alter these thoughts. Similar to the UP (Campbell-Sills & Barlow, 2007), two primary "thinking traps" targeted are (1) overestimation of the likelihood of a negative event occurring ("Everyone is going to laugh at me") and (2) catastrophizing the consequences of the negative event ("I couldn't handle being embarrassed"). Clients learn to ask "detective questions" to assess the accuracy and true probability of these thoughts, as well as how to reframe thoughts to be more realistic. Note that the goal of this module is not to denote these thoughts as "wrong" but rather to allow the adolescent to increase cognitive flexibility and to appraise situations from multiple perspectives. Adolescents are encouraged to use this reappraisal before an emotion-provoking situation occurs (i.e., antecedent-focused reappraisal). In addition to cognitive reappraisal, this module also contains a section on problem solving for situations in which the adolescent feels "stuck" or is having difficulty with decision making. It is particularly recommended that clinicians use problem-solving strategies for interpersonal conflicts and anger regulation during treatment.

The fourth module of treatment extends the generalized emotion exposures from the second module to emotionally evocative situations listed on the patient's EAH, with an overarching goal of encouraging behavioral action tendencies that are incompatible with dysregulated emotion states. In this regard, the fourth module targets the remaining two core components: altering emotion-driven action tendencies (i.e., approach vs. avoidance) and preventing emotional avoidance (i.e., removal of both overt and subtle avoidance attempts). Consistent with a transdiagnostic approach, these exposures are designed to be able to target avoidance strategies across emotions (e.g., fear, sadness, worry). In line with this emotion focus, the goal of the exposures is twofold: (1) approach of the emotion-provoking stimuli or situations and (2) "sitting with" the actual emotion(s) elicited. Adolescents are encouraged to "fully feel" the emotional experiences and refrain from even subtle attempts to avoid emotions (i.e., looking down). Similar to other exposure treatments, patients use subjective units of distress (SUDs) to monitor the level of their emotional intensity. Through this monitoring, the goal of exposures is for adolescents to recognize that the emotional intensity will have a peak and then decrease naturally with time, thus making emotional avoidance unnecessary.

For youth with primary (or secondary) depressive symptoms, the fourth module also contains elements of behavioral activation to improve mood. During behavioral activation, the clinician works with the adolescent to develop a list of pleasurable activities that the client can engage in, particularly during times of low mood. Consistent with the underlying theory of the treatment, behavioral activation is conceptualized as "positive emotion exposures," given the tendency for depressed individuals to avoid or suppress positive emotions (Campbell-Sills et al., 2006).

Furthermore, activation can be conceptualized as incongruent with the action tendency of depressed mood (i.e., behavioral withdrawal). Importantly, this element of the treatment may need to be presented immediately following psychoeducation for primarily depressed adolescents and then reinforced throughout the course of treatment, but it is vital that adolescents attain a basic understanding of the treatment model before proceeding with activation in order to maintain maximal fidelity to planned behavioral engagement strategies.

The fifth module is devoted to skill review and consolidation, relapse prevention, and planning for the future. The clinician and adolescent rerate the client's fear hierarchy and discuss progress made in problem areas. The adolescent is praised for his or her progress and is encouraged to identify which skills of treatment were most helpful. In planning for the future, the clinician should distinguish between "lapse" and "relapse" and, together with the adolescent, determine how the client can use his or her newly developed skills to address a return of symptoms.

Optional Modules

The UP-A contains three optional modules, which can be utilized as needed at any point in treatment. The first optional module concerns dealing with issues of low motivation, which is not atypical for adolescents referred for treatment, especially those with depression (Birmaher et al., 2000). Thus for adolescents with low motivation or those at risk for treatment dropout, the first optional module, which is based on techniques of motivational interviewing (Miller & Rollnick, 2002), may be indicated. Similar motivation enhancement techniques have been shown to be useful in other psychosocial treatments for adolescents (e.g., Gowers & Smyth, 2004).

The second optional module can be utilized in the event of treatment-interfering situations. Such events may include a significant decline in functioning (e.g., worsening of depressive symptoms) or increases in suicidal ideation. In the case of these events, this optional module allows the therapist to work with the adolescent and his or her parent or parents to develop a safety plan, as well as to use any strategies to remain safe. Given that this module can be used at any point in treatment, it gives the therapist flexibility to handle any potential crises, even if relevant treatment material has not yet been covered.

The third optional module can be used to address parenting issues, particularly if treatment-interfering parenting behaviors are evident (e.g., giving frequent reassurance, criticizing the adolescent, permitting avoidant behaviors). Although parents are included throughout treatment, these optional module sessions allow for individual sessions with parents and can be used at any point in treatment. Common uses for these sessions may be to provide a more in-depth treatment rationale and emotion education, including how to avoid common "pitfalls" when parenting anxious and/or depressed adolescents—pitfalls such as being overinvolved/overprotective and modeling anxious and/or depressed behaviors (e.g., avoidance, withdrawal). In promoting more adaptive parenting behaviors, three core components are discussed: independence, consistency, and empathy (ICE). These components are discussed within the section in this chapter that discusses UP-C:ED. Finally, another common target may be parent–child conflict, particularly conflict that is relevant to treatment or interferes with generalization of treatment skills.

UP-A Research Findings

An open trial of the UP-A demonstrated preliminary efficacy with 12 adolescents with any principal anxiety or depressive disorder. In summary, clinical severity ratings (CSRs) for all anxiety and depressive disorders, as assessed using child and parent responses on the Anxiety Disorders Interview Schedule for the DSM-IV, Child and Parent reports (ADIS-IV-C/P; Silverman & Albano, 1996), were reduced significantly from pretreatment to posttreatment (see Ehrenreich, Goldstein, Wright, & Barlow, 2009, for more details). These treatment gains were maintained at 3-month and 6-month follow-up (Ehrenreich et al., 2009). Similarly, both anxiety and depressive symptoms significantly decreased, and in contrast to other CBT protocols (e.g., Suveg et al., 2009), improvements were noted in parent-rated worry, sadness, and anger regulation. Currently, a randomized controlled trial (RCT) with a larger sample comparing immediate treatment of the UP-A to an 8-week wait-list (WL) condition is nearing completion. Among treatment completers, we have observed greater improvements in principal anxiety- or depressive-disorder CSRs for those receiving immediate treatment compared with WL. Furthermore, similar to the open trial, treatment completers have demonstrated improvements in both anxiety and depressive symptoms, as well as numerous indices of adolescent-rated and parent-rated emotion regulation skills. Further analyses using an intent-to-treat (ITT) approach and hierarchical linear modeling (HLM) are planned, and full RCT results will be presented in future papers.

The UP-A: Case Study

Assessment

"Erica"[1] was a 17-year-old female who presented for treatment at our clinic as a potential participant in the UP-A. Erica's intake assessment consisted

---

[1]All relevant case demographics have been altered to ensure patient confidentiality.

of adolescent and parent diagnostic interviews using the ADIS-IV-C/P. In addition, Erica and her mother completed self-report and parent-report questionnaires about Erica's symptoms of anxiety and depression and ER strategies. Erica's primary symptoms included persistent worries about schoolwork, perfectionism, and social impressions, as well as symptoms consistent with panic, including a pounding heart, fears of going crazy, dizziness, and difficulty breathing. Secondary to these worry and panic symptoms, Erica reported symptoms consistent with a current depressive episode, including anhedonia, social withdrawal, and low energy.

Based on information obtained during the ADIS-IV-C/P, coprincipal diagnoses of generalized anxiety disorder (GAD) and panic disorder without agoraphobia (PD) were assigned to account for Erica's anxiety symptoms. Each diagnosis was given a CSR of 5 (range = 0–8, with a 4 indicating a clinical level of interference). Although Erica's depressive symptoms failed to meet a clinical level (with a CSR of 3), her self-report of depressive symptoms, based on the MDD subscale of the Revised Child Anxiety and Depression Scale (RCADS; Chorpita, Yim, Moffitt, Umemoto, & Francis, 2000) was considered elevated (*T*-score = 69). Notably, Erica's comorbid depressive symptoms are common in the clinical presentation of adolescents with GAD and PD (Birmaher & Ollendick, 2004).

Case Conceptualization

In addition to anxious and depressive symptomatology, self-report and parent report of Erica's ER indicated high degrees of both emotional avoidance and suppression, consistent with findings from the literature (Campbell-Sills et al., 2006; Tull & Roemer, 2007). Based on diagnostic information and questionnaire data, her therapist hypothesized that Erica's strong attempts to avoid and suppress uncomfortable emotions (e.g., fear, sadness, anger) underlay her panic, worry, and depressive symptoms. Therefore, a primary treatment goal, in addition to symptom reduction, was to work with Erica to more fully experience and accept a broad range of emotional experiences, both positive and negative.

Treatment

Erica met treatment eligibility and was randomized to the immediate treatment condition, with treatment beginning 2 weeks after the intake assessment. Erica completed the UP-A in 15 weekly 50-minute sessions. Consistent with the theoretical foundation of the protocol, common themes embedded within Erica's treatment included "facing" uncomfortable emotions and adopting a nonjudgmental attitude toward her emotional experiences. In vivo exposures included giving mock speeches in front of confederates instructed to provide nonverbal cues of disapproval, which were intended to target Erica's fears of negative social evaluation. In addition, during these mock speeches Erica was instructed to make mistakes purposely in order to target her perfectionism. In addition to individualized, in vivo exposures, Erica engaged in interoceptive exercises, such as running in place for 1 minute, drawn from treatment for adolescent PD (Pincus, Ehrenreich-May, Whitton, Mattis, & Barlow, 2010) to target somatic sensations of anxiety. Through both in vivo and interoceptive exposures, Erica learned to habituate to anxiety-provoking situations and somatic sensations and to accept her emotions. Behavioral activation strategies designed to increase positive emotions were also incorporated to address her depressive symptoms.

Results

Data gathered from Erica's posttreatment assessment suggested that the UP-A was effective in reducing Erica's anxious and depressive symptoms, as well as emotional avoidance and suppression. Based on the posttreatment ADIS-IV-C/P, conducted by an independent evaluator, Erica's CSRs for both her GAD and PD diagnoses reduced from a 5 at pretreatment to a 2 at posttreatment, indicating subclinical interference. In addition, Erica's posttreatment CSR for MDD decreased from a pretreatment CSR of 3 to a 1. Thus Erica no longer displayed clinical elevations of all of pretreatment diagnoses, suggesting that the UP-A was successful across internalizing symptoms. Similarly, clinician-rated severity of Erica's symptom impairment evidenced reduction, from a pretreatment clinician global impression (CGI) severity score of 4 (moderate severity) to a posttreatment CGI severity score of 2 (slight severity). Finally, gains were maintained at 3-month and 6-month follow-up assessments.

Similarly, decreases in self- and parent report of Erica's emotional avoidance and suppression were also observed. Erica reported a significant decrease in emotional suppression, as evidenced by scores on the Emotion Regulation Questionnaire—Children and Adolescents (ERQ-CA; MacDermott, Betts, Gullone, & Allen, 2008), from pretreatment to posttreatment, with improvements maintained at 3-month and 6-month follow-ups. Using the Children's Emotion Management Scale (CEMS; Zeman, Shipman, & Penza-Clyve, 2001), Erica's mother reported decreases in Erica's dysregulation of anger, sadness, and worry and increases in Erica's ability to cope with these emotions, which were also maintained at 3-month and 6-month follow-ups. These results suggest that (1) the UP-A was effective in reducing Erica's anxiety and depressive symptoms and (2) the UP-A was effective in promoting adaptive emotion regulation strategies across three affective domains (anger, sadness, and worry). These results are promising for adolescents who, like Erica, present with multiple internalizing symptoms and broad deficits in emotion regulation.

The UP-C:ED: Treatment Structure, Content, and Case Study

The UP-C:ED is a downward extension of the UP-A for younger children (ages 7–12) with anxiety disorders, with or without concurrent elevated depressive symptoms. Although the UP-C:ED shares the same theoretical basis and core treatment components as the UP and UP-A, it is developmentally adapted toward younger children, both in the delivery of content and the structure of content. For instance, whereas the UP-A is an individual treatment, the UP-C:ED is a group treatment. The group modality was selected for UP-C:ED to mimic environments in which young children are particularly motivated by fun activities and learn from each other (Santucci, Ehrenreich, Trosper, Bennett, & Pincus, 2009). Furthermore, the treatment components are broken down using a simple mnemonic device and are introduced sequentially as the CLUES skills: Consider how I feel, Look at my thoughts, Use detective questions, Experience my fears and feelings, and Stay healthy and happy. In addition, although parents are included in the UP-A, parental involvement is even greater in the UP-C:ED, as a child group and parent group meet concurrently for each session with separate clinicians. The strong parent component was developed to maximize generalization of treatment skills outside of session. Finally, just as positive reinforcement is used in the UP-A, small rewards are used even more frequently in UP-C:ED to maintain the attention of younger clients and to reinforce learning and appropriate behavior.

UP-C:ED Structure

Unlike the UP-A, which has a modular structure, the UP-C:ED consists of 15 weekly 90-minute sessions that unfold in the same order across participants. With the exception of the sessions dedicated to the "Experience my fears and feelings" skill,[2] each session begins with the parents, children, and clinicians convening to discuss homework and progress from the prior session and the treatment goals for the current session. Then, clinicians lead the child and parent groups in separate rooms for approximately 60 minutes.

UP-C:ED Content

During the "Consider how I feel" sessions of treatment, participants receive general emotion education, including on the purpose and parts

---

[2]During sessions dedicated to the "Experience my fears and feelings" skill, the parent group does not meet, and all of the clinicians are devoted to completing in vivo personalized exposures with the child participants. The parent group reconvenes for the last session, dedicated to the "Stay healthy and happy" skill.

of emotions. UP-C:ED emphasizes the normalization of emotions by engaging participants in activities that demonstrate the universality of emotions. Additionally, participants learn about the nature of avoidance and its negative consequences. During the "Look at my thoughts" portion, participants are introduced to antecedent cognitive reappraisal and begin to practice flexible thinking, or evaluating ambiguous situations from multiple perspectives.

In the "Use detective questions" segment, participants expand on the cognitive skills taught in "Look at my thoughts" and practice reevaluating emotionally charged situations and challenging their automatic interpretations. During the "Experience my fears and feelings" skill, participants engage in both general and individually tailored emotional exposures and approach previously avoided situations. Finally, the "Stay healthy and happy" component provides an opportunity for participants to review the skills they have learned and to reflect on the progress they have made. Participants are encouraged to "become their own therapists" and to list ongoing goals for posttreatment. Table 12.2 describes the skills introduced within each CLUES domain, as well as the corresponding treatment session(s).

To maximize motivation and learning, each child session incorporates both didactic and experiential activities, with skill repetition and positive reinforcement. Experiential activities were designed specifically to reinforce didactic components with the aim of aiding children's memory for skills discussed (Kolb, 1984). For example, during the "Consider

TABLE 12.2. UP-C:ED Structure and Content

Session number(s)	CLUES content	Skills introduced
1–5	Consider how I feel	Emotion education, emotion awareness, somatization, behavioral activation, mindfulness, generalized emotion exposures
6	Look at my thoughts	Identifying automatic thoughts (e.g., probability overestimation, catastrophic thinking)
7–8	Use detective questions	Cognitive reappraisal, problem solving, conflict management
9–14	Experience my fears and feelings	Rationale for emotion exposures, interoceptive exposures, *in vivo* exposures
15	Stay healthy and happy	Relapse prevention, review of skills, wrap-up

how I feel" skill, children learn about the importance of preventing emotional avoidance and fully engaging in emotional experiences. The participants then practice this skill by engaging in "generalized emotion exposures," which are activities that produce low levels of emotions (e.g. watching an emotional film clip). To further encourage generalization of skills, treatment concepts are reviewed using three levels of specificity: abstract, general, and specific. During the "Look at my thoughts" skill, for instance, child participants are introduced to the concept of flexible thinking. To gain experience with this skill, they look at optical illusions and practice generating multiple interpretations of ambiguous pictures. They then generalize this skill to emotions more generally and brainstorm multiple interpretations of emotionally valenced but ambiguous situations (e.g., seeing a group of girls laughing across the street). Finally, they practice applying the skill to specific situations that are personally relevant.

Parental Involvement

While the children practice skills with clinicians in the child group, the parent group meets independently. The overarching goals of the parent group are to teach the parents the skills that the children are practicing and how to best support their children as they navigate the treatment process. Thus, in addition to learning the CLUES skills, parents also learn a set of parenting skills, the "ICE skills," which were originally developed for use in the parent component of the UP-A (Ehrenreich et al., 2008). As noted earlier, the ICE skills include Independence, Consistency, and Empathy.

The "Independence" skill teaches parents techniques to encourage their children to engage in age-appropriate activities that promote autonomy. Anxious children may be especially avoidant of engaging in independence-building activities that involve some level of perceived distress (Hudson & Rapee, 2002). Their parents may be prone to becoming overprotective and overcontrolling of their children; however, such behavior can ultimately accommodate their children's avoidance (Rapee, 2001). The "Consistency" skill teaches parents to consistently use positive reinforcement and other behavioral strategies to encourage appropriate child behavior. Inconsistent discipline is associated with externalizing behaviors, which may undermine treatment (Patterson, 1982). Additionally, evidence suggests that unpredictable parenting may also be associated with depressive symptoms in children (Kim et al., 2003). Children may also particularly benefit from praise and incentives to increase their motivation (Kendall & Gosch, 1994). Finally, the "Empathy" skill provides parents with insight into how to manage their children's distress and to acknowledge progress throughout the treatment process.

In addition to learning the CLUES and ICE skills, parents have time to speak openly about their experiences and seek advice from the clinicians and other parents. This less structured portion of treatment allows clinicians to address any concerns not specifically targeted in treatment and provides the opportunity for parents to connect. Overall, these sessions give parents the skills to help themselves and their children navigate the difficult process of engaging in treatment for internalizing disorders.

After approximately 60 minutes, the two groups reunite and spend the remainder of session reviewing the skills that were covered and discussing homework for the next session. Because this program is in development, it is important that participants are offered multiple opportunities to offer qualitative feedback about their experiences. Therefore, sessions conclude with an opportunity to speak about any concerns or questions regarding an individual child, group procedures, or session content.

UP-C:ED Research Findings

To date, the UP-C:ED has been implemented both as a treatment intervention and within a preventative context. A preliminary investigation examining the application of UP-C:ED as a universal prevention within a recreational camp demonstrated that the UP-C:ED prevention program was associated with high levels of participant satisfaction and a significant reduction in child-reported anxiety symptoms (Ehrenreich-May & Bilek, 2011).

Additionally, a recent open trial of the treatment arm of Emotion Detectives demonstrated the preliminary efficacy of the protocol to address principal anxiety diagnoses, as well as anxious and depressive symptoms (Bilek & Ehrenreich-May, 2012). Specifically, participants in the open trial experienced a significant reduction in CSR ratings for the principal anxiety disorder from pretreatment to posttreatment, as well as a significant reduction in all anxiety and depressive disorder severity ratings. Children reported a significant reduction in anxiety symptoms from pre- to posttreatment, and parents reported a significant reduction in child depressive symptoms following the UP-C:ED. In contrast to findings with anxiety-focused CBT, neither parent- nor child-reported youth depressive symptoms at baseline predicted change in principal anxiety disorder CSR, suggesting that pretreatment depressive symptoms were not associated with poorer outcomes in this investigation. Currently, an RCT is under way to further investigate the efficacy of the UP-C:ED as compared with an active comparison condition (Lyneham, Abbott, Wignall, & Rapee, 2003).

UP-C:ED: Case Study

Assessment

"Mark" was an 11-year-old white, Hispanic male who presented at our clinic as a potential participant in the UP-C:ED. Mark's initial assessment included administration of the ADIS-IV-C/P, as well as self-report and parent-rated anxiety and depressive symptom questionnaires (Screen for Anxiety Related Disorders [SCARED]—Birmaher et al., 1997; Children's Depression Inventory [CDI]—Kovacs, 2001). During the ADIS-IV-C/P, Mark and his mother reported that, despite receiving high marks in all his classes, Mark was experiencing significant anxiety about schoolwork. Specifically, Mark and his mother reported that Mark delayed completing his writing assignments, asked frequent questions when completing schoolwork, and refused to complete his writing assignments without help from others. In addition to Mark's school-related worries, he reported excessive worry about various interpersonal and perfectionistic concerns, which had begun to negatively affect his social and academic functioning. In addition to experiencing significant worries, both Mark and his mother reported that he had been experiencing depressive symptoms, including loss of interest in usual activities, difficulty concentrating, excessive guilt, and irritability, intermittently over the preceding 18 months.

In addition to anxiety and depressive symptoms, Mark's mother also reported that he was previously diagnosed with ADHD—Inattentive Type. At the time of intake, he was taking 25 mg/day of Zoloft and 50 mg/day of Strattera for management of his ADHD and depressive symptoms. Based on data collected in the clinical interview and from the questionnaires, Mark was given a principal diagnosis of GAD (CSR = 6) and a secondary diagnosis of depressive disorder—not otherwise specified (DD-NOS; CSR = 4). Additionally, a diagnosis of ADHD—Inattentive Type was assigned by history.

Case Conceptualization

Mark was suffering from elevated levels of negative affect and physiological arousal, particularly over schoolwork. In line with Gross's model, Mark's maladaptive attempts to regulate these negative emotions manifested in persistent worries about his schoolwork, as well as seeking reassurance from others. In turn, these maladaptive regulation strategies created academic difficulties and interpersonal arguments. In addition, Mark's behavioral withdrawal had resulted in decreased levels of positive affect, which served to maintain Mark's depressed mood. Given Mark's mixed anxious and depressive presentation, the therapist's treatment plan involved helping Mark to develop more effective up-regulation and down-regulation skills to (1) more adaptively cope with negative emotions and physiological arousal and (2) increase levels of positive affect.

Treatment

During the first session of treatment, Mark and his mother identified goals for treatment, including worrying less about schoolwork, reducing depressive symptoms, and improving his relationships with his siblings. During the following sessions, Mark continued to participate readily and was especially interested in learning about the three-component model of emotions. In the parent group, Mark's mother recognized Mark's infrequent participation in pleasurable activities. Mark worked with his individual clinician and his mother to identify activities in which he could participate when he was feeling in a low mood. In subsequent weeks, Mark reported that he had engaged in several pleasurable activities and reported improved mood. Given the success of this initial exercise, Mark's therapist continued to assign behavioral activation homework throughout treatment.

Following behavioral activation, cognitive reappraisal was introduced as "identifying thinking traps" and "using detective thinking" in emotionally evocative situations. Mark identified completing writing assignments as one such situation. He reported that he was afraid that he would not be able to complete the assignment as expected, thus causing him to do poorly and reinforcing his core fear of failing. After learning about thinking traps, Mark identified this fear as "Disaster Dan," or catastrophic thinking. Mark was challenged to reevaluate his catastrophic thinking and examine whether there could be alternative interpretations when he made mistakes on homework or tests. Mark realized that making mistakes could help him identify areas in which he might need help.

Mark and his mother then created an emotional avoidance hierarchy, which included completing writing assignments, making mistakes on homework, and being evaluated negatively by others. These concerns were all addressed through emotional exposures conducted within session and at home. In-session exposure exercises included giving a speech while purposely making mistakes, asking people for the time while wearing a watch visible to others, and completing a writing assignment in session on which he received both negative and positive feedback. For homework, he completed exposure exercises consisting of completing writing assignments without help from his parents and making purposeful mistakes on a homework sheet.

In the final section of treatment, Mark had an opportunity to reflect on the progress that he had made during treatment. Mark's mother told the group that Mark had been able to complete his homework assignments without asking his parents for help. This was a large step for Mark, who had previously required assistance on all of his assignments. Mark's clinician met with Mark and his mother to review ways in which he could continue facing his fears when feeling afraid, as well as continue to engage in pleasurable activities when feeling sad.

Results

Mark attended a total of 13 of the 15 sessions of treatment. Mark and his mother reported decreased anxiety symptoms on the SCARED. Additionally, Mark's mother reported that he was no longer experiencing depressive symptoms at an elevated level. At the posttreatment assessment, Mark's CSR for both his emotional diagnoses had been reduced to a subclinical level. Specifically, his diagnosis of GAD was reduced from a 6 to a 3, and his diagnosis of DD-NOS was reduced from a 4 to a 2. These improvements were maintained at a 3-month follow-up assessment. Additionally, Mark demonstrated improvements on child-reported ER. Specifically, Mark reported an improvement on the ERQ-CA in his emotional reappraisal (increasing from 16 to 18) and a decrease in his suppression of emotional experiences (falling from 8 to 4).

Discussion and Future Research

The high co-occurrence of youth anxiety and depressive diagnoses (Brady & Kendall, 1992) and symptoms (Stark & Laurent, 2001) necessitates treatments that effectively target both domains of internalizing distress. This is especially true given that youth with comorbid diagnoses have historically been underrepresented in treatment trials (e.g., Kendall et al., 2010) and tend to have poorer outcomes when receiving disorder-specific CBT (e.g., Berman et al., 2000; Suveg et al., 2009). The UP-A and UP-C:ED are two emotion-focused, transdiagnostic CBT protocols that focus on common emotional factors in youth anxiety and depression, including higher levels of underlying negative emotionality (e.g., Brown et al., 1998), as well as higher usage of maladaptive strategies (e.g., suppression, avoidance) to regulate a range of negative emotions, including fear, worry, sadness, and anger (e.g., Zeman et al., 2002). As a result, using standard CBT components such as psychoeducation, cognitive reappraisal, problem solving, exposure, and behavioral activation, as well as emotion awareness, experiencing, and expression, more broadly, the UP-A and UP-C:ED seek to positively affect how children and adolescents with anxiety and/or depression experience, think about, and respond to a broad range of negative and positive emotions, rather than disorder-specific emotions (e.g., fear, sadness).

Preliminary results from three research trials, two open trials, and an RCT nearing completion show promise for these two transdiagnostic interventions and may also distinguish them based on prior findings with anxiety-focused or depression-focused treatments. Initial findings suggest that both the UP-A and UP-C:ED demonstrate efficacy in reduction of principal diagnosis severity, as well as total emotional diagnostic severity. Furthermore, both anxiety and depressive symptoms were significantly reduced in the UP-A and UP-C:ED, with comparable effect sizes for anxiety and depression symptom change in each intervention. In contrast to prior anxiety-specific or depression-specific CBT findings, children and adolescents with depressive disorders, or elevated depressive symptoms, have not shown a reduced treatment response when receiving the UP-A or UP-C:ED. Finally, in contrast to prior findings showing positive improvements in only one domain of ER (e.g., worry) with anxiety-focused CBT (Suveg et al., 2009), improvements in worry, sadness, and anger dysregulation have been found with these transdiagnostic protocols, providing evidence that the UP-A and UP-C:ED positively target a broader range of emotional experiences than disorder-specific protocols.

Future research should examine theory-driven mediators of treatment response, including the three core components (e.g., modifying cognitive appraisals, promoting action tendencies incompatible with EDBs, preventing avoidance) targeted in these interventions. In addition, future research should examine potential baseline predictors of treatment response (e.g., levels of negative and positive affect, anxiety sensitivity, emotional awareness) on treatment outcome. Results of such an evaluation, which could be completed in a brief assessment format, would be one avenue for supporting the UP-A's flexible modular treatment approach, whereby assessment could guide the order of skill presentation. Thus this highly individualized intervention would match strengths and weaknesses of each client while incorporating all skill areas over the course of treatment. For example, a child or adolescent who lacks skill with identifying emotions or thoughts might benefit from participating in exposures early in treatment. These experiences might provide concrete, recent, and personal examples the therapist can use to illustrate the other skills.

In addition to examining mediators and predictors of treatment response, a better understanding of how these interventions would fare in community settings is also needed. The flexible structure of these treatments, as well as their transdiagnostic focus, may be particularly attractive to community clinicians. For one, the use of a unified protocol for youth anxiety and depressive disorders may reduce training burden, as practitioners can learn one singular treatment as opposed to multiple disorder-specific manuals. Indeed, inadequate clinician training is considered one of the greatest barriers to effective dissemination and implementation of evidence-based treatments (McHugh & Barlow, 2010). Furthermore, the focus on a broad domain of emotional experiences may also be advantageous, given that community clinicians may often see youth with numerous comorbidities and complex emotional and symptom profiles (Addis & Krasnow, 2000; Weisz, Jensen-Doss, & Hawley, 2006). However, the feasibility and effectiveness of these transdiagnostic interventions, as well as modifications needed within community mental health settings, await empirical testing.

REFERENCES

Addis, M. E., & Krasnow, A. D. (2000). A national survey of practicing psychologists' attitudes toward psychotherapy treatment manuals. *Journal of Consulting and Clinical Psychology, 68,* 331–339.

Allen, N. B., Trinder, J., & Brennan, C. (1999). Affective startle modulation in clinical depression: Preliminary findings. *Biological Psychiatry, 46,* 542–550.

Barlow, D. H., Allen, L. B., & Choate, M. L. (2004). Toward a unified treatment for emotional disorders. *Behavior Therapy, 35,* 205–230.

Beesdo, K., Knappe, S., & Pine, D. S. (2009). Anxiety and anxiety disorders in children and adolescents: Developmental issues and implications for DSM-V. *Psychiatric Clinics of North America, 32*(3), 483–524.

Berman, S. L., Weems, C. F., Silverman, W. K., & Kurtines, W. M. (2000). Predictors of outcome in exposure-based cognitive and behavioral treatments for phobic and anxiety disorders in children. *Behavior Therapy, 31,* 713–731.

Bilek, E. L., & Ehrenreich-May, J. (2012). An open trial investigation of a transdiagnostic group treatment for children with anxiety and depressive symptoms. *Behavior Therapy, 43*(4), 887–897.

Birmaher, B., Brent, D. A., Kolko, D., Baugher, M., Bridge, J., Holder, D., et al. (2000). Clinical outcome after short-term psychotherapy for adolescents with major depressive disorder. *Archives of General Psychiatry, 57,* 29–36.

Birmaher, B., Khetarpal, S., Brent, C., Cully, M., Balach, L., Kaufman, J., et al. (1997). The Screen for Child Anxiety and Related Emotional Disorders (SCARED): Scale construction and psychometric properties. *Journal of the American Academy of Child and Adolescent Psychiatry, 36,* 545–553.

Birmaher, B., & Ollendick, T. H. (2004). Childhood-onset panic disorder. In T. H. Ollendick & J. S. March (Eds.), *Phobic and anxiety disorders in children and adolescents* (pp. 306–333). Oxford, UK: Oxford University Press.

Birmaher, B., Ryan, N. D., Williamson, D. E., & Brent, D. A. (1996). Childhood and adolescent depression: A review of the past 10 years: Part I. *Journal of the American Academy of Child and Adolescent Psychiatry, 35,* 1427–1439.

Brady, E. U., & Kendall, P. C. (1992). Comorbidity of anxiety and depression in children and adolescents. *Psychological Bulletin, 111,* 244–255.

Brent, D. A., Kolko, D. J., Birmaher, B., Baugher, M., Bridge, J., Roth, C., et al. (1998). Predictors of treatment efficacy in a clinical trial of three psychosocial treatments for adolescent depression. *Journal of the American Academy of Child and Adolescent Psychiatry, 37,* 906–914.

Brown, T. A., Chorpita, B. F., & Barlow, D. H. (1998). Structural relationships among dimensions of the DSM-IV anxiety and mood disorders and dimensions of negative affect, positive affect, and autonomic arousal. *Journal of Abnormal Psychology, 107,* 179–192.

Brunstein-Klomek, A., Marrocco, F., Kleinman, M., Schonfeld, I. S., & Gould, M. S. (2007). Bullying, depression, and suicidality in adolescents. *Journal of the American Academy of Child and Adolescent Psychiatry, 46,* 40–49.

Campbell-Sills, L., & Barlow, D. H. (2007). Incorporating emotion regulation into conceptualizations and treatments of anxiety and mood disorders. In J. J. Gross (Ed.), *Handbook of emotion regulation* (pp. 542–559). New York: Guilford Press.

Campbell-Sills, L., Barlow, D. H., Brown, T. A., & Hofmann, S. (2006). Acceptability and suppression of negative emotion in anxiety and mood disorders. *Emotion, 6,* 587–595.

Caspi, A., Moffitt, T. E., Thornton, A., Freedman, D., Amell, J. W., Harrington, H., et al. (1996). The life history calendar: A research and clinical assessment method for collecting retrospective event-history data. *International Journal of Methods in Psychiatric Research, 6,* 101–114.

Chaplin, T. M. (2006). Anger, happiness, and sadness: Associations with depressive symptoms in late adolescence. *Journal of Youth and Adolescence, 35,* 977–986.

Chorpita, B. F., & Barlow, D. H. (1998). The development of anxiety: The role of control in the early environment. *Psychological Bulletin, 124,* 3–21.

Chorpita, B. F., Daleiden, E. L., Moffitt, C., Yim, L., & Umemoto, L. A. (2000). Assessment of tripartite factors of emotion in children and adolescents: I. Structural validity and normative data of an affect and arousal scale. *Journal of Psychopathology and Behavioral Assessment, 22,* 141–160.

Chorpita, B. F., Yim, L., Moffitt, C., Umemoto, L. A., & Francis, S. E. (2000). Assessment of symptoms of DSM-IV anxiety and depression in children: A revised child anxiety and depression scale. *Behaviour Research and Therapy, 38*(8), 835–855.

Costello, E., Mustillo, S., Erkanli, A., Keeler, G., & Angold, A. (2003). Prevalence and development of psychiatric disorders in childhood and adolescence. *Archives of General Psychiatry, 60,* 837–844.

Costello, E., Pine, D. S., Hammen, C., March, J. S., Plotsky, P. M., Weissman, M. M., et al. (2002). Development and natural history of mood disorders. *Biological Psychiatry, 52,* 529–542.

Crawley, S. A., Beidas, R. S., Benjamin, C. L., Martin, E., & Kendall, P. C. (2008). Treating socially phobic youth with CBT: Differential outcomes and treatment considerations. *Behavioural and Cognitive Psychotherapy, 36,* 379–389.

Curry, J., Rohde, P., Simons, A., Silva, S., Vitiello, B., Kratochvil, C., et al. (2006). Predictors and moderators of acute outcome in the Treatment for Adolescents with Depression Study (TADS). *Journal of the American Academy of Child and Adolescent Psychiatry, 45,* 1427–1439.

Ehrenreich, J. T., Buzzella, B. A., Trosper, S. E., Bennett, S. M., Wright, L. A., & Barlow, D. H. (2008). *Unified protocol for the treatment of emotional disorders in youth.* Unpublished treatment manual, University of Miami and Boston University.

Ehrenreich, J., Goldstein, C., Wright, L., & Barlow, D. (2009). Development of a unified protocol for the treatment of emotion disorders in youth. *Child and Family Behavior Therapy, 31,* 20–37.

Ehrenreich-May, J., & Bilek, E. (2009). *Emotion detectives treatment protocol.* Unpublished manuscript.

Ehrenreich-May, J., & Bilek, E. (2011). Universal prevention of anxiety and depression in a recreational camp setting: An initial open trial. *Child Youth Care Forum, 40,* 435–455.

Geller, B., Zimerman, B., Williams, M., Bolhofner, K., & Craney, J. L. (2001). Adult psychosocial outcome of prepubertal major depressive disorder. *Journal of the American Academy of Child and Adolescent Psychiatry, 40,* 673–677.

Gladstone, G. L., Parker, G. B., Mitchell, P. B., Wilhelm, K. A., & Malhi, G. S. (2005). Relationship between self-reported childhood behavioral inhibition and lifetime anxiety disorders in a clinical sample. *Depression and Anxiety, 22,* 103–113.

Gowers, S. G., & Smyth, B. B. (2004). The impact of a motivational assessment interview on initial response to treatment in adolescent anorexia nervosa. *European Eating Disorders Review, 12,* 87–93.

Gross, J. J., & Thompson, R. A. (2007). Emotion regulation: Conceptual foundations. In J. J. Gross (Ed.), *Handbook of emotion regulation* (pp. 3–24). New York: Guilford Press.

Hannesdottir, D. K., & Ollendick, T. H. (2007). The role of emotion regulation in the treatment of child anxiety disorders. *Clinical Child and Family Psychology Review, 10,* 275–293.

Hudson, J., & Rapee, R. (2002). Parent–child interactions in clinically anxious children and their siblings. *Journal of Clinical Child and Adolescent Psychology, 31,* 548–555.

Kabat-Zinn, J. (1994). *Mindfulness meditation for everyday life.* New York: Hyperion.

Keller, M. B., Lavori, P. W., Mueller, T. I., & Endicott, J. (1992). Time to recovery, chronicity, and levels of psychopathology in major depression: A 5-year prospective follow-up of 431 subjects. *Archives of General Psychiatry, 49,* 809–816.

Kendall, P. C., Compton, S. N., Walkup, J. T., Birmaher, B., Albano, A., Sherrill, J., et al. (2010). Clinical characteristics of anxiety disordered youth. *Journal of Anxiety Disorders, 24,* 360–365.

Kendall, P., & Gosch, E. (1994). Cognitive-behavioral interventions. In T. H. Ollendick, N. J. King, & W. Yule (Eds.), *International handbook of phobic and anxiety disorders in children and adolescents* (pp. 415–438). New York: Plenum Press.

Kim, I. J., Ge, X., Brody, G. H., Conger, R. D., Gibbons, F. X., & Simons, R. L. (2003). Parenting behaviors and the occurrence and co-occurrence of depressive symptoms and conduct problems among African American children. *Journal of Family Psychology, 17,* 571–583.

Kolb, D. (1984). *Experiential learning: Experience as the source of learning and development.* Englewood Cliffs, NJ: Prentice-Hall.

Kovacs, M. (2001). *Children's Depression Inventory manual.* North Tonawanda, NY: Multi-Health Systems.

Kovacs, M., Joormann, J., & Gotlib, I. H. (2008). Emotion (dys)regulation and links to depressive disorders. *Child Development Perspectives, 2,* 149–155.

Lewinsohn, P. M., Rohde, P., & Seely, J. R. (1998). Major depressive disorder in older adolescents: Prevalence, risk factors, and clinical implications. *Clinical Psychology Review, 18,* 765–794.

Lonigan, C. J., & Phillips, B. M. (2001). Temperamental influences on the development of anxiety disorders. In M. W. Vasey & M. R. Dadds (Eds.), *The developmental psychopathology of anxiety* (pp. 60–91). New York: Oxford University Press.

Lyneham, H. Abbott, M., Wignall, A., & Rapee, R. M. (2003). *Cool Kids: Family Program* [Manual]. Sydney, NSW, Australia: Macquarie University, Anxiety Research Unit. Retrieved from *www.psy.mq.edu.au/muaru.*

MacDermott, S. T., Betts, J., Gullone, E., & Allen, J. S. (2008). *Emotion regulation in childhood and adolescence: A revised version of the Emotion Regulation Questionnaire (ERQ-CA).* Manuscript submitted for publication.

Masi, G., Favilla, L., Mucci, M., & Millepiedi, S. (2000). Depressive comorbidity in children and adolescents with generalized anxiety disorder. *Child Psychiatry and Human Development, 30,* 205–215.

McHugh, R. K., & Barlow, D. H. (2010). The dissemination and implementation of evidence-based psychological treatments: A review of current efforts. *American Psychologist, 65*(2), 73–84.

Messer, S. C., & Beidel, D. C. (1994). Psychosocial correlates of childhood anxiety disorders. *Journal of the American Academy of Child and Adolescent Psychiatry, 33,* 975–983.

Miller, W. R., & Rollnick, S. (2002). *Motivational interviewing: Preparing people for change* (2nd ed.). New York: Guilford Press.

Narrow, W. E., Rae, D. S., Robins, L. N., & Regier, D. A. (2002). Revised prevalence-based estimates of mental disorders in the United States: Using a clinical significance criterion to reconcile 2 surveys' estimates. *Archives of General Psychiatry, 59,* 115–123.

Ollendick, T. H., Shortt, A. L., & Sander, J. B. (2005). Internalizing disorders of childhood and adolescence. In J. E. Maddux & B. A. Winstead (Eds.), *Psychopathology: Foundations for a contemporary understanding* (pp. 353–376). Mahwah, NJ: Erlbaum.

O'Neil, K. A., & Kendall, P. C. (2012). Role of comorbid depression and co-occurring depressive symptoms in outcomes for anxiety-disordered youth treated with cognitive-behavioral therapy. *Child and Family Behavior Therapy, 34*(3), 197–209.

O'Neil, K. A., Podell, J. L., Benjamin, C. L., & Kendall, P. C. (2010). Comorbid depressive disorders in anxiety-disordered youth: Demographic, clinical, and family characteristics. *Child Psychiatry and Human Development, 41,* 330–341.

Patterson, G. R. (1982). *A social learning approach: Vol. 3. Coercive family process.* Eugene, OR: Castalia.

Penza-Clyve, S., & Zeman, J. (2002). Initial validation of the Emotion Expression Scale for Children (EESC). *Journal of Clinical Child And Adolescent Psychology, 31,* 540–547.

Pérez-Edgar, K., & Fox, N. A. (2005). Temperament and anxiety disorders. *Child and Adolescent Psychiatric Clinics of North America, 14,* 681–706.

Pincus, D. B., Ehrenreich-May, J., Whitton, S. W., Mattis, S. G., & Barlow, D. H. (2010). Cognitive-behavioral treatment of panic disorder in adolescence. *Journal of Clinical Child and Adolescent Psychology, 39,* 638–649.

Pine, D. S. (1994). Child–adult anxiety disorders. *Journal of the American Academy of Child and Adolescent Psychiatry, 33*(2), 32–80.

Rapee, R. M. (2001). The development of generalized anxiety. In M. W. Vasey & M. R. Dadds (Eds.), *The developmental psychopathology of anxiety* (pp. 481–503). New York: Oxford University Press.

Rohde, P., Clarke, G. N., Lewinsohn, P. M., Seeley, J. R., & Kaufman, N. K. (2001). Impact of comorbidity on a cognitive-behavioral group treatment for adolescent depression. *Journal of the American Academy of Child and Adolescent Psychiatry, 40*, 795–802.

Santucci, L. C., Ehrenreich, J. T., Trosper, S. E., Bennett, S. M., & Pincus, D. B. (2009). Development and preliminary evaluation of a one-week summer treatment program for separation anxiety disorder. *Cognitive and Behavioral Practice, 16*, 317–331.

Sheeber, L. B., Davis, B., Leve, C., Hops, H., & Tildesley, E. (2007). Adolescents' relationships with their mothers and fathers: Associations with depressive disorder and subdiagnostic symptomatology. *Journal of Abnormal Psychology, 116*, 144–154.

Silverman, W. K., & Albano, A. M. (1996). *Anxiety Disorders Schedule for DSM-IV: Child and parent versions.* San Antonio, TX: Psychological Corporation.

Sloan, D. M., Strauss, M. E., Quirk, S. W., & Sajatovic, M. (1997). Subjective and expressive emotional responses in depression. *Journal of Affective Disorders, 46*, 135–141.

Sloan, D. M., Strauss, M. E., & Wisner, K. L. (2001). Diminished response to pleasant stimuli by depressed women. *Journal of Abnormal Psychology, 110*, 488–493.

Southam-Gerow, M., & Kendall, P. C. (2000). A preliminary study of the emotion understanding of youths referred for treatment of anxiety disorders. *Journal of Clinical Child Psychology, 29*, 319–327.

Stark, K. D., & Laurent, J. (2001). Joint factor analysis of the Children's Depression Inventory and the Revised Children's Manifest Anxiety Scale. *Journal of Clinical Child Psychology, 30*, 552–567.

Starr, L. R., & Davila, J. (2008). Excessive reassurance seeking, depression, and interpersonal rejection: A meta-analytic review. *Journal of Abnormal Psychology, 117*, 762–775.

Strauss, C. C., Last, C. G., Hersen, M., & Kazdin, A. E. (1988). Association between anxiety and depression in children and adolescents with anxiety disorders. *Journal of Abnormal Child Psychology, 16*, 57–68.

Suveg, C., Sood, E., Comer, J. S., & Kendall, P. C. (2009). Changes in emotion regulation following cognitive-behavioral therapy for anxious youth. *Journal of Clinical Child and Adolescent Psychology, 38*, 390–401.

Suveg, C., & Zeman, J. (2004). Emotion regulation in children with anxiety disorders. *Journal of Clinical Child and Adolescent Psychology, 33*, 750–759.

Tull, M. T., & Roemer, L. (2007). Emotion regulation difficulties associated with the experience of uncued panic attacks: Evidence of experiential avoidance, emotional nonacceptance, and decreased emotional clarity. *Behavior Therapy, 38*, 378–391.

Walkup, J. T., Albano, A., Piacentini, J., Birmaher, B., Compton, S. N., Sherrill, J. T., et al. (2008). Cognitive behavioral therapy, sertraline, or a combination in childhood anxiety. *New England Journal of Medicine, 359*, 2753–2766.

Weissman, M. M., Wolk, S., Goldstein, R. B., Moreau, D., Adams, P., Greenwald, S., et al. (1999). Depressed adolescents grown up. *Journal of the American Medical Association, 281,* 1707–1713.

Weisz, J. R., Jensen-Doss, A., & Hawley, K. M. (2006). Evidence-based youth psychotherapies versus usual clinical care: A meta-analysis of direct comparisons. *American Psychologist, 61,* 671–689.

Zeman, J., Shipman, K., & Penza-Clyve, S. (2001). Development and initial validation of the children's sadness management scale. *Journal of Nonverbal Behavior, 25,* 187–205.

Zeman, J., Shipman, K., & Suveg, C. (2002). Anger and sadness regulation: Predictions to internalizing and externalizing symptoms in children. *Journal of Clinical Child and Adolescent Psychology, 31,* 393–398.

CHAPTER 13

Beyond Disruptive Behavior Disorder Diagnoses

Applications of the Coping Power Program

John E. Lochman, Nicole P. Powell, Caroline L. Boxmeyer, Haley L. Ford, and Jessica A. Minney

The Coping Power program (Lochman, Wells, & Lenhart, 2008; Wells, Lochman, & Lenhart, 2008) takes a transdiagnostic approach to addressing externalizing behavior problems in children. Rather than focusing on specific diagnoses, such as oppositional defiant disorder (ODD) or conduct disorder (CD), the intervention focuses on reducing children's anger and aggression more broadly by targeting specific risk factors and active mechanisms that underlie these problems. The Coping Power program is based on a contextual social-cognitive model of risk for anger and aggression (for review, see Matthys & Lochman, 2010). The aim of the Coping Power intervention is to address the risk factors for children's anger and aggression that are malleable. In doing so, the intervention seeks to improve children's social and emotional coping skills, as well as parents' emotional coping skills and their parenting behavior.

Support for a Transdiagnostic Theory for Disruptive Behaviors

Although problems with anger and aggression can be part of the clinical profile for children with internalizing disorders, as in the irritability displayed by children with depression or when a child with separation anxiety has a tantrum while being dropped off at school, internalizing and externalizing behavior problems are most easily conceptualized as distinct categories. However, research suggests that the initiation and maintenance of internalizing and externalizing behavior problems can be influenced by a common set of risk factors.

Temperament

Children who display "difficult" temperamental features such as irritability, restlessness, irregular patterns of behavior, lack of persistence, and low adaptability are at increased risk for behavior problems (e.g., Caspi, Henry, McGee, Moffitt, & Silva, 1995; Guerin, Gottfried, & Thomas, 1997; Rubin, Burgess, Hastings, & Dwyer, 2003), as well as for internalizing problems (e.g., Booth-LaForce & Oxford, 2008; Keenan, Shaw, Delliquadri, Giovannelli, & Walsh, 1998). Children with "difficult" temperaments appear to be particularly sensitive to their caregiving environments, with increased risk of developing behavioral problems when parenting quality is poor (e.g., Belsky & Pluess, 2009). Similarly, Tschann, Kaiser, Chesney, Alkon, and Boyce (1996) found that preschoolers with "difficult" temperaments were at highest risk for both internalizing and externalizing problems when they lived in high-conflict families.

Family Factors

Research has identified several parenting behaviors that can lead to childhood adjustment problems of both an internalizing and an externalizing nature. Notably, parents who employ harsh discipline practices place their children at risk for conduct problems, as well as for symptoms of anxiety and depression (e.g., Bender et al., 2008). Similarly, low levels of parental warmth and acceptance have been shown to predict externalizing and internalizing problems in children (e.g., Hipwell et al., 2008; Pedersen, 1994). Although parenting practices have been implicated in both internalizing and externalizing problems, some research suggests that certain parenting behaviors may be more characteristic of certain categories of childhood problems. For example, in a review article, Berg-Nielsen, Vikan, and Dahl (2002) concluded that negative parental control appeared more related to internalizing problems, whereas inconsistent discipline practices and low levels of monitoring were associated with conduct problems.

Other family factors that may influence children's emotional and behavioral adjustment include multiple changes in family composition (Ackerman, Brown, D'Eramo, & Izard, 2002), parental alcoholism (e.g., Chassin, Rogosch, & Barrera, 1991), and parental psychiatric problems (e.g., Johnson, Cohen, Kasen, & Brook, 2006). Interestingly, Johnson and colleagues (2006) found that children of parents with externalizing disorders were almost as likely to develop an internalizing disorder as an externalizing disorder, whereas children of parents with internalizing disorders showed only a slightly greater tendency toward developing an internalizing disorder than an externalizing disorder.

Psychosocial Stress

A large body of empirical evidence supports the relation between psychosocial stress and both internalizing and externalizing behaviors in children (Grant et al., 2003). In a review article, McMahon, Grant, Compas, Thurm, and Ey (2003) examined research on the emotional and behavioral effects of different types of psychosocial stress in children, such as exposure to violence, abuse, and exposure to marital conflict. The authors concluded that there was little evidence to suggest that certain categories of stressors are specifically related to either internalizing or externalizing problems. Although there was variability in the findings from different studies, overall most stressors were related to both internalizing and externalizing problems in children. Tiet and colleagues (2001) found that some stressful life events (e.g., school change, parent being jailed) predicted both internalizing and externalizing disorders but that other stressors were associated with specific categories of disorder. For example, stressors involving loss and grief were related to depressive disorders, whereas being a victim of crime, violence, or assault was related to disruptive behavior disorders.

Social-Cognitive Skills

In a review article, Owen (2011) examined empirical research on cognitive processes related to trait anger in adults, concluding that processes relevant to Axis I disorders such as anxiety and depression are similarly related to problems with anger. Selective attention, misinterpretation of others' motives, and a tendency to ruminate were implicated in both the Axis I disorders and trait anger, providing support for a transdiagnostic approach to understanding psychological problems.

Deficiencies and distortions in social-cognitive skills are also associated with both conduct problems and internalizing symptoms in children. The social information processing (SIP; Crick & Dodge, 1994) model was developed to explain aggressive behavior in children but has also been applied to childhood anxiety and depression. Aggressive children have been shown to demonstrate problems at each of the SIP model's six stages. Compared to nonaggressive peers, aggressive children tend to encode fewer relevant details (Lochman & Dodge, 1994) and to be overly attentive to hostile cues (Gouze, 1987); to excessively perceive others' actions as hostile (Lochman & Dodge, 1994); to value dominance and revenge over social affiliation goals (Erdley & Asher, 1996); to generate more action-oriented and aggressive solutions and fewer compromise and verbally assertive solutions (Larson & Lochman, 2011); to evaluate aggression in a positive manner (Crick & Werner, 1998); and to have difficulty enacting prosocial behaviors (Dodge, Pettit, McClaskey, & Brown, 1986). Children with anxiety display problems in the encoding stage by attending to cues signifying danger or threat (Bell-Dolan, 1995) and at the solution evaluation stage by choosing more avoidant response strategies (Barrett, Rapee, Dadds, & Ryan, 1996). Children with depression display problems with solution generation and evaluation, offering and selecting fewer assertive strategies and more ineffective solutions (Goodman, Gravitt, & Kaslow, 1995).

Support for a Transdiagnostic Treatment for Angry and Aggressive Symptoms

Interest in transdiagnostic treatments is growing, as clinicians and researchers search for increasingly effective and efficient intervention approaches (McEvoy, Nathan, & Norton, 2009). Although the existing body of research focuses on internalizing disorders, support for a transdiagnostic approach to treatment across internalizing and externalizing problems can be extrapolated from the literature.

One source of support for a transdiagnostic approach to treatment across internalizing and externalizing disorders comes from nonspecific intervention effects. Empirically supported treatments (ESTs) originally developed to target one category of childhood disorders have been shown to effect positive changes on behaviors in another, presumably distinct, category. For example, parent–child interaction therapy (PCIT; Zisser & Eyberg, 2010) was designed to address oppositional and defiant behaviors in preschool-age children. Consistent with the program's goals, outcome research has demonstrated the effectiveness of PCIT in reducing externalizing behaviors (Zisser & Eyberg, 2010). In addition, PCIT has also been shown to reduce both externalizing and internalizing problems for children with comorbid ODD and separation anxiety disorder (Chase & Eyberg, 2008; Choate, Pincus, Eyberg, & Barlow, 2005). These effects have been attributed to the program's focus on parenting skills, which likely generalize across various child symptoms and behaviors. Another well-supported treatment for disruptive behaviors in children, parent management training (Kazdin, 2010), has similarly documented posttreatment improvements in both externalizing and internalizing behaviors, again likely due to the generalizability of parenting skills taught.

Common treatment elements form a second source of support for transdiagnostic interventions. As noted earlier, parent involvement is a core component of ESTs for childhood anxiety and depression, as well as for disruptive behaviors. Similarities in treatment elements across ESTs for internalizing and externalizing problems also include coping strategies, problem-solving skills, and relaxation training. Interventions containing these elements hold the potential for transdiagnostic application.

Description of Clinical Population

Children are typically referred for inclusion in Coping Power by their parents or through teacher nominations. Parent and teacher concerns may be validated through administration of behavior rating scales that include aggression and externalizing problems, such as the Behavior Assessment System for Children, Second Edition (BASC-2; Reynolds & Kamphaus, 2004). Because anger and aggression are symptoms of a number of clinical concerns, comprehensive evaluation is important to ensure that these problems are the main referral behaviors and not secondary to another condition that warrants the primary focus of treatment. For example, children with depression who display irritability will require treatment of their mood symptoms, and a medication adjustment may be the first treatment option for children presenting with stimulant-induced agitation or dysphoria.

In a clinic setting, children may be identified for the program by virtue of diagnoses such as ODD or CD; however, an explicit disruptive behavior disorder diagnosis is not required. Children who display aggression as part of a range of clinical presentations may benefit, as anger, aggression, and poor behavioral regulation are common to a variety of clinical concerns. For example, Coping Power may be appropriate for children displaying increased anger and aggression related to DSM-5 diagnoses such as adjustment disorder with disturbance of conduct, parent–child relational problem, and sibling relational problem or in cases in which these problems are related to difficulties with peer relationships, temperamental issues, or impulse control problems. The concept of equifinality applies here, as problems with anger and aggression may develop from, and be maintained by, a diverse range of circumstances. However, the Coping Power program's focus is on coping, both with the circumstances that trigger anger and with the angry feelings that arise. As such, the program can be applied to children experiencing any number of issues leading to angry feelings and aggressive behaviors.

In addition to directly targeting processes related to anger and aggression, Coping Power addresses additional problems commonly observed in aggressive children. For instance, aggressive youth frequently have difficulty getting along with peers, and they are often rejected by their peers (Lochman et al., 2012). Furthermore, such youth are at greater risk for developing problems with substance use and violence if their problems with anger and aggression go untreated (Tremblay, 2000). Finally, aggressive youth also encounter problems in the academic domain, including difficulty with reading and mathematics, as well as a lack of skills related to success in school (e.g., motivation, engagement; Lochman et al., 2012).

Description of the Coping Power Intervention

The Coping Power program includes separate child and parent intervention components. Both intervention components are based on cognitive and behavioral treatment principles. The child component includes intervention content for 34 child sessions, which aim to teach a number of core social and emotional competencies. The parent component includes intervention content for 16 parent sessions, which aim to teach specific behavioral parenting skills and to help parents facilitate their children's use of the skills learned in the intervention in their daily lives.

Transdiagnostic Features of Coping Power

There are a number of features inherent in the Coping Power program that can be considered transdiagnostic. The intervention is transdiagnostic across externalizing disorders as a whole in that it does not focus on children with specific diagnoses (e.g., ODD or CD) but rather focuses on targeting malleable risk factors and active mechanisms that underlie anger and aggression. Specific aspects of the intervention that are designed to alter active mechanisms for anger and aggression and are also likely to influence other behavioral outcomes are described next.

Contingency Management

An overarching aim of both the child and parent intervention components is to set and enforce clear contingencies for children's behavior. During the first child intervention session, behavior rules are established, and a token economy is laid out in which children can earn reinforcers for compliant behavior and positive group participation. A systematic method of responding to rule violations is also utilized in each child intervention session. In the parent intervention, parents practice setting clear behavior rules and expectations, giving clear instructions, and assessing child compliance. Parents learn a specific system for providing positive consequences for desired behaviors and utilizing effective punishment strategies for noncompliance and other forms of problem behavior. A primary goal of Coping Power is to reduce parental inconsistency, as intervention-produced improvements in parental consistency have been found to mediate intervention effects on children's externalizing behavior problems (Lochman & Wells, 2002). However, the effective use of contingency management is more broadly transdiagnostic, as it can be used to increase a broad range of desired child behaviors. Creating a more predictable therapeutic environment (through contingency management) may also create a "safe space" within which children can feel comfortable discussing their behavior problems and working to improve their behavior.

Personal Goal Setting

The first several sessions in the child intervention focus on identifying short-term and long-term personal behavioral goals. Therapists solicit input from parents and teachers in advance of child sessions about areas in which each child is in need of behavioral improvement. Therapists then work with children during the initial sessions to help them identify specific behavior goals that they are willing to work on (e.g., resolving problems without fighting, following adults' directions, keeping anger at a medium level or lower). Children continue to set weekly behavior goals throughout the Coping Power program. This intervention activity is intended to serve several purposes, including engaging children in the intervention and making it personally relevant to them, increasing children's motivation to improve their behavior outside of intervention sessions, and facilitating children's receipt of daily feedback about target behaviors and reinforcement for behavioral gains. This intervention activity is inherently transdiagnostic in that it can be adapted to fit each child's specific behavioral needs (based on the therapist's overall case conceptualization) on an ongoing basis throughout the intervention.

Emotional Awareness and Emotion Regulation

The next major unit in the Coping Power child component aims to help children become better at detecting a range of emotions and to recognize the early signs of emotional arousal. Children learn to use a "feelings thermometer" to measure different intensities of common emotions (e.g., happy, sad, scared, mad). Next, they are taught to recognize the physiological, behavioral, and cognitive manifestations of each emotion and how they can use their own thoughts and behavior to reduce negative emotional arousal. Intervention homework assignments are given to help children monitor their own patterns of emotional arousal and to identify common triggers for high levels of anger. Finally, children practice reducing their anger arousal by using a range of coping strategies, including self-instruction, distraction, deep breathing, and relaxation. Children are exposed to increasingly high levels of anger arousal during a series of graded in vivo exposure tasks, and they practice using one or more coping strategies to reduce their anger arousal.

Although the primary emphasis in Coping Power is on helping children learn to manage anger arousal by becoming better at recognizing the early signs of arousal, at paying attention to their thoughts and the impact of their thoughts on their feelings and behavior, and at using coping skills to manage arousal, this sequence of intervention activities may help children manage the arousal associated with other disorders, such as anxiety or depression. Therapists are given the option during these Coping Power sessions to extend the discussion and practice opportunities to address other feeling states, including fear and sadness. These extension activities are particularly recommended when children are exhibiting both externalizing and internalizing symptoms.

Perspective Taking

The next aim of the Coping Power intervention is to help children view situations from others' perspectives. Children practice generating a range of explanations for others' behavior based on hypothetical and real-life interpersonal scenarios. Children also practice attending to a larger range of social cues rather than focusing only on cues that likely convey hostile intent. Although these intervention activities are primarily intended to reduce the hostile attribution bias that frequently occurs in children with anger and aggression problems (Lochman & Dodge, 1994), they also have the potential for transdiagnostic effects. For example, children with social skill deficits or social anxiety may benefit from learning to encode social cues more accurately and learning to view social situations from others' perspectives.

Social Problem Solving

A major unit of the Coping Power intervention teaches children to recognize when they are experiencing a social problem, to generate a range of solutions, to think ahead about the likely consequences of each solution, and to pick the solution with the most positive expected outcome. Children practice the steps in this process, first with hypothetical and then with real-life problem situations, across a number of intervention sessions.

This intervention unit has considerable potential for transdiagnostic application. Programs incorporating social problem-solving strategies have demonstrated effectiveness for children experiencing a range of clinical concerns, including anxiety (Kendall et al., 1997), depression

(Eskin, Ertekin, & Demir, 2008), and impulsivity (Baer & Nietzel, 1991). Although a diverse group, children experiencing emotional and behavioral problems may show similar difficulties in social information processing, such as attending to unhelpful environmental cues, misattributing others' intentions, and failing to generate and consider alternative responses. Orbach, Mikulincer, Blumenson, Mester, and Stein (1999), for example, have posited that suicidal youth resort to self-harm because they feel that their problems are irresolvable in that potential solutions to their problems are undesirable or would result in additional problems.

Social problem-solving strategies can help children with anger or anxiety become aware of problems earlier (before reaching heightened levels of arousal) and can help children identify problems from others' perspectives (rather than being overly self-focused or making misattributions about others' intentions). This process can help impulsive children learn to slow down and think ahead about the consequences of their behavior before acting. Practicing solution enactment can also help children become more adept at using verbal communication strategies (including assertive statements, bargaining, and compromise solutions) and can increase the value children place on verbal solutions. Learning effective problem solving can improve children's relationships with their friends and family members and improve their sense of self-efficacy and may thereby reduce secondary depression in children and perhaps even in their parents.

Coping Power teaches parents to use the same approach to solve family problems. This can help reduce family conflict, increase family cohesion, and help children feel as though they have a "voice" in resolving family problems collaboratively. Finally, learning to enact more than one solution when the first solution does not work out as planned can also help children and parents become more resilient.

Rehearsal and Mastery Opportunities

Every child and parent Coping Power session includes opportunities to practice the specific skill(s) being taught. Homework assignments and personal goal sheets are also utilized to foster rehearsal and generalization of skills outside of Coping Power sessions. The problem-solving unit has a mastery activity in which children produce their own videotaped public-service announcements teaching others how to solve social problems effectively. The children are able to show their completed video to their parents in order to help their parents learn to use the same approach to solve family problems. Thus important transdiagnostic elements of the Coping Power intervention may be (1) its emphasis on clearly defining target behavioral goals; (2) teaching specific social and emotional coping skills to meet these goals; and (3) providing children and parents with frequent opportunities to practice and master new skills, both in and out of therapy sessions.

Adapting Coping Power for Multiple Diagnoses or Problem Sets

The Coping Power activities just described can be adapted as needed to address coexisting diagnoses or problem sets. For example, a comprehensive evaluation may indicate that a child's primary issues result from angry and aggressive behaviors related to a disruptive behavior disorder, that these issues are adversely affecting relationships with teachers and peers, and that, as a result of these problematic interactions, the child is endorsing a mild degree of anxiety in the school setting. In this case, the therapist may make a number of adaptations while implementing the program.

When identifying target behavior goals, the therapist may guide the child toward behavior goals related to anxiety (e.g., "I will volunteer ideas in front of the class"), in addition to aggression (e.g., "I will solve problems without fighting"). To go a step further, the therapist may try to identify an underlying mechanism linking the child's aggression and anxiety and then generate behavior goals that address that mechanism. For example, if the therapist has learned that the child becomes physically or verbally aggressive whenever she feels embarrassed or "singled out" in front of the class, the therapist might help the child generate a goal of taking three deep breaths and using a coping statement whenever she is feeling embarrassed, before deciding what to do next.

During the unit on emotional awareness, the therapist might spend additional time helping the child identify specific physiological signs of anxiety (e.g., sweaty palms, racing thoughts, dry mouth), situations that tend to trigger her anxiety (e.g., being teased by classmates, being redirected by her teacher), and thoughts that cause her anxiety to escalate (e.g., "No one likes me"; "I am such a loser"). The therapist can then help the child practice coping with anxiety by exposing her to scenarios likely to trigger anxiety arousal and helping her practice using coping strategies to reduce her arousal (e.g., taking deep breaths and telling herself "don't worry about what other people think of me"; "it is okay if I get in a little bit of trouble once in awhile, it happens to everyone"). The therapist can conduct exposure tasks for coping with anxiety arousal in addition to the planned exposure tasks for coping with anger arousal.

During the perspective-taking sessions, the therapist may seek to help the child reduce self-directed attributions (e.g., "He looked at me funny because he thinks I am a loser") and practice generating alternate attributions (e.g., "He may have looked at me funny because he lost his glasses," or "He may have been worried about the math test he had coming up"). Finally, during the problem-solving sessions, the therapist may seek to reduce the child's use of avoidant or aggressive solutions and increase the child's use of verbal assertion solutions. Being aware of the child's anxiety symptoms, the therapist may choose to provide additional practice opportunities to help the child become more comfortable resolving problems verbally. The therapist might also provide extra encouragement or rewards when he or she observes the child speaking assertively to others or attempting to do so. It is important to note that, if ongoing evaluation during treatment suggests that it is the child's anxiety that primarily drives his aggression, the therapist may modify the case conceptualization and shift to an evidence-based intervention specifically targeting anxiety (e.g., Coping Cat; Kendall & Hedtke, 2006) while continuing to monitor the aggressive behavior.

This strategy of flexibly using Coping Power to incorporate themes relevant to a variety of clinical issues can also be applied to cases involving depression, impulsivity, or relationship problems. For example, coping self-statements can be developed to address depressive cognitions (e.g., "I have things to look forward to"), perspective-taking exercises can be focused on the child's problematic relationships (e.g., with parents, peers, or siblings), and the importance of thinking through solutions and evaluating potential consequences can be emphasized for impulsive youth.

Empirical Support for Coping Power

The efficacy and effectiveness of Coping Power has been supported by several randomized control trials (RCTs). An initial investigation of the Coping Power program randomized boys who were rated by their teachers as being aggressive to one of three conditions: Coping Power child program only, Coping Power child plus Coping Power parent program, or treatment as usual (Lochman & Wells, 2003). Both of the Coping Power groups had significantly lower rates of delinquency and parent-rated substance abuse relative to the control group at 1-year follow-up (Lochman & Wells, 2004). Furthermore, compared with the control group, both Coping Power groups showed significantly more improvement in teacher-rated behavior at 1-year follow-up. The effects were stronger for the child-plus-parent group, but both groups improved relative to the control group, and significant differences were evident at 1-year postintervention (Lochman & Wells, 2004). These outcomes were mediated by improvements in the children's social cognitive processes and their parents' processes, which supports the theoretical framework of Coping Power (Lochman & Wells, 2002).

Another study evaluated the additive effects of including a universal intervention along with the standard Coping Power program (Lochman & Wells, 2003). The universal intervention included both parent and teacher components but did not intervene directly with the children (Lochman & Wells, 2003). Participating teachers received five in-service training sessions led by Coping Power staff. The in-service sessions focused on equipping teachers with strategies to develop children's academic, social, and emotional competences and increase parents' involvement with the school. Parents of children in the universal intervention classrooms were invited to attend four parent meetings that also focused on improving children's social, academic, and emotional skills, as well as on how parents could prepare their children to transition to middle school (Lochman & Wells, 2003). Relative to an untreated comparison group, the children who received both Coping Power and the universal intervention showed less self-reported substance use and teacher-rated aggression. In addition, children who received both the universal and targeted prevention programs reported higher perceived social competency and were rated by their teachers as having more improvements in classroom behavior. At 1 year postintervention, children who received Coping Power, the universal intervention, or both components had lower rates of delinquent behavior and substance use than children who received no intervention.

Coping Power has also been successfully utilized with clinical populations. Dutch children meeting criteria for at least one disruptive behavior disorder were randomly assigned to clinic treatment as usual or to an abbreviated version of Coping Power. Reductions in disruptive behaviors were evident in both groups; however, the Coping Power group showed significantly greater reductions in overt aggression (van de Wiel et al., 2007; van de Wiel, Matthys, Cohen-Kettenis, & van Engeland, 2003). At 6 months postintervention, both groups had maintained their reductions in disruptive behavior. Four years after treatment, the children in the Coping Power group reported significantly lower rates of tobacco and marijuana use than children who had received clinic treatment as usual (Zonnevylle-Bender, Matthys, Van De Wiel, & Lochman, 2007). In contrast with the experienced therapists conducting treatment as usual, the Coping Power therapists in this study were trained in the manualized intervention but had little clinical experience, yet both groups demonstrated long-term improvements. This suggests that Coping Power can be effectively implemented by less experienced therapists, which may make it an attractive option for community providers and schools (Zonnevylle-Bender et al., 2007).

Developmental Considerations

The contextual social-cognitive model of risk factors (Lochman & Wells, 2002) that serves as a basis for the Coping Power program and the Coping Power Intervention Program and its activities are both developmentally informed. The contextual social-cognitive model describes how distal contextual risk factors and proximal risk factors affect the development and maintenance of children's aggression and conduct problems over time (Matthys & Lochman, 2010). Distal, or background, risk factors predict children's rates of aggressive behaviors and include community and family characteristics. At the community level, children who grow up in impoverished neighborhoods are at greater risk for exhibiting increases in proactive aggressive behavior when they enter into early adolescence in the middle school years (Fite, Wynn, Lochman, & Wells, 2009). Youth who display more proactive aggressive behavior are likely to display severe antisocial behavior such as delinquency and substance use as they proceed through the adolescent years (Fite, Colder, Lochman, & Wells, 2008). Neighborhoods with greater levels of poverty likely have a range of other associated risk factors, such as an active drug trade and violent gangs, which contribute to the youths' development of increasingly serious conduct problems. These broad community-level risk factors are also apparent in the effects of the school environment on children. Aggressive children who are placed into classrooms with high numbers of highly aggressive children are likely to increase their own aggressive behavior across the year, in comparison with similarly aggressive children who are placed in classroom environments with fewer highly aggressive children (Barth, Dunlap, Dane, Lochman, & Wells, 2004).

Family characteristics such as marital conflict, maternal depression, single parenthood, and family poverty predict children's aggressive behavior as well. Many of these background family risk factors influence children's behavior because they disrupt adults' parenting practices. For example, depressed mothers have more inconsistent parenting, and the inconsistent parenting is the mediator, or the direct cause, of children's increased problem behaviors (Barry, Dunlap, Lochman, & Wells, 2009). Thus the inconsistent parenting practices of depressed parents, including their inability to follow through with stated consequences following children's misbehavior, are examples of proximal risk factors contributing to children's aggressive behavior. Other proximal risk factors include children's disrupted peer relations, such as being rejected by one's peers and becoming involved in deviant peer groups (Fite et al., 2008), and the children's acquired social-cognitive and self-regulatory abilities (Matthys & Lochman, 2010).

Interventions such as the Coping Power program can strategically target these proximal risk factors, which are anticipated to be more mutable and open to intervention. This set of distal and proximal risk factors affect children in a developmental cascade, with youth being more prone to experience and possessing multiple risk factors as they get older, leading to the need for increasingly complex and comprehensive interventions for severely antisocial adolescents.

Another developmental process that is very relevant to a transdiagnostic perspective of children's disorder involves the way in which some behavior problems lead to or contribute to other types of emotional or behavioral problems that children may display. Preadolescent and early adolescent aggression has been found to lead to increasing levels of depressive symptoms in subsequent years (Capaldi & Stoolmiller, 1999; Johnson & Lochman, 2011). Later in adolescence, depression has been found to have a bidirectional effect and to lead to increasing levels of conduct problems (Capaldi, 1992; Johnson & Lochman, 2011). Once present, the co-occurrence of conduct problems and depression predisposes youth to earlier onset of other problems, such as substance use (Miller-Johnson, Lochman, Coie, Terry, & Hyman, 1998).

The developmentally appropriate age range for youth to participate in the Coping Power program is 8–14 years of age. Although the program may be able to be adapted for lower functioning youth, Coping Power is most appropriate for children who have at least low average intellectual functioning. The program has been developed to assist children in the latter years of elementary school to acquire improved coping skills as they get ready to transition into middle school. The middle school years are a period of increased risk for youth because of the decreased monitoring and supervision that youth receive in school, the increased array of deviant peers who can influence them, and changes associated with puberty. The program has been adapted for use with children both younger and older than the 8–14 age range. With younger children and with lower functioning preadolescents, program activities and discussion are made more concrete and involve less broad hypothetical reasoning. Activities are more centered around use of puppet role plays and engaging picture books that touch on themes relevant to program objectives. At the other end of developmental adaptation, we are currently engaged with colleagues at Johns Hopkins University in the creation of a version of Coping Power for adolescents. This enhanced version for older adolescents will include a focus on the same objectives as with early adolescents but will also incorporate age-appropriate activities such as journaling, as well as age-appropriate content such as assisting adolescents to repair damaged relationships and to cope with cyberbullying.

Strengths and Challenges

Coping Power is focused on children with aggressive behavior problems, and in that sense it is a disorder-specific intervention. In contrast, transdiagnostic interventions can be defined as interventions that apply the same underlying treatment principles across different disorders (Clark & Taylor, 2009). However, as Clark and Taylor (2009) note, the difference between transdiagnostic and disorder-specific protocols can be a matter of degree. Thus disorder-specific interventions, such as Coping Power, may have certain key transdiagnostic elements. Research has found that disorder-specific interventions for panic disorder and for posttraumatic stress disorder have produced reductions in comorbid depression (Clark & Taylor, 2009). Even a focused intervention such as Coping Power, targeted on certain risk factors, can influence other outcomes (besides aggression) because (1) some other outcomes follow from aggression (e.g., secondary depression in the child, and perhaps even in the parent), and changes in aggression or conduct problems can influence those outcomes; (2) there are some common active mechanisms that can influence multiple outcomes (e.g., social problem solving can affect aggression and depression), and thus activities (social problem-solving training) designed to affect that targeted mechanism can affect the related outcomes; and (3) aggressive children can commonly have co-occurring problems (reactive aggressive children can have co-occurring anxiety, as well as aggression) that can be influenced by well-planned adaptations of the intervention (the use of Coping Power with an aggressive-anxious child). We perceive that Coping Power frequently operates in these types of hybrid transdiagnostic ways.

A primary challenge is deciding whether and when a co-occurring set of anxiety or depression symptoms is so severe that the common treatment effect from the Coping Power activities may not be sufficient to address the co-occurring problems. In that case, use of a disorder-specific intervention such as Coping Power requires a clinical decision about whether there should be a pause in the Coping Power sessions in order to introduce a disorder-specific intervention for a period of time to address the co-occurring anxiety or depression, or whether several sessions directed at the co-occurring problem can be imported into the Coping Power sequence. The latter approach, which relies on "traveling sessions," is a key feature of the integrated set of disorder-specific, but easily integrated, program modules developed by the Integrated Psychotherapy Consortium (e.g. Wells, Lochman, Goldman, & the Integrated Psychotherapy Consortium, 2007).

Future Directions

Future directions for refinement and research on Coping Power include a focus on several transdiagnostic-related changes to the basic program, including testing an adaptive, or tailored, version of Coping Power and incorporating other specific intervention elements into Coping Power to directly enhance its potential for transdiagnostic effects. In addition, it will be critical to test the comparative efficacy of transdiagnostic interventions and disorder-specific protocols (Clark & Taylor, 2009).

Manualized interventions such as the Coping Power program (Lochman & Wells, 2003) have been effective in reducing children's proactive aggression and subsequent delinquency but have been less successful in quickly reducing children's reactive aggression. These results suggest that the anger management portions of cognitive-behavioral interventions such as Coping Power could be adapted to better address children's reactive aggression and associated fearfulness and anxiety. Two promising approaches to assisting children to better self-regulate their physiological arousal when in socially problematic situations are yoga and mindfulness training (e.g., Duncan, Coatsworth, & Greenberg, 2009). Mindfulness training assists individuals in bringing their attention to internal and external experiences occurring in the present moment and has been found to feasibly address multiple anxiety and depression disorders (Baer, 2003; Burke, 2009). We would like to examine whether the Coping Power program, augmented with mindfulness training (CP-MT), could influence biomarkers and emotional reactions associated with reactive aggression and anxiety, in comparison with Coping Power and treatment as usual. We plan to develop a new manualized CP-MT protocol that will include translational tools and mindfulness components designed to assist children to better self-regulate their arousal (yoga, mindful attention and awareness, meditation, deep breathing) in both the parent and the child components of Coping Power.

It will be useful to explore how a structured, manualized program such as Coping Power can be provided in an adaptive, tailored way to address the specific risk factors and comorbid behavioral-emotional problems of individual children and their parents. With colleagues at Johns Hopkins University and the University of Missouri, we are beginning to explore how a motivational interviewing approach such as the Family Check-Up (Dishion & Kavanagh, 2003) can lead families to choose which program elements are most fitting for their particular pattern of problem behaviors. Adaptive versions of Coping Power could be structured to include additional program elements to make the program more transdiagnostic, with the aim of directly addressing the co-occurring depression and anxiety of aggressive children.

REFERENCES

Ackerman, B. P., Brown, E. D., D'Eramo, K. S., & Izard, C. E. (2002). Maternal relationship instability and the school behavior of children from disadvantaged families. *Developmental Psychology, 38,* 694–704.

Baer, R. A. (2003). Mindfulness training as a clinical intervention: A conceptual and empirical review. *Clinical Psychology: Science and Practice, 10,* 125–143.

Baer, R. A., & Nietzel, M. T. (1991). Cognitive and behavioral treatment of impulsivity in children: A meta-analytic review of the outcome literature. *Journal of Clinical Child Psychology, 20,* 400–412.

Barrett, P. M., Rapee, R. M., Dadds, M. R., & Ryan, S. M. (1996). Family enhancement of cognitive style in anxious and aggressive children: Threat bias and the FEAR effect. *Journal of Abnormal Child Psychology, 24,* 187–203.

Barry, T. D., Dunlap, S., Lochman, J. E., & Wells, K. C. (2009). Inconsistent discipline as a mediator between maternal distress and aggression in boys. *Child and Family Behavior Therapy, 31,* 1–19.

Barth, J. M., Dunlap, S. T., Dane, H., Lochman, J. E., & Wells, K. C. (2004). Classroom environment influences on aggression, peer relations, and academic focus. *Journal of School Psychology, 42,* 115–133.

Bell-Dolan, D. J. (1995). Social cue interpretation of anxious children. *Journal of Clinical Child Psychology, 24,* 2–10.

Belsky, J., & Pluess, M. (2009). Beyond diathesis–stress: Differential susceptibility to environmental influences. *Psychological Bulletin, 135,* 885–908.

Bender, H. L., Allen, J. P., McElhaney, K. B., Antonishak, J., Moore, C. M., Kelly, H. O., et al. (2008). Use of harsh physical discipline and developmental outcomes in adolescence. *Development and Psychopathology, 19,* 227–242.

Berg-Nielsen, T. S., Vikan, A., & Dahl, A. A. (2002). Parenting related to child and parental psychopathology: A descriptive review of the literature. *Clinical Child Psychology and Psychiatry, 7,* 529–552.

Booth-LaForce, C., & Oxford, M. L. (2008). Trajectories of social withdrawal from grades 1 to 6: Prediction from early parenting, attachment, and temperament. *Developmental Psychology, 44,* 1298–1313.

Burke, C. A. (2009). Mindfulness-based approaches with children and adolescents: A preliminary review of current research in an emergent field. *Journal of Child and Family Studies, 19,* 133–144.

Capaldi, D. M. (1992). Co-occurrence of conduct problems and depressive mood in early adolescent boys: II. Two-year follow-up at 8th grade. *Development and Psychopathology, 4,* 125–144.

Capaldi, D. M., & Stoolmiller, M. (1999). Co-occurrence of conduct problems and depressive symptoms in early adolescent boys: III. Prediction to young adult adjustment. *Development and Psychopathology, 11,* 59–84.

Caspi, A., Henry, B., McGee, R. O., Moffitt, T. E., & Silva, P. A. (1995). Temperamental origins of child and adolescent behavior problems: From age three to age fifteen. *Child Development, 66,* 55–68.

Chase, R. M., & Eyberg, S. M. (2008). Clinical presentation and treatment outcome for chidren with comorbid externalizing and internalizing symptoms. *Journal of Anxiety Disorders, 22,* 273–282.

Chassin, L., Rogosch, F., & Barrera, M. (1991). Substance use and symptomatology among adolescent children of alcoholics. *Journal of Abnormal Psychology, 100,* 449–463.

Choate, M. L., Pincus, D. B., Eyberg, S. M., & Barlow, D. H. (2005). Parent–child interaction therapy for treatment of separation anxiety disorder in young children: A pilot study. *Cognitive and Behavioral Practice, 12,* 126–135.

Clark, D. A., & Taylor, S. (2009). The transdiagnostic perspective on cognitive-behavioral therapy for anxiety and depression: New wine for old wineskins? *Journal of Cognitive Psychotherapy: An International Quarterly, 23,* 60–66.

Crick, N. R., & Dodge, K. A. (1994). A review and reformulation of social-information processing mechanisms in children's social adjustment. *Psychological Bulletin, 115,* 74–101.

Crick, N. R., & Werner, N. E. (1998). Response decision processes in relational and overt aggression. *Child Development, 69,* 1630–1639.

Dishion, T. J., & Kavanagh, K. (2003). *Intervening in adolescent problem behavior: A family-centered approach.* New York: Guilford Press.

Dodge, K. A., Pettit, G. S., McClaskey, C. L., & Brown, M. M. (1986). Social competence in children. *Monographs of the Society for Research in Child Development, 51,* 1–85.

Duncan, L. G., Coatsworth, J. D., & Greenberg, M. T. (2009) A model of mindful parenting: Implications for parent–child relationships and prevention research. *Clinical Child and Family Psychology Review, 12,* 255–270.

Erdley, C. A., & Asher, S. R. (1996). Children's social goals and self-efficacy perceptions as influences on their responses to ambiguous provocation. *Child Development, 67,* 1329–1344.

Eskin, M., Ertekin, K., & Demir, H. (2008). Efficacy of a problem-solving therapy for depression and suicide potential in adolescents and young adults. *Cognitive Therapy and Research, 32,* 227–245.

Fite, P. J., Colder, C. R., Lochman, J. E., & Wells, K. C. (2008). Developmental trajectories of proactive and reactive aggression from fifth to ninth grade. *Journal of Clinical Child and Adolescent Psychology, 37,* 412–421.

Fite, P. J., Wynn, P., Lochman, J. E., & Wells, K. C. (2009). The effect of neighborhood disadvantage on proactive and reactive aggression. *Journal of Community Psychology, 37,* 542–546.

Goodman, S. H., Gravitt, G. W., & Kaslow, N. J. (1995). Social problem solving: A moderator of the relation between negative life stress and depression symptoms in children. *Journal of Abnormal Child Psychology, 23,* 473–485.

Gouze, K. R. (1987). Attention and social problem solving as correlates of aggression in preschool males. *Journal of Abnormal Child Psychology, 15,* 181–197.

Grant, K. E., Compas, B. E., Stuhlmacher, A. F., Thurm, A. E., McMahon, S. D., & Halpert, J. A. (2003). Stressors and child and adolescent psychopathology: Moving from markers to mechanisms of risk. *Psychological Bulletin, 129,* 447–466.

Guerin, D. W., Gottfried, A. W., & Thomas, C. W. (1997). Difficult temperament and behaviour problems: A longitudinal study from 1.5 to 12 years. *International Journal of Behavioral Development, 21,* 71–90.

Hipwell, A., Keenan, K., Kasza, K., Loeber, R., Stouthamer-Loeber, M., & Bean, T. (2008). Reciprocal influences between girls' conduct problems and depression, and parental punishment and warmth: A six-year prospective analysis. *Journal of Abnormal Child Psychology, 36,* 663–677.

Johnson, B. S., & Lochman, J. E. (2011, August). *The co-morbidity of depression and conduct problems in the transition to adolescence.* Paper presented at the annual Berkeley McNair Scholar Symposium, Berkeley, CA.

Johnson, J. G., Cohen, P., Kasen, S., & Brook, J. S. (2006). A multiwave multi-informant study to the specificity of the association between parental and offspring psychiatric disorders. *Comprehensive Psychiatry, 47,* 169–177.

Kazdin, A. E. (2010). Problem-solving skills training and parent management training for oppositional defiant disorder and conduct disorder. In J. R. Weisz & A. E. Kazdin (Eds.), *Evidence-based psychotherapies for children and adolescents* (2nd ed., pp. 211–226). New York: Guilford Press.

Keenan, K., Shaw, D., Delliquadri, E., Giovannelli, J., & Walsh, B. (1998). Evidence for the continuity of early problem behaviors: Application of a developmental model. *Journal of Abnormal Child Psychology, 26,* 441–452.

Kendall, P. C., Flannery-Schroeder, E., Panichelli-Mindell, S. M., Southam-Gerow, M., Henin, A., & Warman, M. (1997). Therapy for youths with anxiety disorders: A second randomized clinical trial. *Journal of Consulting and Clinical Psychology, 65,* 366–380.

Kendall, P. C., & Hedtke, K. A. (2006). *Coping Cat Workbook* (2nd ed.). Ardmore, PA: Workbook Publishing.

Larson, J., & Lochman, J. E. (2011). *Helping schoolchildren cope with anger: A cognitive-behavioral intervention* (2nd ed.). New York: Guilford Press.

Lochman, J. E., Boxmeyer, C. L., Powell, N. P., Siddiqui, S., Stromeyer, S. L., & Kelly, M. (2012). Anger and aggression: School-based cognitive-behavioral interventions. In R. B. Mennuti, R. W. Christner, & A. Freeman (Eds.), *Cognitive-behavioral interventions in educational settings: A handbook for practice* (2nd ed., pp. 305–338). New York: Routledge.

Lochman, J. E., & Dodge, K. A. (1994). Social-cognitive processes of severely violent, moderately aggressive and nonaggressive boys. *Journal of Consulting and Clinical Psychology, 62,* 366–374.

Lochman, J. E., & Wells, K. C. (2002). Contextual social-cognitive mediators and child outcome: A test of the theoretical model in the Coping Power program. *Development and Psychopathology, 14,* 945–967.

Lochman, J. E., & Wells, K. C. (2003). Effectiveness of the Coping Power program and of classroom intervention with aggressive children: Outcomes at a 1-year followup. *Behavior Therapy, 34,* 493–515.

Lochman, J. E., & Wells, K. C. (2004). The Coping Power program for preadolescent aggressive boys and their parents: Outcome effects at the 1-year follow-up. *Journal of Consulting and Clinical Psychology, 72,* 571–578.

Lochman, J. E., Wells, K. C., & Lenhart, L. A. (2008). *Coping Power: Child group program, facilitator guide.* New York: Oxford University Press.

Matthys, W., & Lochman, J. E. (2010). *Oppositional defiant disorder and conduct disorder in childhood.* Oxford, UK: Wiley-Blackwell.

McEvoy, P. M., Nathan, P., & Norton, P. J. (2009). Efficacy of transdiagnostic treatments: A review of published outcome studies and future research directions. *Journal of Cognitive Psychotherapy, 23,* 20–33.

McMahon, S. D., Grant, K. E., Compas, B. E., Thurm, A. E., & Ey, S. (2003). Stress and psychopathology in children and adolescents: Is there evidence of specificity? *Journal of Child Psychology and Psychiatry, 44,* 107–133.

Miller-Johnson, S., Lochman, J. E., Coie, J. D., Terry, R., & Hyman, C. (1998). Comorbidity of conduct and depressive problems at sixth grade: Substance use outcomes across adolescence. *Journal of Abnormal Child Psychology, 26,* 221–232.

Orbach, I., Mikulincer, M., Blumenson, R., Mester, R., & Stein, D. (1999). The subjective experience of problem irresolvability and suicidal behavior: Dynamics and measurement. *Suicide and Life-Threatening Behavior, 29,* 150–164.

Owen, J. M. (2011). Transdiagnostic cognitive processes in high trait anger. *Clinical Psychology Review, 31,* 193–202.

Pedersen, W. (1994). Parental relations, mental health, and delinquency in adolescents. *Adolescence, 29,* 975–990.

Reynolds, C. R., & Kamphaus, R. W. (2004). *Behavior Assessment System for Children–Second Edition (BASC-2).* Circle Pines, MN: AGS.

Rubin, K. H., Burgess, K. B., Hastings, P. D., & Dwyer, K. M. (2003). Predicting preschoolers' externalizing behaviors from toddler temperament, conflict, and maternal negativity. *Developmental Psychology, 39,* 164–176.

Tiet, Q. Q., Bird, H. R., Hoven, C. W., Moore, R., Wu, P., Wicks, J., et al. (2001). Relationship between specific adverse life events and psychiatric disorders. *Journal of Abnormal Child Psychology, 29,* 153–164.

Tremblay, R. E. (2000). The development of aggressive behaviour during childhood: What have we learned in the past century? *International Journal of Behavioral Development, 24,* 129–141.

Tschann, J. M., Kaiser, P., Chesney, M. A., Alkon, A., & Boyce, W. T. (1996). Resilience and vulnerability among preschool children: Family functioning, temperament, and behavior problems. *Journal of the American Academy of Child and Adolescent Psychiatry, 35,* 184–192.

van de Wiel, N. M. H., Matthys, W., Cohen-Kettenis, P., Maassen, G. H., Lochman, J. E., & van Engeland, H. (2007). The effectiveness of an experimental treatment when compared to care as usual depends on the type of care as usual. *Behavior Modification, 31,* 298–312.

van de Wiel, N. M. H., Matthys, W., Cohen-Kettenis, P., & van Engeland, H. (2003). Application of the Utrecht Coping Power program and care as usual to children with disruptive behavior disorders in outpatient clinics: A comparative study of cost and course of treatment. *Behavior Therapy, 34,* 421–436.

Wells, K., Lochman, J., Goldman, E., & the Integrated Psychotherapy Consortium. (2007). *Project Liberty Enhanced Services Program: Disruptive behavior symptoms intervention manual.* New York: Columbia University.

Wells, K. C., Lochman, J. E., & Lenhart, L. A. (2008). *Coping Power parent group program: Facilitator guide.* New York: Oxford University Press.

Zisser, A., & Eyberg, S. M. (2010). Parent–child interaction therapy and the treatment of disruptive behavior disorders. In J. R. Weisz & A. E. Kazdin (Eds.), *Evidence-based psychotherapies for children and adolescents* (2nd ed., pp. 179–193). New York: Guilford Press.

Zonnevylle-Bender, M. J. S., Matthys, W., Van De Wiel, N. M. H., & Lochman, J. E. (2007). Preventive effects of treatment of disruptive behavior disorder in middle childhood on substance use and delinquent behavior. *Journal of the American Academy of Child and Adolescent Psychiatry, 46,* 33–39.

CHAPTER 14

Multisystemic Therapy

Sonja K. Schoenwald

Interventions that aim to retain theoretically cogent and empirically supported case conceptualization and clinical procedures while allowing for individualization to client attributes have been described as falling into three categories: transdiagnostic, modular, and principle-based treatments (McHugh, Murray, & Barlow, 2009). These approaches aim to leverage the evidence base on the efficacy and effectiveness of diagnosis-specific treatment protocols, evidence regarding the similarities within some classes of disorders among clinical features and maintaining mechanisms, and practitioner capacity to deploy effective treatment approaches without having to master multiple, distinct, evidence-based treatment protocols (Chorpita & Daleiden, 2009; Ehrenreich, Goldstein, Wright, & Barlow, 2009; McHugh et al., 2009). An additional aim is to accommodate flexibility within fidelity, at least where evidence indicates such accommodation can occur without attendant degradation in client outcomes. Retaining clinician focus on the client—with respect to outcomes and as the basis for flexibility—is paramount. As emphasized in a recent treatise on the compatibility of evidence-based, measurement-based, and individualized care: "Conflict between personalized care and evidence-based care arises only if we are personalizing care to meet the needs of providers. That is, unfortunately, sometimes the case" (Simon, 2011, p. 701).

The extent to which transdiagnostic, modular, or principle-based approaches to intervention offer efficient means by which to extend the reach of effective treatments to consumers or to realize the effective personalization of such treatments (i.e., personalization that maintains or enhances positive outcomes achieved under distinct protocols) is an empirical question. Answers to the question may turn out to vary by approach (e.g., transdiagnostic, modular, principle-based) and/or target population. The focus of this chapter is on multisystemic therapy (MST; Henggeler, Schoenwald, Borduin, Rowland, & Cunningham, 2009). MST could be characterized as principle based, measurement based, and flexible. There is extensive evidence of the effectiveness of MST with juvenile offenders, the target population for which it was originally developed. Modifications of MST for use with other challenging populations have also been developed and rigorously evaluated. This chapter describes the unified approach MST takes to clinical conceptualization and intervention across target populations and the processes used to determine when a target population is sufficiently distinctive to warrant the integration and evaluation of novel therapeutic techniques into MST.

Description of the MST Intervention

MST uses a short-term (3–5 months) intensive home- and community-based model of service delivery to implement comprehensive treatment that specifically targets factors in each system in the youth's social ecology (family, peers, school, neighborhood, and community). Clinicians are organized into teams of two to four therapists and a clinical supervisor. MST therapists carry a caseload of four to six families at a time and vary the frequency and duration of treatment contacts to the circumstances, needs, and strengths of each family throughout the treatment episode. Nine treatment principles and a specified analytical process guide the clinical formulation process and MST assessment and intervention strategies. Interventions typically focus on improving caregiver discipline and monitoring practices, reducing family conflict, improving affective relations among family members, decreasing youth association with deviant peers, increasing association with prosocial peers, improving school or vocational performance, and developing an indigenous support network of family, friends, and neighbors to support treatment progress and help the family sustain treatment gains. Specific treatment techniques are integrated into a social ecological framework for understanding behavior from those therapies that have the most empirical support, including behavioral and behavioral parent training, cognitive behavioral, and pragmatic family therapies.

Research and Theory Underlying MST

Research findings from large correlational and longitudinal studies show that delinquency is predicted by a combination of risk factors within and between the key systems in which children are embedded—family (supervision, discipline strategies, consistency of parenting, parental support, affective relations, conflict) peer (association with deviant peers), school (poor performance, poor family–school linkage), and neighborhood (transience, high crime). Among seminal longitudinal studies are those conducted by Elliott (e.g., Elliott, 1994), Loeber (e.g., Loeber, Farrington, Stouthamer-Loeber, & Van Kammen, 1998), and Thornberry (Thornberry & Krohn, 2003). Although some differences in risk factors for different populations (e.g., males vs. females, whites vs. African Americans, early vs. late adolescence) have emerged, findings from these and other studies of antisocial behavior in adolescents have been remarkably consistent throughout the past decades. Antisocial behavior in adolescents is multiply determined by factors within the youth and across his or her social ecology (i.e., family, peers, school, and neighborhood) (Biglan, Brennan, Foster, & Holder; 2004; Hoge, Guerra, & Boxer, 2008). Delinquency interventions, however, historically focused on only one or a small set of these risk factors and were largely ineffective (Howell, 2003).

Theory of Social Ecology

The fundamental tenet of the social ecological framework (Bronfenbrenner, 1979) is that individuals are embedded in multiple systems that have direct and indirect influences on behavior. This conceptualization provides an excellent fit with the known determinants of antisocial behavior in children and adolescents in family, peer, school, and community. Moreover, as first emphasized by Bell (1968), interactions among these systems are reciprocal in nature. For example, adolescents influence their parents, and, in turn, parents influence their children. Hence behavior is embedded within systems of reciprocal influence.

Pragmatic Family Therapies

The development of MST was also informed by the work of strategic (Haley, 1976) and structural (Minuchin, 1974) family therapy theorists. Several aspects of MST are based on commonalities of these approaches. The models (1) are problem focused and change oriented, (2) recognize the principle of equifinality (i.e., that many different paths can lead to the same outcomes), (3) assume that the therapist should take an active role in treatment, (4) develop interventions within the context of the presenting problem, and (5) view changing interpersonal transactions as essential to long-term behavior change.

Specification via Principles

The focus of MST on the interaction of a comprehensive array of risk factors in the social ecology, as well as the individualization of treatment to each youth and family, defies its specification in step-by-step or session-by-session format. An intermediary step between describing MST largely through extended case examples (Henggeler & Borduin, 1990) and the specification of MST in manuals for therapists (Henggeler, Schoenwald, Borduin, Rowland, & Cunningham, 1998; Henggeler, Schoenwald, et al., 2009) was the development of treatment principles. This principle-based approach to treatment specification was based on the example set by Fred Piercy (1986) in research on brief family therapy.

The nine principles of MST, which follow, were designed to balance specification of key aspects of the model with responsiveness to the needs and strengths of each youth and family. These principles organize therapists' case conceptualizations and the development and implementation of intervention strategies.

- *Principle 1*: The primary purpose of assessment is to understand the "fit" between the identified problems and their broader systemic context.
- *Principle 2*: Therapeutic contacts should emphasize the positive and should use systemic strengths as levers for change.
- *Principle 3*: Interventions should be designed to promote responsible behavior and decrease irresponsible behavior among family members.
- *Principle 4*: Interventions should be present-focused and action oriented, targeting specific and well-defined problems.
- *Principle 5*: Interventions should target sequences of behavior within and between multiple systems that maintain the identified problems.
- *Principle 6*: Interventions should be developmentally appropriate and fit the developmental needs of the youth.
- *Principle 7*: Interventions should be designed to require daily or weekly effort by family members.
- *Principle 8*: Intervention efficacy is evaluated continuously from multiple perspectives, with providers assuming accountability for overcoming barriers to successful outcomes.
- *Principle 9*: Interventions should be designed to promote treatment generalization and long-term maintenance of therapeutic change by empowering caregivers to address family members' needs across multiple systemic contexts.

The MST principles embody the specificity of problem definition and the present-focused and action-oriented emphases of behavioral and cognitive-behavioral treatment techniques; the contextual emphases of pragmatic family systems therapies; and the importance of client–clinician collaboration and treatment generalization emphasized in the system of care and consumer philosophies. In MST, however, these evidence-based interventions, which have historically focused on a limited aspect of the youth's social ecology (e.g., the cognitions or problem-solving skills of the individual youth, the discipline strategies of a parent, or family interactions but not interactions between family and other systems, such as schools or youth peer networks), are integrated into a social-ecological framework. Moreover, MST interventions are delivered where the problems and their potential solutions are found: at home, at school, and in the neighborhood, rather than in a therapist's office.

In contrast with "combined" (Kazdin, 1996) and multicomponent (Liddle, 1996) approaches to treatment, MST interventions are not delivered as separate elements. Instead, they are strategically selected and integrated in ways hypothesized to maximize synergistic interaction. For example, parents who follow permissive parenting practices often need instrumental and emotional support from spouses, kin, and/or friends to change their parenting practices in the face of significant protests from the youth. Thus therapist and parent might need to work together to mend fences between the parent and an estranged relative before trying to implement new rules and consequences for a youth so that the relative can actively support the parent when she or he first tries to implement new rules and consequences.

Analytical Process

In addition to the MST principles, a scientific method of hypothesis testing, referred to as the MST analytical process (a.k.a. the "Do-Loop"; Figure 14.1) encourages clinicians to generate specific hypotheses about the combination of factors that sustain a particular problem behavior, to provide evidence to support the hypotheses, to test the hypotheses by intervening, to collect data to assess the impact of the intervention, and to use that data to begin the assessment process again. The sources of information from which hypotheses are drawn are, first, the knowledge base on the individual, family, peer, school, and neighborhood factors that contribute to serious clinical problems and, second, observations and reports of the youth, family members, and key members of the social context.

The MST analytical process, or "Do-Loop," entails interrelated steps that connect the ongoing assessment of the "fit" of referral problems (e.g., criminal activity, fighting with peers, verbal and physical aggression with family members, school expulsion) with the development, implementation, and evaluation of interventions. From initial case formulation through discharge from treatment, therapists are encouraged to engage in hypothesis testing as they try to identify the causes and correlates of a particular problem, the reasons that improvements have occurred, and barriers to change. Therapists refine the initial conceptualization of the

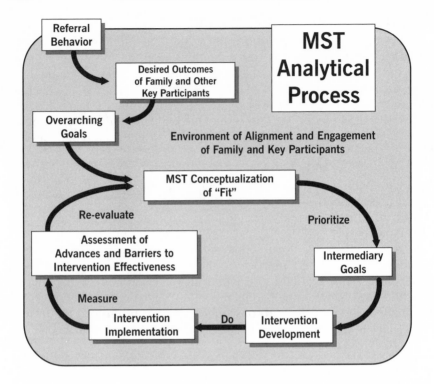

FIGURE 14.1. MST analytical process (Do-Loop). From Henggeler, Schoenwald, Borduin, Rowland, and Cunningham (2009). Copyright 2009 by The Guilford Press. Reprinted with permission.

fit of the referral problems on the basis of information and observations about the strengths and weaknesses in all systems of the social ecology, develop intermediary treatment goals that represent logical steps toward achieving the overarching goals, and identify and implement intervention modalities. Assessment of the effects of interventions and of factors presenting barriers to their effectiveness is ongoing (e.g., marital discord, parental depression, and low social support interfere with parental rule setting and youth monitoring). Each of these factors, in turn, may be influenced by a combination of case-specific, clinician-specific, and supervision-specific issues. For example, a clinician may have missed a proximal and powerful influence on a particular behavior, may have failed to ensure that caregivers had sufficient practice in sessions with a behavioral intervention for the youth to implement it adequately, or may have aborted an effort to reduce marital conflict when verbal aggression between spouses escalated. A supervisor, in turn, may not have ensured that the therapist was adequately skilled to diffuse such aggression. Thus the MST treatment process is self-reflexive for clinicians and supervisors, who continuously consider how their own behaviors contribute to intervention success and failure.

MST Quality Assurance/Quality Improvement System

The MST quality assurance and improvement (QA/QI) system is designed to support the sustainable implementation with fidelity of MST at multiple levels of the clinical context. The three broad components of the MST QA/QI system are: (1) clinician training and ongoing support in the form of weekly onsite group clinical supervision, remote (telephone) consultation from an MST expert, and quarterly booster training; (2) organizational support; and (3) implementation measurement and reporting. Each component consists of several elements, which are integrated into a feedback loop that includes data about MST implementation at the level of the family, therapist, supervisor, expert consultant, and organization operating the MST program. Optimizing youth outcomes is the focus of all elements of the system. Findings supporting linkages among adherence at each level of the practice context and youth outcomes have emerged from randomized trials and from a 43-site National Institute of Mental Health (NIMH)-funded study of the transportability of MST and are summarized elsewhere (Schoenwald, 2008; Schoenwald, Sheidow, & Chapman, 2009). The MST QA/QI system is depicted and described in detail in several publications (see, e.g., Henggeler, Schoenwald, et al., 2009; Schoenwald, 2008) and Internet sites (*www.mstinstitute.org*) and is deployed through MST Services, LLC (MSTS), and 21 Network Partner organizations.

Evidence for Effectiveness of MST

MST has been evaluated in 21 published outcome studies (19 randomized trials and two quasi-experimental studies) and identified in government, scholarly, and meta-analytic reviews as an effective treatment for adolescents with serious behavioral problems that include delinquency, substance abuse, and comorbidity of these conditions and other problems. A comprehensive review by Scott Henggeler (2011) of the processes and science involved in the development and validation of MST includes an extensive table presenting information on the design, measures, and results of published MST outcome studies. MST has been found consistently to reduce recidivism, out-of-home placement, and substance abuse of juvenile offenders cost effectively in both the short and long term and to improve family functioning, including parenting practices associated with youth outcomes. The results of randomized trials of adaptations of

MST for target populations with other challenging clinical problems are briefly presented in a subsequent section of this chapter.

Empirical Tests of the MST Theory of Change

Three lines of research provide support for the MST theory of change and the theory of social ecology on which MST is based.

Results from MST Clinical Trials

Randomized clinical trials with juvenile offenders have shown that MST can significantly reduce youth antisocial behavior (i.e., criminal offending, substance use) in comparison with other types of interventions (see Henggeler, 2011). Importantly for examining the MST theory of change, many of these same studies also showed that MST was effective in changing key family (e.g., improved parenting) and peer (e.g., decreased association with deviant peers) variables that are linked with adolescent antisocial behavior. Some of these findings are described next. Although the findings do not demonstrate that improved family relations and decreased association with deviant peers directly caused the reductions in youth antisocial behavior, such findings are consistent with this possibility.

Direct Tests of MST Mechanisms of Change

A second line of research tests the MST theory of change directly through advanced statistical methods. Using data from separate MST clinical trials with serious juvenile offenders (Henggeler, Melton, Brondino, Scherer, & Hanley, 1997) and substance-abusing offenders (Henggeler, Pickrel, & Brondino, 1999), Huey and colleagues (Huey, Henggeler, Brondino, & Pickrel, 2000) showed that, across both studies, therapist adherence to MST was associated with improved family relations and decreased association with delinquent peers, which, in turn, were associated with reductions in delinquent behavior. Findings from a randomized trial of MST with juvenile sexual offenders (Henggeler, Letourneau, et al., 2009) showed that favorable MST effects on reducing youth antisocial behavior were mediated by increased follow-through on discipline practices, as well as decreased caregiver disapproval of and concern about the youth's deviant peers, over a 12-month follow-up. These findings suggest that MST empowered caregivers to better identify friends that were having a negative influence on their adolescents, to advise the youth to stop associating with such friends, and to follow through on planned discipline. These behaviors, in turn, led to decreased antisocial behavior of the juvenile sexual offenders.

Similar findings emerged from a randomized trial testing the effects of juvenile drug courts relative to traditional family courts, MST, and the integration of contingency management procedures into MST (Schaeffer et al., 2010). Specifically, increased parental supervision was associated with reduced delinquent behavior and marijuana and polydrug use, and reduction in polydrug use was associated with more consistent parental discipline. Decreased association of youth with delinquent peers and with drug-using peers was associated with reduced delinquent behavior and reduced use of alcohol, marijuana, and polydrugs. Finally, increased youth association with conventional peers predicted decreased delinquent behavior, alcohol use, and polydrug use.

The similar results across these trials are consistent with the MST theory of change. MST (or adherence to MST) altered key family and peer risk factors for criminal behavior, and these changes in risk factors resulted in decreased adolescent antisocial behavior.

Mechanisms of Change for Other Evidence-Based Treatments of Youth Antisocial Behavior

The third line of research supporting the MST theory of change pertains to the few studies that have examined mechanisms of change for other evidence-based treatments of youth antisocial behavior. In a study of multidimensional treatment foster care (MTFC; Chamberlain, 2003) in which juvenile offenders received either MTFC or group home care, Eddy and Chamberlain (2000) showed that the positive effects of MTFC on adolescent criminal activity were mediated by caregiver behavior management practices and adolescent association with deviant peers. Similarly, in an indicated prevention trial of the Coping Power Program with at-risk preadolescent boys, Lochman and Wells (2002) found that inconsistent parental discipline was a key mediator of subsequent youth antisocial behavior outcomes.

MST Adaptations

As the effectiveness of MST in treating serious juvenile offenders became known to the policy, practice, and research communities, several groups of investigators began to use standard MST as a platform for the development of adaptations to treat other serious problems, including substance abuse and dependence, chronic psychiatric problems that place youth at high risk for hospitalization, juvenile sex offending, child abuse and neglect, and chronic health conditions such as diabetes, obesity, asthma, and HIV infection. However, interest in testing the feasibility and effects of MST with populations of youth presenting serious problems in addition to delinquency has existed since the early years of model development. For example, the feasibility and effects of using standard MST to treat juvenile sex offenders and their families (Borduin, Henggeler, Blaske, & Stein, 1990) and families in which child abuse and neglect occurred (Brunk, Henggeler, & Whelan, 1987) had been tested with small samples in the mid-1980s. Subsequently, larger scale, community-based, randomized effectiveness trials of MST were conducted with specific adaptations for each of these populations.

A common feature of all MST adaptations is their focus on populations of youth whose serious and complex problems trigger involvement with one or more service systems with legal mandates related to public health or safety. The target populations are not defined by a specific diagnostic criterion or disorder but rather by, first, the topography of the behavioral and functional challenges the youth evidences across multiple contexts—home, school, and community—and, second, the consequences to the youth, family, and public of that constellation of challenges.

In the programs of research focused on MST adaptations, the MST principles for assessment and intervention, analytical process (Do-Loop), home-based model of service delivery, and training and quality assurance procedures are retained. The addition and integration of select clinical procedures for each adaptation is informed by research on the specific aspects of clinical presentation and social ecology pertinent to the specific target problem (i.e., substance abuse/dependence, psychiatric crises, sex offending, abuse/neglect, chronic health problems). The procedures are specified in manuals and training sessions that augment but do not supplant the standard MST manual and training process. There are currently 13 adaptations of MST progressing through stages of adaptation pilot testing, efficacy and effectiveness trials, transportability pilot testing, mature transport, and proactive dissemination. A four-page document that summarizes the process, identifies the primary developers of the adaptations, discusses the stage of adaptation development and testing, and provides cursory information about key enhancements of adaptationAcan be downloaded from the MST Services website (*www.mstservices. com*).

Four adaptations are described here: (1) MST augmented with contingency management components for adolescent substance abuse and dependence (MST–Substance Abuse); (2) MST with Psychiatric Supports (MST–Psychiatric, or MST-PSYCH) for youth ages 9–17 at risk of out-of-home placement (including psychiatric hospitalization) due to serious behavioral problems and co-occurring mental health symptoms such as thought disorder, bipolar affective disorder, depression, anxiety, and impulsivity; (3) MST–Child Abuse and Neglect (MST-CAN) for families involved with the child welfare system due to physical abuse and/or neglect of a child ages 6–17; and (4) MST for chronic health conditions

(MST–Health Care), a category that includes distinct protocols for the effective management of juvenile diabetes, asthma, and obesity, and for adolescents with HIV/AIDS.

These adaptations were selected for four reasons.

1. The results of randomized trials testing their effectiveness are published, and their transport and implementation in community settings is well under way.
2. They highlight variation in the client populations and service contexts that may prompt the modification of an empirically supported intervention model, even one as relatively broad in scope and flexible in implementation as MST—and, potentially, transdiagnostic and modular approaches to treatment.
3. Some components in these adaptations build on components developed for other adaptations (e.g., safety planning protocols, psychiatrist intervention).
4. They can be conceptualized along a continuum of modification extensiveness.

Other adaptations are equally well suited to illustrate these points, but owing to space constraints, they are not described. For example, MST for juvenile sex offenders (the majority of whom also commit nonsexual offenses), known as MST–Problem Sexual Behavior (MST-PSB), has been specified in a manual (Borduin, Letourneau, Henggeler, Saldana, & Swenson, 2005); includes some elements (i.e., safety planning, clarification, and ownership of responsibility for abuse instances) that resemble MST-PSYCH or MST-CAN elements and others that are unique; has been found effective in two randomized trials (Borduin, Schaeffer, & Heiblum, 2009; Henggeler, Letourneau, et al., 2009); and is being transported to community settings.

MST–Substance Abuse (Formerly MST-Contingency Management)

MST for substance abuse with components of contingency management is designed to treat adolescents whose substance abuse and dependence problems co-occur with serious behavior problems. In several prior publications, including those cited in this section, this adaptation was known as MST–Contingency Management (MST-CM). However, as service systems sought to import this adaptation and government agencies developed catalogues of evidence-based treatments, it became clear the "CM" moniker did not adequately convey to stakeholders and consumers the focus of the treatment on substance abuse. In addition, other MST adaptations are identified in terms of the target populations they serve. Hence, MST–Substance Abuse is replacing MST-CM as the term for this adaptation.

Rationale for Adaptation

The initial impetus for this adaptation might be characterized as a quest to improve on positive findings. Findings from two randomized trials of MST with violent and chronic juvenile offenders, published in a single report (Henggeler et al., 1991), showed posttreatment decreases in youth self-reported alcohol and drug use, as well as long-term decreases in substance-related arrests. A subsequent randomized trial was designed to test the effects of standard MST with juvenile offenders meeting criteria for substance abuse or dependence. Results showed that MST was more effective than usual services at reducing youth substance use and out-of-home placement (50% reduction) but not recidivism (19% reduction, not significant; Henggeler, Pickrel, & Brondino, 1999). At 4-year follow-up MST participants evidenced significantly reduced violent crime and marijuana abstinence (Henggeler, Clingempeel, Brondino, & Pickrel, 2002). In the interim, however, the quest to improve the recidivism as well as substance use outcomes for substance-abusing and -dependent youth had begun, in the form of the integration of clinical procedures used in contingency management (CM; Donohue & Azrin, 2001) and the closely related community reinforcement approach (CRA; Budney & Higgins, 1998) to substance use treatment for adults.

Several similarities between standard MST and the CM and CRA approaches to substance abuse treatment facilitated their integration: (1) strong commitment to empirical validation; (2) the use of functional analysis to identify the proximal determinants of identified problems and guide intervention design; (3) the use of pragmatic and goal-oriented intervention strategies; (4) a broad-based view of treatment that specifically addresses risk and protective factors in the client's social ecology; and (5) a programmatic commitment to remove barriers to service access (Cunningham et al., 2003).

In addition, research on risk and protective factors for adolescent substance use and antisocial behavior (e.g., Dishion & Kavanagh, 2003) indicates that the majority of risk factors that exert direct and indirect influence on adolescent substance use and other antisocial behaviors are similar. As noted in a recent discussion of that research (Sheidow & Henggeler, 2008), some variables, such as parental substance abuse and dependence, place a youth at greater risk for substance use disorders; but this effect occurs primarily through the impact of the caregivers' substance use on their parenting ability and family management practices. In addition, association with drug-using peers influences youth drug use via multiple channels (access to drugs, modeling, norms for use, beliefs, status).

Clinical Additions and Adaptations

Several aspects of CM were integrated into MST.

• *Functional analyses.* In standard MST, functional analyses may be conducted as part of the "fit" assessment for some cases. Within this adaptation, functional analyses are: (1) required for each instance of substance use or nonuse and (2) conducted in a prescribed, step-by-step manner.

• *Self-management plans.* In standard MST, therapists develop interventions that address drivers for drug use; in MST–Substance Abuse, therapists develop, write, and revise a specific kind of plan for the youth to follow to avoid substance use, called a "Self-Management Plan."

• *Drug-refusal skills.* In standard MST, the therapist and caregivers may teach a youth specific drug-refusal skills as necessary. In this adaptation, the teaching of drug-refusal skills (1) is required for all youth in the program; (2) is conducted using a specific structure; and (3) includes extensive role play of the drug-refusal strategies with the youth.

• *Designing voucher systems and providing incentives.* Although providing incentives specifically for nondrug use is sometimes a part of standard MST, doing so is a required component of MST–Substance Abuse. This component is specified contractually with the youth and caregivers and partially funded by and through the program.

• *Drug testing.* Although drug screens are often conducted in standard MST, random drug screens are required in this adaptation, obtained by the MST–Substance Abuse program and collected with the frequency required to detect the youth's drug of choice.

The length of treatment, therapist caseload, team size, and supervision and consultation process and frequency are the same in MST–Substance Abuse as in standard MST.

Administrative Additions and Adaptations

The inclusion of drug testing and of voucher systems that include incentives requires additional resources for program operations. Accordingly, costs of incentives and of urine drug screen, alcohol scans, and laboratory testing (as appropriate) are included in the operating budget for MST–Substance Abuse programs.

Training and Support

In addition to the standard 5-day orientation required in standard MST, a 1-day training on the integration of CM procedures is required. An expert trained in MST–Substance Abuse provides the weekly consultation and quarterly booster training for teams implementing MST–Substance Abuse. The booster training may focus on standard MST topics and/or CM, depending on the needs of the team. The duration of treatment and the duration and frequency of supervision and consultation are the same for MST and MST–Substance Abuse.

Randomized Trial Results

The results of randomized trials evaluating the effects of standard MST and MST–Substance Abuse for substance-using adolescents conducted in the context of juvenile drug courts showed both MST and MST–Substance Abuse to be more effective than drug court and community drug treatment alternatives in reducing substance use and that the integration of CM accelerated the decrease in substance use achieved by MST. Youth receiving MST–Substance Abuse showed significant decreases in marijuana, alcohol, and polysubstance use at discharge and maintained improvement at 12 months after referral (Henggeler et al., 2006).

MST with Psychiatric Supports (MST-Psychiatric)

MST with psychiatric supports is designed to treat youths ages 9–17 whose serious behavioral and co-occurring mental health problems place them at risk of out-of-home placements that may include psychiatric hospitalization. The goal of MST–Psychiatric (MST-PSYCH) is to improve mental health symptoms, suicidal behaviors, and family relations while allowing youth to spend more time in school and in the home. Although delinquent youth were expected to be among this target population, the adaptation was developed for youth and families expected to differ in several important respects from juvenile offenders, and even juvenile offenders with co-occurring substance use problems, as described next.

Rationale

The modification of MST for youth demonstrating significant psychiatric impairment in the mid-1990s was prompted by several forces, including the federal government's System of Care (SOC) initiative, health-care finance reform efforts, the lack of data to support the effectiveness of psychiatric hospitalization, and MST's strong track record in treating serious juvenile offenders. In 1995, NIMH funded a randomized trial comparing MST and psychiatric hospitalization for youth in psychiatric crises (Henggeler, Rowland, et al., 1999). At the time, research increasingly indicated that, in addition to individual biological and cognitive factors, various caregiver, family, peer, and school factors played a role in predicting or sustaining internalizing conditions (e.g. depression, suicidal behavior, anxiety, and posttraumatic stress disorder [PTSD]), as well as disorders with an externalizing component (e.g., ADHD and bipolar affective disorder). This research was reviewed in a volume describing the development, use, and evaluation of psychiatrically supported MST (Henggeler, Schoenwald, Rowland, & Cunningham, 2002). At the same time, the research literature suggested that youth with psychiatric impairments and their families would differ from those referred primarily for serious antisocial behavior and their families with respect to prevalence of bipolar affective disorder, thought disorder, serious depression, anxiety, and other internalizing problems; gender and age; and prevalence of psychiatric disorders among parents and relatives.

Clinical Additions

The modifications of MST crafted for use as an alternative to the psychiatric hospitalization of youth experiencing psychiatric crises were described in a published manual for therapists (Henggeler, Schoenwald, et al., 2002). Subsequent refinements were made on the basis of experiences from a replication trial (Rowland et al., 2005) and in community-based transport (Rowland & Westlake, 2006). Key features of psychiatrically supported MST follow.

- *Therapeutic strategies.* Clinical protocols are used that focus on safety, crisis intervention, substance abuse treatment, and psychiatric impairments in youth and caregivers.

- *Standardized safety assessment.* A standardized assessment of the home is made using an ecologically based safety planning process.

- *Safety plan.* A safety plan is developed with the family and supportive members of the family ecology to eliminate the potential for risks or self-harm to youth.

- *Crisis intervention protocol.* To better equip therapists to address the needs of youth in psychiatric crisis and their families, salient aspects of research on the predictors, prevention, and treatment of youth and adult suicidal, homicidal, and psychotic behavior are incorporated into a crisis intervention protocol.

- *Substance abuse treatment for caregivers and youth.* Substance abuse or dependence among caregivers and youth is treated using components of CM.

- *Evidence-based assessment and management of youth and caregiver mental illness.* Delivery and management of appropriate psychiatric interventions is ensured, including the implementation of evidence-based pharmacological algorithms.

- *Treatment team.* A half-time *psychiatrist* is formally incorporated into the delivery of MST. The psychiatrist meets with the therapists and supervisors on a regular basis (generally weekly) and before and after each psychiatrist visit with a youth or caregiver to collaborate in planning the intervention steps warranted in light of the psychiatric consultation and in planning adjustments to psychiatric interventions warranted in light of psychosocial intervention success and setbacks. The psychiatrist is also regularly on call to provide advice to therapists and the supervisor.

The role of the *crisis caseworker* was developed to enhance the therapist's ability to achieve treatment goals with families experiencing multiple crises. The crisis caseworker is a bachelor's-level mental health professional who assists the therapist with specific crisis interventions and provides practical, clinical, and administrative support of therapist interventions. For example, caseworkers are trained to perform safety assessments, to coordinate access to crisis services (e.g., police, ambulance), and to provide clinical support to therapists during crisis situations (e.g., to calm siblings, to monitor youth). They also execute tasks that can be categorized as case management, such as finding housing and employment resources. In standard MST, the therapist typically carries out such tasks.

• *Average caseload and treatment duration.* The average length of treatment is approximately 6 months but ranges from 4 to 8 months. Therapists carry a caseload of four families.

Training and Ongoing Support

A 1.5-day training focused on safety and the integration of psychiatry into MST is added to the standard 5-day orientation training. A 1-day training on CM is provided early in the first quarter of implementation but does not have to occur within the orientation training. The psychiatrist attends the first day of standard orientation training, and the 1.5-day training focused on the integration of psychiatry into MST. As in standard MST, booster sessions take place quarterly.

In contrast with supervisors of standard MST teams, the supervisor for MST-PSYCH is typically a doctoral-level practitioner. The supervisor is dedicated to that position full time. Weekly group supervision lasts 1–1.5 hours. The psychiatrist meets with the supervisor a minimum of 1 hour per week for mutual updates on case conceptualization, priorities for treatment, and intervention details. Weekly consultation ranges from 1 to 1.5 hours and is conducted by a trained expert consultant and a trained MST expert psychiatrist.

Randomized Trial Results

Results of the randomized trial of MST-PSYCH as an alternative to hospitalization for psychiatric crisis stabilization were positive. Significant short-term reductions were found in hospitalization and other out-of-home placements (Schoenwald, Ward, Henggeler, & Rowland, 2000) and in youth externalizing behaviors, and improvements were found in family relations, school attendance, and consumer satisfaction (Henggeler, Rowland, et al., 1999). Reductions in youth suicide attempts were also greater and more rapid for youth receiving MST-PSYCH at 16-month postrecruitment follow-up (Huey et al., 2004). At longer term follow-up, however, the placement findings dissipated. The adaptation was replicated and refined in a randomized trial testing the feasibility and effects of an intensive MST–Continuum of Care for youth in Hawaii whose multiple inadequately treated clinical problems had given rise to a class action suit against the state (Rowland et al., 2005). Hawaii had previously imported standard MST for juvenile offenders and collaborated in the design, implementation, and funding (along with the Annie E. Casey Foundation) of the randomized trial of the MST-Continuum. Psychiatrically supported MST was provided within the continuum. Youth in the MST-Continuum experienced significantly decreased symptoms and days in out-of-home placement relative to youth in the comparison condition (Rowland et al., 2005). The transport and evaluation of MST-PSYCH is ongoing at several sites.

MST for Child Abuse and Neglect

As noted previously, a test of the efficacy of MST with maltreating families was first conducted in the mid-1980s (Brunk et al., 1987). The sample of 33 families had been referred for abuse or neglect. Findings showed that MST was more effective than behavioral parent training in improving aspects of parent–child interaction associated with child maltreatment. The subsequent specification of MST for use with families of physically abused adolescents was undertaken by Cynthia Cupit Swenson and colleagues and evaluated in a community-based effectiveness trial (Swenson, Schaeffer, Henggeler, Faldowski, & Mayhew, 2010).

Rationale for Adaptation

Child physical abuse is associated with a broad array of adverse short-term (trauma symptoms, substance abuse, mental health and health problems) and long-term (increased risk in adulthood of anxiety, depression) outcomes. In contrast to the referral issues and service pathways that bring to treatment delinquent youth or youth at risk of placement due to psychiatric crises, it is typically the behavior of caregivers (physical abuse, neglect) and the response of the child welfare system to that behavior that bring youth who are physically abused and neglected and their families to treatment. Treatment goals are, therefore, to prevent recurrence of caregiver abuse and to address the behavioral, emotional, and health problems in their children. Research indicates that the physical abuse of youth is multidetermined, with risks of abuse accruing as a function of characteristics of the individual youth (noncompliant behavior), individual parent (negative perceptions of child, low involvement with child, mental health problems), and family (high stress, low social support, social isolation; Swenson et al., 2010).

Clinical Additions

MST-CAN adaptations are fully specified in a manual (Swenson, Penman, Henggeler, & Rowland, 2010). Key additions and adaptations follow.

- *Therapeutic strategies.* Therapeutic activities in MST-CAN include the following:
  1. Detailed safety planning based on functional analyses of physical abuse incidents.
  2. Use of a clarification process to help the parent apologize and take responsibility for abusive or neglectful behaviors, relieve the child and family of fault for the parent's behavior, and support the development of the comprehensive safety plan.
  3. Prolonged exposure therapy (Foa, Hembree, & Rothbaum, 2007) for parents experiencing PTSD symptoms and trauma-focused CBT for youth (Cohen, Mannarino, & Deblinger, 2006).
  4. Increased use of CBT specifically for deficits in anger management of the parent and youth, as indicated.
  5. Use of reinforcement-based treatment (Tuten, Jones, Schaeffer, Wong, & Stitzer, 2011) for parental substance abuse.
  6. Close collaboration of the MST team with child protective services agency (rather than with juvenile justice agencies, as in standard MST) personnel to align CPS decision making with evidence regarding clinical need and treatment progress.

- *Treatment duration.* To address the serious child safety concerns and severity of parental difficulties in families of physically abused youth, the length of treatment ranges from 6 to 9 months.

- *Treatment team.* MST-CAN is delivered by a team of three therapists, a case manager, a full-time clinical supervisor, and a psychiatrist dedicated to the team at 20% time. The full-time rather than part-time availability of the clinical supervisor was designed to accommodate the crisis-driven nature of the referrals and relative complexity of problems presented by the families. The psychiatrist provides evidence-based psychopharmacology to youth and parents when warranted and consultation on psychiatric emergencies.

Training and Support

To the standard MST training and support system, MST-CAN adds 4 days of training on the clinical adaptations. An expert trained in MST-CAN provides weekly consultation, and the onsite supervisor is also trained in MST-CAN. Supervision sessions typically last 2 hours per week, and consultation sessions last 1.5 hours.

Randomized Trial Results

In an effectiveness trial (Swenson et al., 2010), 86 youth and families referred by the child protective system for treatment participated in MST-CAN or enhanced outpatient treatment that included a structured, group-based parent training program for caregivers and an array of mental health and substance abuse treatment services for the youth and for caregivers as needed. Both conditions were implemented in a community-based mental health center. MST-CAN was more effective than the enhanced outpatient condition in reducing youth mental health symptoms (including PTSD symptoms), reducing caregiver and parenting behaviors associated with maltreatment (including assault incidents), and increasing caregiver social support. At 16 months postbaseline, youth in the MST-CAN condition were less likely to be placed out of the home and spent 63% fewer days in placement. Although youths in the MST-CAN condition experienced a lower rate of re-abuse (4.5% vs. 11.9% for the comparison), this difference was not statistically significant.

MST for Youth with Chronic Health Conditions

Since the late 1990s, a program of research led by pediatric psychologists Deborah Ellis, Sylvie Naar-King, and colleagues at Wayne State University, in which MST researchers at the Medical University of South Carolina collaborated, has focused on adaptation of MST for children with diabetes, asthma, obesity, and HIV-AIDS. Because the medical indicators and effective medical management procedures for each condition vary, this section does not present the content of clinical additions made for each population. Instead, examples are provided of the type of clinical content added to MST for the adaptations for specific medical conditions.

Rationale for Adaptation

The impetus for the pursuit of MST adaptations for pediatric health conditions lay in the evidence that effective management via medication, diet, and exercise regimens often declines in adolescence and that a consequence of poor illness management for particularly high-risk youth, such as those with chronically poor metabolic control or severe regimen adherence difficulties, is repeated hospitalizations. Research has implicated a combination of child, family, peer, school, and health-care-provider factors as contributing to poor adherence and metabolic control for diabetes (Ellis et al., 2005).

Details of the adaptation for chronic illness management in adolescents are reported elsewhere (Ellis, Naar-King, Frey, Rowland, & Greger, 2003). To summarize, MST interventions targeted problems related to medical regimen adherence within the family system, peers, schools, and the health-care system. With respect to youth with Type I diabetes, the issues of insulin administration, blood glucose testing, and/or dietary management were addressed, depending on whether the youth had difficulty adhering to this particular regimen component. The intervention targeted family factors such as low levels of parental supervision of diabetes care, peer factors such as low support for health behaviors, school factors such as lack of communication between parents and school personnel regarding the youth's health care needs, and health-care-system factors such as barriers to appointment keeping. The standard training and quality assurance procedures used to support the transport and implementation of MST in community settings was used, and the 5-day initial training and boosters were adapted by the research team to include formal diabetes education for therapists, as well as education regarding factors that are predictive of poor treatment adherence and metabolic control. Illness-specific education components were similarly adapted for asthma, obesity, and HIV-AIDS.

Numerous publications have reported the results of randomized trials evaluating the implementation and outcomes of the adaptations of MST for chronic health conditions in youth, specifically diabetes, asthma, obesity, and HIV-AIDS (see review and Table 1 in Henggeler, 2011). Across these studies, the results were favorable to the MST adaptation in question, as evidenced by improvements in youth and caregiver medical management and youth medical status with respect to the condition targeted by the adaptation (i.e., diabetes, asthma, obesity, HIV-AIDS), and decreased service use and costs (e.g., hospitalization, medical costs).

Discernment in the Transport and Implementation of MST and Its Adaptations

The implementation and outcomes of an evidence-based treatment model can degrade when a mismatch exists between the population for which treatment effectiveness was established and the populations with which it is implemented. For youth at risk of out-of-home placement, their families, and the systems mandated to provide services to them, the price of treatment failure is high. In this high-stakes context, the comprehensive and individualized nature of MST can sometimes be perceived or portrayed as a panacea. Yet the use of either standard MST or unplanned adaptations to treat populations with overlapping but distinct risk and protective profiles can hold both promise and peril for youth, families, and service systems. In the journey from the early development of MST to its larger scale transport, exploring the boundary conditions of standard MST for other populations has been a collaborative process involving numerous service system and provider organization partners. The adequate specification of the treatment and service delivery model and of the quality assurance and improvement process used to transport and implement standard MST in community settings facilitated this collaboration and the development and testing of MST adaptations. As detailed elsewhere (Schoenwald, 2010), at least two different approaches characterized this process: (1) purposeful net widening in several locales to see whether standard MST would prove adequate for case mixes that included delinquent and seriously emotionally disturbed youth; and (2) collaboration in the implementation and funding of randomized trials testing modifications for specific target populations. Both avenues have been fruitful with respect to the ultimate development, testing, and transport of standard MST and its adaptations.

Implications for Transdiagnostic, Modular, and Principle-Based Approaches

Transdiagnostic, modular, and other principle-based approaches to treatment seek to incorporate a broader array of treatment operations and sequencing options than is available in many standard, manualized treatment protocols for specific disorders. The flexibility and potential robustness of such approaches could be expected to stimulate demand for their transport among stakeholders in mental health—consumers, practitioners, and public and private payers. The avenues taken in the transport and evaluation of MST and its adaptations may prove fruitful for evaluating the boundary conditions of the effectiveness and transportability of these approaches. For example, in response to requests to extend the use of a particular approach to clients with a broader array of presenting problems, researchers might suggest collaborating in an evaluation to illuminate characteristics of target populations expected to affect outcomes. Depending on the design and scope of the evaluation, sufficient funding for it may be obtained from sources making the request. The evaluation results can be used to guide and document a systematic net widening process and to protect against the potential ill effects (poor outcomes) of premature widening of the net. Similarly, well-crafted evaluations can signal when implementation failure rather than intervention failure is responsible for decrements in expected outcomes and which aspects of implementation matter most to the successful deployment and thus should be codified for future deployment. When adequately designed, such evaluations produce data that can be used in real time to inform decision making about populations to be served and aspects of implementation that require adjustment and that contribute to the knowledge base regarding the boundary conditions of the intervention approach and aspects of its implementation that affect its potency in diverse practice contexts.

Conclusion

The clinical and scientific journey from the initial development and validation of MST to its larger scale transport has produced evidence to support the MST treatment theory and unified approach to clinical conceptualization and intervention. That theory and approach, along with effectiveness evidence from clinical trials of standard MST, provided the platform for the development, testing, and transport of adaptations of MST for several clinical populations. MST provides an example of both the potentially expanded clinical reach and the boundary conditions of intervention approaches built on theory and evidence about etiological factors and therapeutic mechanisms of action common across somewhat distinctive clinical populations.

ACKNOWLEDGMENTS

Support for preparation of this chapter was provided by Grant No. 96.2013 from the Annie E. Casey Foundation (Sonja K. Schoenwald, Principal Investigator), National Institute of Mental Health (NIMH) Research Grant No. P30 MH074778 (John Landsverk, Principal Investigator), and NIMH research grant No. 1P20MH0784458 (Marc Atkins, Principal Investigator). The content is solely the responsibility of the author and does not necessarily represent the official view of the Annie E. Casey Foundation or National Institutes of Mental Health. Sonja K. Schoenwald is a Board Member and stockholder in MST Services, LLC, which has the exclusive licensing agreement through the Medical University of South Carolina for the dissemination of MST technology. I thank Charles Borduin, Phillippe Cunningham, Richard Munschy, Joanne Penman, Jeff Randall, Melisa Rowland, and Cynthia Cupit Swenson for their help with queries about the brief summaries of MST adaptations in this chapter and Scott Henggeler for the decades of scholarly and clinical leadership and collaboration that spawned much of the work described in this chapter.

REFERENCES

Bell, R. Q. (1968). A reinterpretation of the direction of effects in studies of socialization. *Psychological Review, 75*, 81–95.

Biglan, A., Brennan, P. A., Foster, S. L., & Holder, H. D. (2004). *Helping adolescents at risk: Prevention of multiple problem behaviors.* New York: Guilford Press.

Borduin, C. M., Henggeler, S. W., Blaske, D. M., & Stein, R. (1990). Multisystemic treatment of adolescent sexual offenders. *International Journal of Offender Therapy and Comparative Criminology, 35*, 105–114.

Borduin, C. M., Letourneau, E. J., Henggeler, S. W., Saldana, L., & Swenson, C. C. (2005). *Treatment manual for multisystemic therapy with juvenile sexual offenders and their families.* Charleston: Medical University of South Carolina, Department of Psychiatry and Behavioral Sciences.

Borduin, C. M., Schaeffer, C. M., & Heiblum, N. (2009). A randomized clinical trial of multisystemic therapy with juvenile sexual offenders: Effects on youth social ecology and criminal activity. *Journal of Consulting and Clinical Psychology, 77*, 26–37.

Bronfenbrenner, U. (1979). *The ecology of human development: Experiments by design and nature.* Cambridge, MA: Harvard University Press.

Brunk, M., Henggeler, S. W., & Whelan, J. P. (1987). A comparison of multisystemic therapy and parent training in the brief treatment of child abuse and neglect. *Journal of Consulting and Clinical Psychology, 55*, 171–178.

Budney, A. J., & Higgins, S. T. (1998). *A community reinforcment plus vouchers approach: Treating cocaine addiction.* Rockville, MD: U.S. Department of Health and Human Services, National Institutes of Health, National Institute on Drug Abuse.

Chamberlain, P. (2003). *Treating chronic juvenile offenders: Advances made through the Oregon multidimensional treatment foster care model.* Washington, DC: American Psychological Association.

Chorpita, B. F., & Daleiden, E. L. (2009). Mapping evidence-based treatments for children and adolescents: Application of the distillation and matching model to 615 treatments from 322 randomized trials. *Journal of Consulting and Clinical Psychology, 77*, 566–579.

Cohen, J. A., Mannarino, A. P., & Deblinger, E. (2006). *Treating trauma and traumatic grief in children and adolescents.* New York: Guilford Press.

Cunningham, P. B., Donohue, B., Randall, J., Swenson, C. C., Rowland, M. D., Henggeler, S. W., et al. (2003). *Integrating contingency management into multisystemic therapy.* Charleston: Medical University of South Carolina, Department of Psychiatry and Behavioral Sciences, Family Services Research Center.

Dishion, T. J., & Kavanagh, K. (2003). *Intervening in adolescent problem behavior: A family-centered approach.* New York: Guilford Press.

Donohue, B., & Azrin, N. H. (2001). Family behavior therapy. In E. F. Wagner & H. B. Waldron (Eds.), *Innovations in adolescent substance abuse interventions* (pp. 205–227). New York: Pergamon Press.

Eddy, J. M., & Chamberlain, P. (2000). Family management and deviant peer association as mediators of the impact of treatment condition on youth antisocial behavior. *Journal of Consulting and Clinical Psychology, 68*, 857–863.

Ehrenreich, J. T., Goldstein, C. R., Wright, L. R., & Barlow, D. H. (2009). Development of a unified protocol for the treatment of emotional disorders in youth. *Child and Family Behavior Therapy, 31,* 20–37.

Elliott, D. S. (1994). Serious violent offenders: Onset, developmental course, and termination. *Criminology, 32,* 1–21.

Ellis, D. A., Naar-King, S., Frey, M. A., Rowland, M., & Greger, N. (2003). Case study: Feasibility of multisystemic therapy as a treatment for urban adolescents with poorly controlled type 1 diabetes. *Journal of Pediatric Psychology, 28,* 287–293.

Ellis, D. A., Frey, M. A., Naar-King, S., Templin, T., Cunningham, P. B., & Cakan, N. (2005). The effects of multisystemic therapy on diabetes stress in adolescents with chronically poorly controlled type I diabetes: Findings from a randomized controlled trial. *Pediatrics, 116,* e826–e832.

Foa, E. B., Hembree, E. A., & Rothbaum, B. O. (2007). *Prolonged exposure therapy for PTSD: Emotional processing of traumatic experiences.* New York: Oxford University Press.

Haley, J. (1976). *Problem solving therapy.* San Francisco: Jossey-Bass.

Henggeler, S. W. (2011). Efficacy studies to large-scale transport: The development and validation of multisystemic therapy programs. *Annual Review of Clinical Psychology, 7,* 351–381.

Henggeler, S. W., & Borduin, C. M. (1990). *Family therapy and beyond: A multisystemic approach to treating the behavior problems of children and adolescents.* Pacific Grove, CA: Brooks/Cole.

Henggeler, S. W., Borduin, C. M., Melton, G. B., Mann, B. J., Smith, L., Hall, J., et al. (1991). Effects of multisystemic therapy on drug use and abuse in serious juvenile offenders: A progress report from two outcome studies. *Family Dynamics of Addiction Quarterly, 1,* 40–51.

Henggeler, S. W., Clingempeel, W. G., Brondino, M. J., & Pickrel, S. G. (2002). Four-year follow-up of multisystemic therapy with substance abusing and dependent juvenile offenders. *Journal of the American Academy of Child and Adolescent Psychiatry, 41,* 868–874.

Henggeler, S. W., Halliday-Boykins, C. A., Cunningham, P. B., Randall, J., Shapiro, S. B., & Chapman, J. E. (2006). Juvenile drug court: Enhancing outcomes by integrating evidence-based treatments. *Journal of Consulting and Clinical Psychology, 74,* 42–54.

Henggeler, S. W., Letourneau, E. J., Chapman, J. E., Borduin, C. M., Schewe, P., & McCart, M. R. (2009). Mediators of change for multisystemic therapy with juvenile sexual offenders. *Journal of Consulting and Clinical Psychology, 77,* 451–462.

Henggeler, S. W., Melton, G. B., Brondino, M. J., Scherer, D. G., & Hanley, J. H. (1997). Multisystemic therapy with violent and chronic juvenile offenders and their families: The role of treatment fidelity in successful dissemination. *Journal of Consulting and Clinical Psychology, 65,* 821–833.

Henggeler, S. W., Pickrel, S. G., & Brondino, M. J. (1999). Multisystemic treatment of substance abusing and dependent delinquents: Outcomes, treatment fidelity, and transportability. *Mental Health Services Research, 1,* 171–184.

Henggeler, S. W., Rowland, M. D., Randall, J., Ward, D., Pickrel, S. G., Cunningham, P. B., et al. (1999). Home-based multisystemic therapy as an alternative to the hospitalization of youth in psychiatric crisis: Clinical outcomes. *Journal of the American Academy of Child and Adolescent Psychiatry, 38,* 1331–1339.

Henggeler, S. W., Schoenwald, S. K., Borduin, C. M., Rowland, M. D., & Cunningham, P. B. (1998). *Multisystemic treatment of antisocial behavior in children and adolescents.* New York: Guilford Press.

Henggeler, S. W., Schoenwald, S. K., Borduin, C. M., Rowland, M. D., & Cunningham, P. B. (2009). *Multisystemic therapy for antisocial behavior in children and adolescents* (2nd ed.). New York: Guilford Press.

Henggeler, S. W., Schoenwald, S. K., Rowland, M. D., & Cunningham, P. B. (2002). *Serious emotional disturbance in children and adolescents: Multisystemic therapy.* New York: Guilford Press.

Hoge, R. D., Guerra, N. G., & Boxer, P. (Eds.). (2008). *Treating the juvenile offender.* New York: Guilford Press.

Howell, J. C. (2003). *Preventing and reducing juvenile delinquency: A comprehensive framework.* Thousand Oaks, CA: Sage.

Huey, S. J., Henggeler, S. W., Brondino, M. J., & Pickrel, S. G. (2000). Mechanisms of change in multisystemic therapy: Reducing delinquent behavior through therapist adherence and improved family and peer functioning. *Journal of Consulting and Clinical Psychology, 68,* 451–467.

Huey, S. J., Henggeler, S. W., Rowland, M. D., Halliday-Boykins, C. A., Cunningham, P. B., Pickrel, S. G., et al. (2004). Multisystemic therapy effects on attempted suicide by youth presenting psychiatric emergencies. *Journal of the American Academy of Child and Adolescent Psychiatry, 43,* 183–190.

Kazdin, A. E. (1996). Problem solving and parent management in treating aggressive and antisocial behavior. In E. D. Hibbs & P. S. Jensen (Eds.), *Psychosocial treatments for child and adolescent disorders: Empirically based strategies for clinical practice* (pp. 377–408). Washington, DC: American Psychological Association.

Liddle, H. A. (1996). Family-based treatment for adolescent problem behaviors: Overview of contemporary developments and introduction to the special section. *Journal of Family Psychology, 10,* 3–11.

Lochman, J. E., & Wells, K. C. (2002). Contextual social-cognitive mediators and child outcome: A test of the theoretical model in the Coping Power program. *Development and Psychopathology, 14,* 945–967.

Loeber, R., Farrington, D. P., Stouthamer-Loeber, M., & Van Kammen, W. B. (1998). *Antisocial behavior and mental health problems: Explanatory factors in childhood and adolescence.* Mahwah, NJ: Erlbaum.

McHugh, R. K., Murray, H. W., & Barlow, D. H. (2009). Balancing fidelity and adaptation in the dissemination of empirically supported treatments: The promise of transdiagnostic interventions. *Behaviour Research and Therapy, 11,* 946–953.

Minuchin, S. (1974). *Families and family therapy.* Cambridge, MA: Harvard University Press.

Piercy, F. P. (1986). *Training manual: Purdue brief family therapy.* West Lafayette, IN: Center for Instructional Services.

Rowland, M. D., Halliday-Boykins, C. A., Henggeler, S. W., Cunningham, P. B., Lee, T. G., Kruesi, M. J. P., et al. (2005). A randomized trial of multisystemic therapy with Hawaii's Felix Class youths. *Journal of Emotional and Behavioral Disorders, 13,* 13–23.

Rowland, M. D., & Westlake, L. A. (2005). *Mental health multisystemic therapy: Psychiatry resource book.* Charleston: Medical University of South Carolina, Department of Psychiatry and Behavioral Sciences, Family Services Research Center.

Schaeffer, C. M., Henggeler, S. W., Chapman, J. E., Halliday-Boykins, C. A., Cunningham, P. B., Randall, J., et al. (2010). Mechanisms of effectiveness in juvenile drug court: Altering risk processes associated with delinquency and substance abuse. *Drug Court Review, 7,* 57–94.

Schoenwald, S. K. (2008). Toward evidence-based transport of evidence-based treatments: MST as an example. *Journal of Child and Adolescent Substance Abuse, 17*(3), 69–91.

Schoenwald, S. K., (2010). From policy pinball to purposeful partnership: The policy contexts of multisystemic therapy (MST) transport and dissemination. In J. R. Weisz & A. E. Kazdin (Eds.), *Evidence-based psychotherapies for children and adolescents* (pp. 538–553). New York: Guilford Press.

Schoenwald, S. K., Sheidow, A. J., & Chapman, J. E. (2009). Clinical supervision in treatment transport: Effects on adherence and outcomes. *Journal of Consulting and Clinical Psychology, 77,* 410–421.

Schoenwald, S. K., Ward, D. M., Henggeler, S. W., & Rowland, M. D. (2000). MST vs. hospitalization for crisis stabilization of youth: Placement 4 months postreferral. *Mental Health Services Research, 2,* 3–12.

Sheidow, A. J., & Henggeler, S. W. (2008). Multisystemic therapy with substance using adolescents: A synthesis of the research. In A. Stevens (Ed.), *Crossing frontiers: International developments in the treatment of drug dependence* (pp. 11–35). Brighton, UK: Pavilion.

Simon, G. E. (2011). Promoting evidence-based and measurement-based care. *Psychiatric Services, 62,* 701.

Swenson, C. C., Penman, J., Henggeler, S. W., & Rowland, M. D. (2010). *Multisystemic therapy for child abuse and neglect.* Charleston: Medical University of South Carolina, Department of Psychiatry and Behavioral Sciences, Family Services Research Center.

Swenson, C. C., Schaeffer, C. M., Henggeler, S. W., Faldowski, R., & Mayhew, A. M. (2010). Multisystemic therapy for child abuse and neglect: A randomized effectiveness trial. *Journal of Family Psychology, 24,* 497–507.

Thornberry, T. P, & Krohn, M. D. (Eds.). (2003). *Taking stock of delinquency: An overview of findings from contemporary longitudinal studies.* New York: Kluwer/Plenum Press.

Tuten, L. M., Jones, H. E., Schaeffer, C. M., Wong, C. J., & Stitzer, M. L. (2011). *Reinforcement-based treatment (RBT): A practical guide for the behavioral treatment of drug addiction.* Washington, DC: American Psychological Association.

CHAPTER 15

Integrated Treatment of Traumatic Stress and Substance Abuse Problems among Adolescents

Liza M. Suárez, B. Heidi Ellis, and Glenn N. Saxe

Given the documented links between traumatic stress and substance abuse among adolescents, integrated approaches to treatment are needed. This chapter begins by reviewing how common trauma and substance abuse are in adolescence and describes the range of problems experienced by this population, as well as some common psychological, biological, and social processes that shed light on the link between these problems. Following a brief review of current available treatment approaches, an integrated treatment program is summarized, and implementation details are illustrated through a case example.

Prevalence and Comorbidity

Trauma exposure, PTSD, and substance abuse problems are common among adolescents. Findings from the Great Smoky Mountains Study (a longitudinal study of psychopathology and use of medical services in childhood) found that two-thirds of children and adolescents experienced a traumatic event by the time they were 16 years old (Copeland, Keeler, Angold, & Costello, 2007). Additionally, every year, approximately one in five American adolescents between the ages of 12 and 17 engages in abusive/dependent or problematic use of drugs or alcohol (Knight et al., 2007; Substance Abuse and Mental Health Services Administration [SAMHSA], 2006). Data from the National Survey of Adolescents suggest that comorbidity is the norm rather than the exception among youth diagnosed with PTSD. Nearly three-fourths of adolescents with PTSD had at least one comorbid diagnosis, with 29.7% of boys and 24.2% of girls with PTSD also meeting criteria for substance abuse or dependence (Kilpatrick et al., 2003). This co-occurrence is even higher in adolescent clinical samples (Deykin & Buka, 1997; Funk, McDermeit, Godley, & Adams, 2003), and findings suggest that as traumatic stress levels increase, the level of substance abuse also increases (Stevens, Murphy, & McKnight, 2003).

A Complex Clinical Picture

Adolescents with trauma histories typically experience a wide range of difficulties. After undergoing trauma exposure, teenagers may develop PTSD, characterized by intense emotional and physical responses triggered by reminders of the event (American Psychiatric Association, 2013). Individuals who experience interpersonal traumas (e.g., sexual assault, physical abuse, victimization) have a greater risk of developing PTSD relative to those experiencing traumas that are not interpersonal (e.g., accidents, natural disasters) (Charuvastra & Cloitre, 2008). Although not all traumatized children and adolescents develop PTSD, it is common for affected youth to have problems in at least one of the four major symptom areas: intrusion, avoidance, negative alterations in cognitions and mood, and alterations in arousal and reactivity. In addition, many adolescents exposed to trauma experience a wide range of emotional and behavioral problems. Traumatized youth often have difficulties in regulating affect and are more likely to suffer from mood disturbances such as depression, anxiety, anger, and aggression (Clark & Kirisci, 1996; Heim & Nemeroff, 1999; Pollock et al., 1990).

Teenagers who have experienced trauma and subsequently developed PTSD or other emotional problems may have additional difficulties that affect everyday functioning. For example, adolescents who have experienced maltreatment are more likely to have problems with peers or to engage in antisocial behavior, including violent offenses and arrests (Smith, Ireland, & Thornberry, 2005). They may avoid school or have increased academic difficulty (Reinherz, Giaconia, Lefkowitz, Pakiz, & Frost, 1993). Individuals who have experienced trauma also report greater somatic complaints in response to distress (Walker, McLaughlin, & Greene, 1988). Finally, the Adverse Childhood Experiences (ACE) study has produced evidence of the long-term sequelae of childhood difficulties (e.g., psychological, physical, or sexual abuse; violence against mother;

living with household members who were substance abusers, mentally ill, suicidal, or ever imprisoned) that are associated with the occurrence of numerous subsequent health problems among adults (Felitti et al., 1998).

Similarly, adolescents with substance use problems experience a wide range of co-occurring issues. In addition to the development of specific substance use disorders (SUDs), (American Psychiatric Association, 2013), adolescents with substance abuse problems are more likely to display poorer academic achievement and more school adjustment difficulties relative to nonabusers (Clark & Kirisci, 1996; Reinherz et al., 1993). Early substance use is also associated with youth engagement in criminal activity and risky sexual behaviors (Diamond et al., 2006; Gordon, Kinlock, & Battjes, 2004). Substance-abusing youth also tend to have higher severity of mental distress. In fact, studies show that co-occurring disorders and trauma histories are prevalent among adolescents seeking substance abuse treatment (Diamond et al., 2006).

Given the evidence just discussed, it is not surprising to learn that adolescents with co-occurring substance abuse problems and exposure to trauma exhibit problems in more areas than do youth with only one of those conditions (Giaconia et al., 2000; Suárez, Belcher, Briggs, & Titus, 2012). These additional problems, which may include poor academic functioning, involvement in the juvenile justice system, social problems, and increased health concerns, present further challenges in providing care to this population. Despite the higher level of need, teenagers with trauma and substance abuse often do not receive integrated treatment or coordinated care.

Common Psychological, Biological, and Social Processes

Transdiagnostic approaches to the understanding and treatment of psychological disorders typically pay unique attention to commonalities in psychological and biological processes (Harvey et al., 2004). The amygdala, a brain structure associated with learning, memory, and the processing of emotions, has been implicated in both PTSD (Rauch et al., 2000) and SUDs (Koob, 2006). This brain structure seems to be responsible for storing the emotional content of conditioned reactions (Koob & LeMoal, 1997), including information about the context of drug and alcohol use (Boening, 2001), as well as for processing emotionally laden stimuli, such as trauma reminders (Charney, Deutch, Krystal, Southwick, & Davis, 1993). Connections between the prefrontal cortex and the amygdala play a role in the modulation of affective, cognitive, and behavioral dysregulation (Tarter et al., 1999), and challenges in the regulation of biological stress response systems in these areas have been described in both PTSD and SUDs (Dawes et al., 2000; DeBellis, 2002). Furthermore, dysregulation of biological stress response systems can increase vulnerability for PTSD in youth, and the negative affect resulting from this condition can increase the risk for the development of early onset alcohol problems or SUDs (DeBellis, 2002).

In both PTSD and SUDs, an internal or external stimulus or "trigger" may lead to the experience of intense psychological and physiological arousal. When faced with situations, places, people, or things that evoke past traumatic events (known as "trauma reminders"), individuals with trauma histories often experience intense psychological arousal, including hypervigilance, an exaggerated startle response, and difficulty concentrating (Orr, Metzger, & Pitman, 2002). Similarly, individuals with SUDs experience cravings for their substance(s) of abuse when exposed to stimuli associated with use (e.g., context similar to where they use, substance-using peers, objects typically associated with use). Substance use cue reactivity associated with the craving response involves physiological changes such as increased heart rate, salivation, and arousal, as well as anxiety (McCusker & Brown, 1995; Monti et al., 1987).

Research in this area has suggested that among individuals with co-occurring trauma and substance abuse, substance use cravings also increase with exposure to cues of the traumatic event (Coffey et al., 2002; Saladin et al., 2003). Saladin and colleagues' (2003) research on individuals with co-occurring PTSD and drug dependence suggests that negative emotional states associated with PTSD augment craving and that this in turn promotes further drug use. Stasiewicz and Maisto's (1993) two-factor learning model helps to elucidate the classic conditioning processes at work, in which a traumatized individual develops conditioned emotional responses (CERs), such as hyperarousal, from the connection between a "neutral" stimulus (e.g., loud voices) and painful events (e.g., emotional and physical abuse). Conditioned avoidant responses (e.g., substance abuse) develop when individuals try to eliminate or reduce the negative emotion resulting from the experience of CERs. The avoidance of negative emotion resulting from substance abuse, in turn, continues to reinforce and maintain ongoing use (Saladin et al., 2003).

Findings from several treatment outcome studies shed further light on the relationship between trauma cues, negative emotion, and substance use cravings. A large body of research has demonstrated that exposure therapy, and in particular imaginal exposure to trauma cues, leads to reduced emotional reactivity regarding trauma-related stimuli, which in turn leads to a reduction in PTSD symptomatology among adults (Foa, Rothbaum, Riggs, & Murdock, 1991; Marks, Lovell, Noshirvani, Livanou, & Thrasher, 1998; McDonagh et al., 2005; Tarrier et al., 1999) and children (Cohen, Deblinger, Mannarino, & Steer, 2004; Deblinger, Lippman, & Steer, 1996; King et al., 2000; Stein et al., 2003). Some have advised caution in the use of trauma-cue exposure with individuals with co-occurring PTSD and substance abuse and dependence, emphasizing the possibility that trauma triggers might lead to additional dysregulation and exacerbation of alcohol or drug use (Pitman et al., 1991). Integrated adult treatment programs for PTSD and SUDs, however, have found that exposure sessions are well tolerated in this population, and treatment outcome studies have not found an increase in substance use during this portion of treatment (Brady, Danksy, Back, Foa, & Carroll, 2001; Coffey, Schumacher, Brimo, & Brady, 2005). In fact, emerging research in this area has shown that exposure may lead to a reduction in trauma-related negative emotion, which in turn may reduce substance use craving among adults with co-occurring alcohol dependence and PTSD (Coffey, Stasiewicz, Hughes, & Brimo, 2006). In this study by Coffey and colleagues (2006), participants assigned to the imaginal exposure condition showed a decrease in PTSD symptoms and alcohol cravings, whereas those in the imagery-based relaxation condition showed no change. According to the authors, these results suggest negative emotion to be a potential mechanism driving substance use cravings in the context of trauma cues.

In addition to understanding biological and behavioral processes associated with traumatic stress, emotional dysregulation, and substance use problems, it is important to consider the role of social processes within the environmental context. Youth with trauma and substance use share a set of vulnerabilities across important domains that can have a significant impact on youth development and functioning. There is a large body of research examining the environmental risk and protective factors associated with youth substance abuse, as well as contextual factors characterizing youth exposed to trauma.

The family environment is a particularly important part of the social context. Healthy patterns of affect regulation, for example, are more likely to develop when a responsive caregiver is available to the youth (Lieb et al., 2000). Disruptions in the parental bond can negatively affect the healthy development of children's sense of control, as well as their confidence in their ability to affect the world around them, which can lead to development of anxiety and mood problems, particularly in the face of additional stressors (Suárez, Bennett, Goldstein, & Barlow, 2009). Furthermore, when faced with external pressures, adolescents with a stronger sense of attachment to their parents are less likely to engage in risky behaviors such as drug and alcohol use (Kostelecky, 2005).

Challenges in the family environment may limit a caregiver's ability to help youth with traumatic stress and substance abuse problems manage distress. Characteristics in the home environment that lead to poorer youth outcomes include a broken family structure, the presence of many people in the home, psychopathology in the family, parental substance use, family conflict, low parental involvement and monitoring, and problems managing youth behavior (Anderson & Henry, 1994; Brook, Brook,

Arencibia-Mireles, Richter, & Whiteman, 2001; Chassin, Pillow, Curran, Molina, & Berrera, 1993; Hoffman & Cerbone, 2002; Kilpatrick et al., 2000; Merikangas et al., 1998; Needle et al., 1986; Weist, Acosta, & Youngstrom, 2001; Westermeyer, Wahmanholm, & Thuras, 2001). Therefore, treatment programs for youth with multiple problems should incorporate strategies that target family, social, and contextual needs and challenges.

Current Treatment Approaches

Although much progress has been made in the development and empirical validation of psychosocial treatments for trauma-related problems (Silverman et al., 2008) and in the adolescent substance abuse field (Waldron & Turner, 2008), integrated treatment programs for youth with both concerns are scarce. Few treatment programs directly address the environmental and contextual factors that exacerbate emotional and behavioral problems in youth, and even fewer programs explicitly target both environmental needs and emotional regulation. Integrated treatment programs for trauma and substance abuse that have been adapted from adult models lack substantial parental involvement, family treatment components, or attention to environmental and contextual problems common among youth (e.g., Najavits, Gallop, & Weiss, 2006). Furthermore, little is known about the effectiveness of treatment for this population when trauma and substance abuse services are delivered in parallel. Randomized clinical trials among traumatized youth rarely report substance abuse outcomes, and in fact many of these studies typically exclude youth with substance abuse problems (Cohen, Mannarino, Zhitova, & Capone, 2003). However, findings from several adolescent substance abuse treatment outcome studies suggest that trauma histories and co-occurring PTSD are associated with negative treatment outcomes (Funk et al., 2003; Grella & Joshi, 2003; Titus, Dennis, White, Scott, & Funk, 2003). Similarly, substance abuse treatment outcome studies with adults report higher relapse rates among individuals with trauma histories (Read, Brown, & Kahler, 2004). Additionally, initial PTSD severity has been identified as a significant predictor of relapse (Brown, 2000; Ouimette, Brown, & Najavits, 1998). These findings suggest that without the tools to manage distress associated with traumatic stress, individuals receiving substance abuse treatment will have great difficulty achieving and maintaining sobriety.

In a review of treatment outcome studies for PTSD and substance abuse problems in adolescents, Cohen and colleagues (2003) suggest that treatment for this population should incorporate elements from empirically supported treatments for both PTSD and substance abuse in adolescents. The components mentioned in the review included (1) establishment of a collaborative working relationship with the youth and family,

(2) stress management skills, (3) affect modulation, (4) cognitive restructuring, (5) skill building, (6) gradual exposure, (7) parental involvement, (8) psychoeducation, (9) random urine screens, (10) psychopharmacology, and (11) participation in self-help groups, such as Alcoholics Anonymous.

Integrated Treatment Approach

Trauma systems therapy for adolescent substance abuse (TST-SA; Suárez, Saxe, Ehrenreich, & Barlow, 2006) is an integrated treatment program that incorporates empirically supported strategies for traumatic stress and substance abuse problems. TST-SA was adapted from trauma systems therapy (Saxe, Ellis, & Kaplow, 2006), a comprehensive treatment program for children and adolescents with traumatic stress that enhances individually based approaches to trauma by specifically addressing social and environmental factors influencing traumatic stress problems.

TST-SA is a comprehensive treatment approach that aims to address the magnitude of difficulties often experienced by trauma-exposed adolescents struggling with substance use problems. This approach was designed for adolescents with complex trauma histories, primarily of an interpersonal nature (e.g., physical abuse, sexual assault, victimization), who are experiencing emotional and/or behavioral distress as a result of the trauma exposure and are also abusing alcohol or other drugs. The treatment combines a joint focus on environmental stability (e.g., addressing threats to safety, increasing parental ability to help and protect youth, soliciting help from relevant service systems) and emotional–behavioral regulation (e.g., improving youths' ability to manage distress, impulses, and behavior). TST-SA integrates established intervention strategies targeting both substance abuse and traumatic stress that have been previously empirically validated with adolescents, including cognitive-behavior therapy (Cohen et al., 2004), motivational interviewing (Miller & Rollnick, 2002; Sampl & Kadden, 2001), and family-focused behavioral and systemic interventions (Henggeler, Clingempeel, Brondino, & Pickrel, 2002; Liddle et al., 2001). TST-SA is a flexible treatment approach in which interventions are tailored to address the specific needs of each adolescent and family based on the dual assessment of environmental stability (e.g., stable, distressed, and threatening) and level of emotional dysregulation (e.g., regulated, dysregulation of emotion, dysregulation of emotions and behavior) described in Table 15.1. During the assessment process, clinicians use the assessment grid to categorize youth and determine the starting treatment phase, which in turn will determine the selection of treatment modules and specific intervention strategies within them, which are then applied according to problem severity. Youth with the greatest severity across both domains begin treatment in more intense and acute

TABLE 15.1. Assessment of Self-Regulation and the Social Environment

Emotion regulation	Social environmental stability		
	Stable	Distressed	Threatening
Regulated	Phase 5: Transcending	Phase 4: Understanding	Phase 3: Enduring
Emotionally dysregulated	Phase 4: Understanding	Phase 3: Enduring	Phase 2: Stabilizing
Behaviorally dysregulated	Phase 3: Enduring	Phase 2: Stabilizing	Phase 1: Surviving

phases that target stability and safety and progress through the treatment to less intensive phases. Because treatment modules are selected based on the initial severity assessment illustrated in Table 15.1, only youth with the greatest severity receive all modules. The initial stabilization phases focus on strengthening family and community contexts by reducing threats to safety and increasing environmental supports through crisis management, connecting the youth to services, and diminishing triggers that exacerbate symptoms. During the stabilization phase, services are offered in the home several times a week. As treatment progresses, youth learn and apply skills to manage dysregulated states and are guided in processing traumatic memories. Treatment ends with encouragement to build the foundation of hope for a brighter future through the development of meaning-making skills. Clinicians select treatment modules as needed in accordance with the corresponding treatment phase as described in Table 15.2. Boxes shaded in dark gray depict *essential* modules to administer within each treatment phase, boxes shaded in light gray correspond to modules that are *often helpful* to implement in each phase, and boxes that are not shaded are *not used* for those phases (e.g., cognitive processing of the trauma would be contraindicated in the "Surviving" phase but essential in the "Understanding" phase). Treatment modules include Stabilization-on-Site, Advocacy, Skill-Based Psychotherapy (e.g., emotional regulation skills training, trauma processing, and meaning-making skills training), and Psychopharmacology. Because the number of treatment modules selected depends on the level of severity, treatment length can range from 3 to 9 months.

In TST-SA, symptoms associated with traumatic stress and substance abuse are conceptualized as dysregulated emotional and behavioral states that occur in the context of a potentially unstable, and at times threatening, environment. This transdiagnostic approach to care recognizes that traumatized youth often display a diverse set of responses when faced

TABLE 15.2. Selection of TST Treatment Modules

Module	Phase				
	Surviving	Stabilizing	Enduring	Understanding	Transcending
Stabilization-on-site	• Crisis management • Connection to services • Diminish triggers	• Parenting skills • Connection to services • Diminish triggers	–	–	–
Services Advocacy	• Services advocacy	• Services advocacy	• Services advocacy	–	–
Skill-Based Psychotherapy	• Emotion regulation	• Emotion regulation	• Emotion regulation	• Cognitive processing	• Meaning making
Psychopharmacology	• Psycho-pharmacology	• Psycho-pharmacology	• Psycho-pharmacology	• Psycho-pharmacology	• Psycho-pharmacology

Note. Dark gray shading, essential; light gray shading, often helpful; no shading, not used.

with distress in their social environment (e.g., trauma reminders). With this multidimensional focus in mind, environmental interventions are intended to maximize family, peer, school, and service system supports (e.g., improving family communication, increasing opportunities for prosocial interactions, connecting family with needed services), whereas emotion-regulation interventions are meant to help the child learn better ways to cope in a less-than-perfect world through skill building to manage trauma reminders and substance abuse cues (Saxe et al., 2006). Thus, this treatment approach is able to more comprehensively address mood and behavioral regulation problems (which extend far beyond PTSD and SUD symptomatology to include tendencies toward self harm, aggression, and risk-taking) as well as interpersonal (e.g., lack of trust) and socioenvironmental (e.g., threats to personal safety) challenges, which are so salient for this population.

The application of TST to adolescent substance abuse includes several modifications to the original intervention. Motivational interviewing strategies are included to engage youth in treatment and to reduce ambivalence about reduced substance abuse. Throughout the treatment, youth and caregivers are educated about the interaction between substance abuse and symptoms of traumatic stress, and they are taught to identify and manage response patterns commonly observed in youth with co-occuring PTSD and substance use problems. PTSD, mood regulation, and substance abuse treatment strategies are fully integrated in this approach and are organized based on symptom severity and functional impairment, as well as level of environmental stability. For example, throughout the treatment, youth learn skills to manage both trauma reminders and substance abuse cues. Additionally, interpersonal skills such as problem solving and assertiveness training are applied to situations involving trauma reminders and emotional distress, as well as substance use.

TST-SA incorporates a strong emphasis on parent behavior management strategies, including increased monitoring and appropriate limit setting, particularly concerning drug use and high-risk behaviors. The model also incorporates substance abuse treatment strategies such as improving parent–teen communication skills, recognizing and planning for substance abuse cues or trigger situations, cognitive restructuring and interpersonal problem solving, and relapse-prevention techniques. Careful attention is given to the connection between substance abuse cravings and the negative emotions associated with the experience of trauma. Skill-building strategies focus on helping youth manage emotional and behavioral distress, as well as trauma reminders and substance abuse cravings.

Findings from an open trial of TST (Saxe, Ellis, Fogler, Hansen, & Sorkin, 2005) demonstrated a significant reduction in trauma symptoms and improvements in emotional and behavioral regulation among children, as well as a more stable social environment after 3 months of treatment, based on clinician ratings using the Child and Adolescent Needs and Strengths–Trauma Exposure and Adaptation Version. TST contributed significantly to youths' readiness to transition from more intensive to less intensive phases of treatment. In addition, reductions in psychiatric symptoms and increased environmental stability were correlated with clinicians' assessment of improvements in child functioning after 3 months. A more recent 15-month follow-up outcomes study of TST (Ellis et al., 2012) showed significant improvements in emotion regulation, social-environmental stability, and child functioning, while improvement in child functioning and in social-environmental stability significantly contributed to overall improvement in emotion regulation.

Implementing TST-SA

TST and TST-SA provide a framework in which to conceptualize presenting problems and organize care. The intervention plan is guided by an assessment strategy dually focused on the stability of the social environment and the youth's emotion-regulation capacity. Interventions are tailored to individual and family needs based on the level of severity. The TST approach pays careful attention to multiple domains of individual emotional and behavioral functioning and its relationship to the broader context. TST prescribes the general approaches to use at each phase of treatment and provides a "menu" of interventions to choose from. Providers using this approach apply the TST framework to organize care and target the most acute problems first, but they also have the flexibility to select modular interventions that are best suited to meet the needs of youth and families.

The TST approach includes five modules of treatment. These have been adapted in TST-SA by integrating treatment strategies taken from evidence-based programs for adolescents that target traumatic stress, emotional regulation, and substance abuse. These modules follow.

Ready–Set–Go

Ready–Set–Go (RSG) allows the clinician to build the foundation for the treatment alliance by establishing a shared understanding of the presenting problems and potential solutions. This module is implemented with all youth at the start of treatment, regardless of which treatment phase or level of severity was determined during the assessment. During the RSG module, teens, parents, and team members reach an agreement on the goals of treatment and the needed interventions and define everybody's role in meeting these goals. Barriers that interfere with treatment participation are also addressed. The RSG module in TST-SA includes Motivational enhancement strategies (Miller & Rollnick, 2002) to maximize engagement and facilitate readiness for change among substance-abusing youth.

Stabilization-on-Site

Stabilization-on-Site (SOS) includes home- and community-based interventions, where services are made more accessible to families during times of acute need (e.g., threats to environmental safety, potential for self harm). In TST-SA, this module incorporates strategies common to both traumatic stress and substance abuse treatment approaches, focusing on enhancing family communication, improving caregivers' ability to manage youth behavior, and promoting prosocial behavior in youth.

Services Advocacy

Services Advocacy (SA) aims to activate resources available within the community to meet the service advocacy needs of each family. The treatment team applies tools included in the treatment program to prioritize advocating for needed resources that are likely to lead to improved youth and family functioning and maximize youth and family participation in treatment. These could include advocacy with child protection agencies to ensure proper supervision when visitation with birth parents may be unsafe, connecting youth with specialized services at school or in the community, or addressing barriers to treatment attendance, such as child care or transportation.

Skill-Based Psychotherapy

This module includes emotional regulation, cognitive processing, and meaning-making skill building. *Emotional regulation skills training* provides youth and families with specific tools to manage episodes of emotional and behavioral dysregulation. In TST-SA, youth and families learn to recognize emotion regulation patterns resulting from exposure to trauma and substance abuse cues. This is followed by applying specific emotion-regulation skills (as needed), which are categorized as improving affect management, competency building, and emotion identification and acceptance. Cognitive-behavioral strategies for traumatic stress, anxiety, mood management, and substance abuse are integrated throughout the module. *Cognitive processing skills* guide youth through the exposure to the trauma narrative. Cognitive restructuring strategies are used to address unhealthy thinking patterns associated with past traumatic experiences. Because substance abuse cravings might increase initially during this period, the trauma narrative exposure is done after the youth has demonstrated commitment to change and experienced success in managing substance abuse cravings. Through the development of *meaning-making skills*, youth and families are encouraged to look beyond their traumatic experiences to find personal meaning and establish a new direction for the future. These skills are based on the notion that positive change can result amidst very stressful life circumstances (e.g., posttraumatic growth), leading to increased appreciation for life, discovery of personal strengths, and the development of meaningful interpersonal relationships (Frankl, 1992; Tedeschi & Calhoun, 2004; Woodward & Joseph, 2003). Meaning-making skills enable youth to create new ways of viewing the trauma and its consequences, as well as instilling hope and encouraging the pursuit of a brighter future. Additionally, the TST-SA adaptation incorporates relapse prevention strategies during this portion of treatment.

Psychopharmacology

This module is provided when psychotropic medication is needed to address dysregulated emotional and behavioral states. In TST-SA, this module incorporates a focus on health problems associated with substance use, as well as possible interactions between psychotropic medication and substances of abuse.

Developmental Considerations

Adolescents experience risks that set them apart from younger children and adults. Initiation of substance use during the adolescent years increases the likelihood of developing substance abuse or dependence later in life and has been associated with lifelong negative consequences (DeWit, Adlaf, Offord, & Ogborne, 2000). Additionally, substance use during adolescence may disrupt normal brain development and interfere with processes associated with critical thinking, planning, impulse control, and emotional regulation (DeBellis et al., 2005; Zeigler et al., 2005). TST-SA was developed to address the specific needs of this age group. Adolescent adaptations are summarized next.

Youth and Family Engagement

Substance-using teenagers rarely initiate treatment voluntarily. They are often identified by concerned parents, teachers, or school counselors, or they may enter treatment through disciplinary channels such as drug courts or juvenile justice. For this reason, *motivational interviewing* and *motivational enhancement strategies* (Miller & Rollnick, 2002) were included in TST-SA to maximize youth participation in treatment and to promote commitment to change. TST-SA also applies engagement strategies to maximize parent and family participation.

"Teen-Friendly" Content

TST-SA materials include themes relevant to teenagers and have been adapted to their developmental level. This includes encouraging the use of personal examples and presenting material in simple language without sounding "too young." The TST-SA approach incorporates the use of adolescent and parent workbooks to facilitate psychoeducation, skill building, and active participation in treatment. These supplemental materials have been created to illustrate TST-SA interventions using language that is appropriate for teenagers and caregivers. Psychoeducational materials have been designed to be interactive in order to enhance learning.

Peer Relationships

Peer relationships can exert a tremendous influence on youth functioning and well-being. Youth who have experienced interpersonal traumas are likely to show deficits in this area. For these reasons, it is very important for interventions to incorporate themes relevant to the peer and social world. Interpersonal skills taught in TST-SA include conflict resolution, assertiveness training, and the application of assertiveness skills to drug refusal situations.

Community Integration

Youth with traumatic stress and substance abuse problems often gravitate to less desirable social activities that increase the chance of engaging in risky behaviors (e.g., being involved with negative peers, becoming truant, spending time in unsafe settings, driving under the influence, having unprotected sex). For this reason, TST-SA prioritizes the need to increase prosocial integration in the community by promoting healthier alternatives. Efforts include working with the family and the community to find prosocial activities that the teenager is willing to engage in, that are within the means of the family and existing community resources (e.g., sports and recreation, mentoring, life-skill or vocational training), and that are incompatible with drug use and risky behavior.

Parental Participation in Treatment

Caregiver participation is essential in all phases of TST-SA, beginning with treatment planning and engagement. During the initial phases of treatment, caregivers participate in parent or family sessions focused on increasing stability and safety in the home environment and helping caregivers understand and support their adolescent children in times of distress. Parents receive psychoeducation about the relationship between environmental triggers and the symptoms of traumatic stress and substance abuse, and they are taught to reinforce coping skills learned by youth during treatment sessions. Additionally, TST-SA specifically targets parent–teen communication and teaches behavior management strategies (e.g., monitoring, consistent limit setting). The supplemental parent workbook serves as a guide for parents throughout treatment. Depending on the phase of treatment and specific issues being addressed, parents may be the sole focus of a session, may be present in a family session, or may participate in a weekly check-in at the start or end of a session with the youth.

TST-SA Case Example

Rosie is a 16-year-old who was brought up in a home affected by neglect, domestic violence, and parental alcohol abuse. She was sexually abused by her stepfather from the age of 5 until the age of 10, when she and her younger sister were removed from the home and eventually adopted by extended relatives. Over the years, Rosie developed symptoms of PTSD and has been bothered by ongoing flashbacks and intrusive memories of her troubled past. Rosie experienced depression and anxiety for most of her life and thought about death and dying during times of increased stress. She began to use alcohol and marijuana sporadically at age 14 and progressed to using marijuana daily and alcohol on weekends. Rosie had to move to a different neighborhood when she was removed from her birth parents' home, but as soon as she learned how to use public transportation, she began to visit her old group of friends and spend time around the park where she used to play during most of her childhood. Rosie felt very strongly about maintaining her old ties, even though she had to travel through several unsafe neighborhoods to get there. She would often appear agitated and distressed when she returned home from these visits, and increased alcohol and marijuana use would follow. Eventually, Rosie confided to her younger sister that she came across her abusive stepfather on several occasions when she visited her friends in her old neighborhood and that she became very frightened and upset. At first her adoptive parents were not aware of this, and Rosie was very afraid that they would become upset and refuse to let her visit her friends if they knew. Seeing her stepfather and subsequently facing the possibility of seeing him again while visiting her old neighborhood brought back many terrible memories and led to constant worry about her own safety. During visits with her friends, Rosie coped by drinking and smoking more, but when she got home she became overwhelmed and tried to distract herself from unwanted memories and flashbacks of past abuse by cutting on her arms and legs.

Although Rosie felt positive feelings toward her adoptive parents, she often became extremely upset after minor arguments. Whenever they raised their voices, and during times when they expressed disappointment in her behavior or her efforts, Rosie was reminded of past experiences with her birth parents when she was spoken to harshly. Specifically, Rosie had clear memories of her birth parents telling her that she would never amount to much. When her adoptive parents complained that she wasn't trying hard enough at school or that her behavior at home was unacceptable, these early memories would automatically emerge, leading Rosie to further engage in self-mutilation and substance use. Rosie's example illustrates the complex picture typical of youth with co-occurring substance abuse problems, and underscores the importance of applying a transdiagnostic approach that extends beyond a set of emotional and behavioral concerns.

Surviving

Rosie presented for treatment with acute needs. The TST evaluation framework suggested that her self-injurious and risky behaviors represented high levels of emotional and behavioral dysregulation. In addition, her encounters with her stepfather suggested the possibility of a real threat to her safety and the potential for sexual revictimization. Furthermore, her responses to conflict with caregivers were indicative of another important area of concern. Using the assessment of self-regulation and the social environment outlined in Table 15.1, clinicians placed Rosie in the Surviving phase, the most acute level of care in TST-SA. The guide to selection of treatment modules provided in Table 15.2 suggests beginning treatment with the Stabilization-on-Site and Advocacy modules once the RSG engagement module is complete. At the start of treatment, social-environmental interventions in the Surviving phase for Rosie included a focus on assessing safety and advocating for environmental changes that could result in improved functioning. The treatment team, in collaboration with Rosie's adoptive caregivers, promoted more open communication and increased caregiver involvement in order to assess the degree to which she was at risk of being harmed by her stepfather. Advocacy and connections with the child protection agency aimed to ensure that steps were taken to maximize her safety and minimize possibility of contact with stepfather. Additionally, the treatment team developed a safety plan to minimize self-injurious behaviors (increasing her support when she was upset, increasing monitoring of her, and reducing her access to sharp objects). During the surviving phase, services were provided at home two to three times a week, and frequency decreased as Rosie transitioned from Surviving to Stabilizing.

Stabilizing

During the Stabilizing phase, Stabilization-on-Site and work with adoptive caregivers focused on helping the family to understand the connection between negative family interactions and reminders of past abuse and neglect for Rosie. Caregivers were taught how to provide feedback and make requests using an approach that felt more nurturing to Rosie. Additionally, caregivers received assistance with implementing strategies to improve communication and provide effective monitoring and limit setting. In this phase, services advocacy focused on managing environmental needs (e.g., maximizing opportunities for Rosie to participate in prosocial activities with more adult supervision). Careful attention was paid to understanding thoughts and memories linking current stressors with dysregulated responses.

Enduring

The Enduring phase began by providing more detailed information to Rosie and her family about the connection between trauma reminders, environmental triggers, emotional dysregulation, and substance use. For example, the therapist guided Rosie and her caregivers in observing how being in her old neighborhood after seeing her stepfather led to increased distress, increased substance abuse, and self-harm. Her parents received assistance in learning to recognize when Rosie was at risk of becoming upset and impulsive during everyday interactions at home, and they were guided in how to support her during changes in emotional states in order to minimize self-harm and reduce risky behaviors and substance use. As the Enduring phase continued, Rosie received additional tools to manage emotional distress (e.g., relaxation, pleasant activity scheduling, positive self-talk) and substance use cravings (emotional acceptance, assertiveness, and drug refusal skills). During the Enduring phase, caregivers were provided information on various skills that were particularly useful to Rosie so that they could support her and encourage her to use the skills at home.

Understanding

The Understanding phase began once Rosie achieved mastery in managing distress and was able to abstain from self-injurious and substance-abusing behaviors. This phase involved cognitive processing sessions that included exposure to the trauma narrative and the application of cognitive restructuring strategies to address unhealthy thinking patterns associated with past traumatic experiences. During this phase, treatment focused on addressing Rosie's low self-worth and feelings of guilt and self-blame. It was also important to help Rosie recognize that her past traumatic experiences created an expectation of harm from others, which led to decreased trust and increased conflict with family members and peers.

Transcending

During Transcending, the final phase of treatment, Rosie was encouraged to look beyond her traumatic experiences to find new meaning and establish a new direction for the future. Rosie indicated that she felt stronger now than she was before and was able to identify specific things she has learned from her past experiences. She also discovered that she found joy in the opportunity to help others overcome similar challenges, and she was often sought out by her friends for her willingness and ease in providing support.

Practice and Service System Implications

Although much advancement has been made in the development and empirical validation of youth treatment approaches for traumatic stress and substance use (Silverman et al., 2008; Waldron & Turner, 2008), a substantial number of these programs apply a unidimensional, single-problem focus to care. Moreover, clinicians lack guidance in learning how to apply multiple elements from different treatment programs (Dos, 2005) when working with youth with multiple problems and complex trauma histories. Additionally, mental health and substance abuse services are often fragmented, and youth rarely receive coordinated treatment across service systems, let alone integrated care within a single treatment program (Suárez et al., 2012). Our current diagnostic classification systems, coupled with the separation between mental health and substance abuse service systems and funding streams, also contribute to the compartmentalization of care. For youth like Rosie, however, ongoing challenges with traumatic stress and substance use are interconnected and equally affected by environmental distress, and they call for an integrated approach to care.

TST-SA represents an attempt to offer a comprehensive treatment approach that can flexibly address the magnitude of difficulties often experienced by this population through careful evaluation of emotional regulation and environmental stability and an increased understanding of the connection between the two. The treatment framework provides a set of guidelines that can help to prioritize and organize care. More research is needed to determine the effectiveness of this and other integrated treatment approaches for youth with co-occurring PTSD and SUDs. In addition, future studies should evaluate the feasibility of implementing multicomponent programs in diverse settings such that available resources are maximized. Furthermore, an increased focus on evaluating and validating transdiagnostic approaches to treatment and services might present a more desirable alternative to single-problem focused treatment approaches, thereby increasing the acceptability of evidence-based practices.

ACKNOWLEDGMENTS

The development, implementation and dissemination of Trauma Systems Therapy for Adolescent Substance Abuse was supported by the Center for Mental Health Services, U.S. Substance Abuse and Mental Health Services Administration (Grant No. SM56225 for the Adolescent Traumatic Stress and Substance Abuse Treatment Center at Boston University, and Grants No. SM59297 and SM061260 for the Urban Youth Trauma Center at the University of Illinois, Chicago), as part of the National Child Traumatic Stress Network Initiative.

REFERENCES

American Psychiatric Association. (2013). *Diagnostic and statistical manual of mental disorders* (5th ed.). Arlington, VA: American Psychiatric Association.

Anderson, A. R., & Henry, C. S. (1994). Family system characteristics and parental behaviors as predictors of adolescent substance use. *Adolescence, 29*, 405–420.

Barlow, D. H., Allen, L. B., & Choate, M. L. (2004). Toward a unified treatment for emotional disorders. *Behavior Therapy, 35*, 205–230.

Boening, J. A. L. (2001) Neurobiology of an addiction memory. *Journal of Neural Transmission, 108*, 755–765.

Bolton, C., Gooding, P., Kapur, N., Barrowclough, C., & Tarrier, N. (2007) Developing psychological perspectives of suicidal behaviour and risk in people with a diagnosis of schizophrenia: We know they kill themselves but do we understand why? *Clinical Psychology Review, 27*, 511–536.

Brady, K. T., Dansky, B. S., Back, S. E., Foa, E. B., & Carroll, K. M. (2001). Exposure therapy in the treatment of PTSD among cocaine-dependent individuals: Preliminary findings. *Journal of Substance Abuse Treatment, 21*, 47–54.

Bronfenbrenner, U. (1979). *The ecology of human development: Experiments by nature and design.* Cambridge, MA: Harvard University.

Brook, J. S., Brook, D. W., Arencibia-Mireles, O., Richter, L., & Whiteman, M. (2001). Risk factors for adolescent marijuana use across cultures and across time. *Journal of Genetic Psychology, 162*, 357–374.

Brown, P. J. (2000). Outcome in female patients with both substance use and post-traumatic stress disorders. *Alcoholism Treatment Quarterly, 18*, 127–135.

Charney, D. S., Deutch, A. Y., Krystal, J. H., Southwick, S. M., & Davis, M. (1993). Psychobiologic mechanisms of posttraumatic stress disorder. *Archives of General Psychiatry, 50*, 295–305.

Charuvastra, A., & Cloitre, M. (2008). Social bonds and posttraumatic stress disorder. *Annual Review of Psychology, 59*, 301–328.

Chassin, L., Pillow, D. R., Curran, P. J., Molina, B. S., & Barrera, M. (1993). Relation of parental alcoholism to early adolescent substance use: A test of three mediating mechanisms. *Journal of Abnormal Psychology, 102*, 3–19.

Clark, D. B., & Kirisci, L. (1996). Posttraumatic stress disorder, depression, alcohol use disorders, and quality of life in adolescents. *Anxiety, 2*, 226–233.

Cohen, J. A., Deblinger, E., Mannarino, A. P., & Steer, R. A. (2004). A multisite randomized controlled study of sexually abused, multiply traumatized children with PTSD: Initial treatment outcome. *Journal of the American Academy of Child and Adolescent Psychiatry, 43*, 393–402.

Cohen, J. A., Mannarino, A. P., Zhitova, A. C., & Capone, M. E. (2003). Treating child-abuse related posttraumatic stress and comorbid substance abuse in adolescents. *Child Abuse and Neglect, 27*, 1345–1365.

Coffey, S. F., Saladin, M., Drobes, D. J., Brady, K. T., Dansky, B. S., & Kilpatrick, D. G. (2002). Trauma and substance cue reactivity in individuals with comorbid posttraumatic stress disorder and cocaine or alcohol dependence. *Drug and Alcohol Dependence, 65*, 115–127.

Coffey, S. F., Schumacher, J. A., Brimo, M. L., & Brady, K. T. (2005). Exposure therapy for substance abusers with PTSD: Translating research to practice. *Behavior Modification, 29*, 10–38.

Coffey, S. F., Stasiewicz, P. R., Hughes, P. M., & Brimo, M. L. (2006). Trauma-focused imaginal exposure for individuals with comorbid posttraumatic stress disorder and alcohol dependence: Revealing mechanisms of alcohol craving in a cue reactivity paradigm. *Psychology of Addictive Behaviors, 20,* 425–435.

Copeland, W. E., Keeler, G., Angold, A., & Costello, E. J. (2007). Traumatic events and posttraumatic stress in childhood. *Archives of General Psychiatry, 64,* 577–584.

Dawes, M. A., Antelman, S. M., Vanyukov, M. M., Giancola, P., Tarter, R. E., Susman, E. J., et al. (2000). Developmental sources of variation in liability to adolescent substance use disorders. *Drug and Alcohol Dependence, 61,* 3–14.

DeBellis, M. D. (2002). Developmental traumatology: A contributory mechanism for alcohol and substance use disorders. *Psychoneuroendocrinology, 27,* 155–170.

DeBellis, M. D., Narasimhan, A., Thatcher, D. L., Keshavan, M. S., Soloff, P., & Clark, D. B. (2005). Prefrontal cortex, thalamus, and cerebellar volumes in adolescents and young adults with adolescent-onset alcohol use disorders and comorbid mental disorders. *Alcoholism: Clinical and Experimental Research, 29,* 1590–1600.

Deblinger, E., Lippman, J., & Steer, R. (1996). Sexually abused children suffering posttraumatic stress symptoms: Initial treatment outcome findings. *Child Maltreatment, 1,* 310–321.

DeWit, D. J., Adlaf, E. M., Offord, D. R., & Ogborne, A. C. (2000). Age at first alcohol use: A risk factor for the development of alcohol disorders. *American Journal of Psychiatry, 157,* 745–750.

Deykin, E. Y., & Buka, S. L. (1997). Prevalence and risk factors for posttraumatic stress disorder among chemically dependent adolescents. *American Journal of Psychiatry, 154,* 752–757.

Diamond, G., Panichelli-Mindel, S. M., Shera, D., Dennis, M., Tims, F., & Ungemack, J. (2006). Psychiatric syndromes in adolescents with marijuana abuse and dependency in outpatient treatment. *Journal of Child and Adolescent Substance Abuse, 15,* 37–54.

Dos, A. J. (2005). Is comorbidity really a problem for the dissemination of evidence-based treatments for youth? *Behavior Therapist, 28,* 160–161.

Ellis, B. H., Fogler, J., Hansen, S., Forbes, P., Navalta, C. P., & Saxe, G. (2012). Trauma systems therapy: 15-month outcomes and the importance of effecting environmental change. *Psychological Trauma: Theory, Research, Practice, and Policy, 4,* 624–630.

Fairburn, C. G., Cooper, Z., & Shafran, R. (2003). Cognitive behaviour therapy for eating disorders: A transdiagnostic theory and treatment. *Behaviour Research and Therapy, 41,* 509–528.

Felitti, V. J., Anda, R. F., Nordenberg, D., Williamson, D. F., Spitz, A. M., Edwards, V., et al. (1998). Relationship of childhood abuse and household dysfunction to many of the leading causes of death in adults: The Adverse Childhood Experiences (ACE) study. *American Journal of Preventive Medicine, 14,* 245–258.

Foa, E. B., Rothbaum, B. O., Riggs, D., & Murdock, T. B. (1991). Treatment of posttraumatic stress disorder in rape victims: A comparison between cognitive-behavioral procedures and counseling. *Journal of Consulting and Clinical Psychology, 59,* 715–723.

Frankl, V. E. (1992). *Man's search for meaning: An introduction to logotherapy.* Boston: Beacon Press.

Funk, R. R., McDermeit, M., Godley, S. H., & Adams, L. (2003). Maltreatment issues by level of adolescent substance abuse treatment: The extent of the problem at intake and relationship to early outcomes. *Child Maltreatment, 8,* 36–45.

Giaconia, R. M., Reinherz, H. Z., Hauf, A. C., Paradis, A. D., Wasserman, M. S., & Langhammer, D. M. (2000). Comorbidity of substance use and post-traumatic stress disorder in a community of adolescents. *American Journal of Orthopsychiatry, 70,* 253–262.

Gordon, M. S., Kinlock, T. W., & Battjes, R. J. (2004). Correlates of early substance use and crime among adolescents entering outpatient substance abuse treatment. *American Journal of Drug and Alcohol Abuse, 30,* 39–59.

Grella, C. E., & Joshi, V. (2003). Treatment processes and outcomes among adolescents with a history of abuse who are in drug treatment. *Child Maltreatment, 8,* 7–18.

Harvey, A., Watkins, E., Mansell, W., & Shafran, R. (2004). *Cognitive behavioural processes across psychological disorders: A transdiagnostic approach to research and treatment.* Oxford, UK: Oxford University Press.

Heim, C., & Nemeroff, C. B. (1999). The impact of early adverse experiences on brain systems involved in the pathophysiology of anxiety and affective disorders. *Biological Psychiatry, 46,* 1509–1522.

Henggeler, S. W., Clingempeel, W. G., Brondino, M. J., & Pickrel, S. G. (2002). Four-year follow-up of multisystemic therapy with substance-abusing and substance-dependent juvenile offenders. *Journal of the American Academy of Child and Adolescent Psychiatry, 41,* 868–874.

Hoffmann, J. P., & Cerbone, F. G. (2002). Parental substance use disorder and the risk of adolescent drug abuse: An event history analysis. *Drug and Alcohol Dependence, 66,* 255–264.

Kilpatrick, D. G., Acierno, R., Saunders, B., Resnick, H. S., Best, C. L., & Schnurr, P. P. (2000). Risk factors for adolescent substance abuse and dependence: Data from a national sample. *Journal of Consulting and Clinical Psychology, 68,* 19–30.

Kilpatrick, D. G., Ruggiero, K. J., Acierno, R., Saunders, B. E., Resnick, H. S., & Best, C. L. (2003). Violence and risk of PTSD, major depression, substance abuse/dependence, and comorbidity: Results from the National Survey of Adolescents. *Journal of Consulting and Clinical Psychology, 71,* 692–700.

King, N. J., Tonge, B. J., Mullen, P., Myerson, N., Heyne, D., Rollings, S., et al. (2000). Treating sexually abused children with posttraumatic stress symptoms: A randomized clinical trial. *Journal of the American Academy of Child and Adolescent Psychiatry, 39,* 1347–1355.

Knight, J. R., Harris, S. K., Sherritt, L., Van Hook, S., Lawrence, N., Brooks, T., et al. (2007). Prevalence of positive substance abuse screen results among adolescent primary care patients. *Archives of Pediatric Adolescent Medicine, 161,* 1035–1041.

Koob, G. F. (2006). The neurobiology of addiction: A neuroadaptational view relevant for diagnosis. *Addiction, 101,* 23–30.

Koob, G. F., & Le Moal, M. (1997). Drug abuse: Hedonic homeostatic dysregulation. *Science, 278,* 52–58.

Kostelecky, K. L. (2005). Parental attachment, academic achievement, life events and their relationship to alcohol and drug use during adolescence. *Journal of Adolescence, 28,* 665–669.

Lieb, R., Wittchen, H. U., Höfler, M., Fuetsch, M., Stein, M. B., & Merikangas, K. R. (2000). Parental psychopathology, parenting styles, and the risk of social phobia in offspring: A prospective-longitudinal community study. *Archives of General Psychiatry, 57,* 859–866.

Liddle, H. A., Dakof, G. A., Diamond, G. S., Parker, G. S., Barrett, K., & Tejeda, M. (2001). Multidimensional family therapy for adolescent substance abuse: Results of a randomized clinical trial. *American Journal of Drug and Alcohol Abuse, 27,* 651–687.

Marks, I., Lovell, K., Noshirvani, H., Livanou, M., & Thrasher, S. (1998). Treatment of posttraumatic stress disorder by exposure and/or cognitive restructuring: A controlled study. *Archives of General Psychiatry, 55,* 317–325.

Miller, W. R., & Rollnick, S. (2002). *Motivational interviewing: Preparing people for change* (2nd ed.). New York: Guilford Press.

McCusker, C. G., & Brown, K. (1995). Cue-exposure to alcohol-associated stimuli reduces autonomic reactivity, but not craving and anxiety, in dependent drinkers. *Alcohol and Alcoholism, 30,* 319–327.

McDonagh, A., Friedman, M., McHugo, G., Ford, J., Sengupta, A., Mueser, K., et al. (2005). Randomized trial of cognitive-behavioral therapy for chronic posttraumatic stress disorder in adult female survivors of childhood sexual abuse. *Journal of Consulting and Clinical Psychology, 73,* 515–524.

Merikangas, K. R., Stolar, M., Stevens, D. E., Goulet, J., Preisig, M. A., Fenton, B., et al. (1998). Familial transmission of substance use disorders. *Archives of General Psychiatry, 55,* 973–979.

Miller, W. R., & Rollnick, S. (2002). *Motivational interviewing: Preparing people for change* (2nd ed.). New York: Guilford Press.

Monti, P. M., Binkoff, J. A., Abrams, D. B., Zwick, W. R., Nirenberg, T. D., & Liepman, M. R. (1987). Reactivity of alcoholics and nonalcoholics to drinking cues. *Journal of Abnormal Psychology, 96,* 122–126.

Najavits, L. M., Gallop, R. J., & Weiss, R. D. (2006). Seeking Safety therapy for adolescent girls with PTSD and substance abuse: A randomized controlled trial. *Journal of Behavioral Health Services and Research, 33,* 453–463.

Needle, R., McCubbin, H., Wilson, M., Reineck, R., Lazar, A., & Mederer, H. (1986). Interpersonal influences in adolescent drug use: The role of older siblings, parents, and peers. *International Journal of the Addictions, 21,* 739–766.

Norton, P. J. (2008). An open trial of a transdiagnostic cognitive-behavioral group therapy for anxiety disorder. *Behavior Therapy, 39,* 242–250.

Norton, P. J., & Philipp, L. M. (2008). Transdiagnostic approaches to the treatment of anxiety disorders: A quantitative review. *Psychotherapy: Theory, Research, Practice, Training, 45,* 214–226.

Ouimette, P. C., Brown, P. J., & Najavits, L. M. (1998). Course and treatment of patients with both substance use and posttraumatic stress disorders. *Addictive Behaviors, 23,* 785–795.

Orr, S. P., Metzger, L. J., & Pitman, R. K. (2002) Psychophysiology of posttraumatic stress disorder. *Psychiatric Clinics of North America, 25,* 271–293.

Pitman, R. K., Altman, B., Greenwald, E., Longpre, R. E., Macklin, M. L., Poire,

R. E., et al. (1991). Psychiatric complications during flooding therapy for posttraumatic stress disorder. *Journal of Clinical Psychiatry, 52,* 17–20.

Pollock, V. E., Briere, J., Schneider, L., Knop, J., Mednick, S. A., & Goodwin, D. W. (1990). Childhood antecedents of antisocial behavior: Parental alcoholism and physical abusiveness. *American Journal of Psychiatry, 147,* 1290–1293.

Rauch, S. L., Whalen, P. J., Shin, L. M., McInerney, S. C., Macklin, M. L., Lasko, N. B., et al. (2000). Exaggerated amygdala response to masked facial stimuli in posttraumatic stress disorder: A functional MRI study. *Biological Psychiatry, 47,* 769–776.

Read, J. P., Brown, P. J., & Kahler, C. W. (2004). Substance use and posttraumatic stress disorders: Symptom interplay and effects on outcome. *Addictive Behaviors, 29,* 1665–1672.

Reinherz, H. Z., Giaconia, R. M., Lefkowitz, E. S., Pakiz, B., & Frost, A. K. (1993). Prevalence of psychiatric disorders in a community population of older adolescents. *Journal of the American Academy of Child and Adolescent Psychiatry, 32,* 369–377.

Saladin, M. E., Drobes, D. J., Coffey, S. F., Dansky, B. S., Brady, K. T., & Kilpatrick, D. G. (2003). PTSD symptom severity as a predictor of cue-elicited drug craving in victims of violent crime. *Addictive Behaviors, 28,* 1611–1629.

Sampl, S., & Kadden, R. (2001). *Motivational Enhancement Therapy and Cognitive Behavioral Therapy (MET-CBT-5) for adolescent cannabis users.* Rockville, MD: Center for Substance Abuse Treatment, Substance Abuse and Mental Health Services Administration.

Saxe, G., Ellis, B. H., Fogler, J., Hansen, S., & Sorkin, B. (2005). Comprehensive care for traumatized children: An open trial examines treatment using Trauma Systems Therapy. *Psychiatric Annals, 35,* 443–448.

Saxe, G. N., Ellis, B. H., & Kaplow, J. B. (2006). *Collaborative treatment of traumatized children and teens: The trauma systems therapy approach.* New York: Guilford Press

Silverman, W. K., Ortiz, C. D., Viswesvaran, C., Burns, B. J., Kolko, D. J., Putnam, F. W., et al. (2008). Evidence-based psychosocial treatments for children and adolescents exposed to traumatic events. *Journal of Clinical Child and Adolescent Psychology, 37,* 156–183.

Smith, C. A., Ireland, T. O., & Thornberry, T. P. (2005). Adolescent maltreatment and its impact on young adult antisocial behavior. *Child Abuse and Neglect, 29,* 1099–1119.

Stasiewicz, P. R., & Maisto, S. A. (1993). Two-factor avoidance theory: The role of negative affect in the maintenance of substance use and substance use disorder. *Behavior Therapy, 24,* 337–356.

Stein, B. D., Jaycox, L. H., Kataoka, S. H., Wong, M., Tu, W., Elliott, M. N., et al. (2003). A mental health intervention for schoolchildren exposed to violence. *Journal of the American Medical Association, 290,* 603–611.

Stevens, S. J., Murphy, B. S., & McKnight, K. (2003). Traumatic stress and gender differences in relationship to substance abuse, mental health, physical health, and HIV risk behavior in a sample of adolescents enrolled in drug treatment. *Child Maltreatment, 8,* 46–57.

Suárez, L. M., Belcher, H. M. E., Briggs, E. C., & Titus, J. C. (2012). Supporting the need for an integrated system of care for youth with co-occurring traumatic stress and substance abuse problems. *American Journal of Community Psychology, 49*, 430–440.

Suárez, L. M., Bennett, S., Goldstein, C., & Barlow, D. H. (2009). Understanding anxiety disorders from a "triple vulnerability" framework. In M. M. Anthony & M. B. Stein (Eds.), *Oxford handbook of anxiety and related disorders* (pp. 153–172). New York: Oxford University Press.

Suárez, L. M., Saxe, G., Ehrenreich, J., & Barlow, D. (2006). *Trauma systems therapy for adolescent substance abuse.* Unpublished treatment manual, Boston University, Center for Anxiety and Related Disorders.

Substance Abuse and Mental Health Services Administration. (2006). *Results from the 2005 National Survey on Drug Use and Health: National findings* (DHHS Publication No. SMA 06-4194). Rockville, MD: U.S. Department of Health and Human Services, Office of Applied Studies.

Tarrier, N., Pilgrim, H., Sommerfield, C., Faragher, B., Reynolds, M., Graham, E., et al. (1999). A randomized trial of cognitive therapy and imaginal exposure in the treatment of chronic posttraumatic stress disorder. *Journal of Consulting and Clinical Psychology, 67*, 13–18.

Tarter, R. E., Vanyukov, M. M., Giancola, P., Dawes, M., Blackson, T., Mezzich, A., et al. (1999). Etiology of early age onset substance use disorder: A maturational perspective. *Developmental Psychopathology, 11*, 657–683.

Tedeschi, R. G., & Calhoun, L. G. (2004). Posttraumatic growth: Conceptual foundations and empirical evidence. *Psychological Inquiry, 15*, 1–18.

Titus, J. C., Dennis, M. L., White, W. L., Scott, C. K., & Funk, R. R. (2003). Gender differences in victimization severity and outcomes among adolescents treated for substance abuse. *Child Maltreatment, 8*, 19–35.

Waldron, H. B., & Turner, C. W. (2008). Evidence-based psychosocial treatments for adolescent substance abuse. *Journal of Clinical Child and Adolescent Psychology, 37*, 238–261.

Walker, L. S., McLaughlin, F. J., & Greene, J. W. (1988). Functional illness and family functioning: A comparison of healthy and somaticizing adolescents. *Family Process, 27*, 317–325.

Weist, M. D., Acosta, O. M., & Youngstrom, E. A. (2001). Predictors of violence exposure among inner-city youth. *Journal of Clinical Child Psychology, 30*, 187–198.

Westermeyer, J., Wahmanholm, K., & Thuras, P. (2001). Effects of childhood physical abuse on course and severity of substance abuse. *American Journal on Addictions, 10*, 101–110.

Woodward, C., & Joseph, S. (2003). Positive change processes and post-traumatic growth in people who have experienced childhood abuse: Understanding vehicles of change. *Psychology and Psychotherapy: Theory, Research and Practice, 76*, 267–283.

Zeigler, D. W., Wang, C. C., Yoast, R. A., Dickinson, B. D., McCaffree, M. A., Robinowitz, C. B., et al. (2005). The neurocognitive effects of alcohol on adolescents and college students. *Preventitive Medicine, 40*, 23–32.

Family-Based Treatment
for Adolescent Eating Disorders

Daniel Le Grange and Katharine L. Loeb

Transdiagnostic Conceptualizations of Eating Disorders

The eating disorders section in the *Diagnostic and Statistical Manual of Mental Disorders* (DSM-5; American Psychiatric Association, 2013) delineates four diagnoses: anorexia nervosa (AN), bulimia nervosa (BN), binge eating disorder (BED), avoidant/restrictive food intake disorder (RFID), and feeding or eating disorder not elsewhere classified (EDNEC). The cardinal features of AN include refusal to maintain a normal body weight, disturbance in the experience of shape and weight (e.g., regarding oneself as fat despite emaciation), and extreme fear of weight gain. BN is characterized by recurrent binge eating and unhealthy compensatory behaviors (e.g., purging) in the context of a self-concept that is heavily influenced by shape and weight. DSM-IV EDNOS, a residual category of eating disturbance, encompasses subthreshold and atypical variants of AN and BN, as well as distinct disorders such as binge-eating disorder (BED), which has been codified as a primary eating disorder in the new DSM-5 (American Psychiatric Association, 2013). Notably, DSM-IV EDNOS is markedly more prevalent in clinical samples than either AN, BN, or the two combined (Ricca et al., 2001; Turner & Bryant-Waugh, 2004), and there has been much debate in the field as to how to best parse this broad but clinically significant category (Crow, 2007; Fairburn & Cooper, 2007; Fairburn et al., 2007; Waller, 2008; Wilfley, Bishop, Wilson, & Agras, 2007). Disagreement about the optimal disposition of DSM-IV EDNOS in general and of the specific clinical descriptions therein is embedded in a larger controversy regarding the nosology of eating disorders, with many proposed alternatives to the DSM-IV system taken into consideration for the current DSM-5 system (Wonderlich, Joiner, Keel, Williamson, & Crosby, 2007), including dimensional conceptualizations (e.g., Stice, Killen, Hayward, & Taylor, 1998) explicitly adopting or implicitly supporting a transdiagnostic perspective.

Eating disorders as diagnostic entities lend themselves to a transdiagnostic framework in several ways (Fairburn, 2008; Fairburn, Cooper, & Shafran, 2003). First, the bounds that distinguish AN, BN, and EDNOS from one another are blurred, both in the manner in which DSM-IV-TR criteria capture present state and temporally in the migration between diagnostic categories over the course of illness (Eddy et al., 2008; Fichter & Quadflieg, 2007; Milos, Spindler, Schnyder, & Fairburn, 2005). For instance, binge eating appears across the eating disorders, and it is common for patients to cross over from AN, restricting type (AN-R), to AN, binge/purge type (AN-BP), and from AN-BP to BN (Eddy et al., 2008; Fichter & Quadflieg, 2007; Fichter, Quadflieg, & Hedlund, 2006; Milos et al., 2005; Tozzi et al., 2005; Wentz, Gillberg, Gillberg, & Rastam, 2001), with only time, weight status, and clinical judgment determining the point at which AN-BP in partial remission becomes BN. In fact, what defines and differentiates AN, BN, and EDNOS has changed with each iteration of DSM, with only DSM-5 for eating disorders to some extent reflecting a statistically derived classification system such as taxometric or latent class analysis (Wonderlich, Crosby, Mitchell, & Engel, 2007; Wonderlich, Joiner, et al., 2007). A classic example of this is the classification of individuals who binge-eat in the absence of inappropriate compensatory mechanisms, such as purging, who would have received a diagnosis of bulimia in DSM-III (American Psychiatric Association, 1980), no clear diagnosis in DSM-III-R (American Psychiatric Association, 1987), a designation of BED under EDNOS in DSM-IV-TR (American Psychiatric Association, 2000), and a formal diagnosis of BED as a fully recognized independent eating disorder in DSM-5 (American Psychiatric Association, 2013). Several additional changes in the eating disorders section in DSM-5 capture prior cases of EDNOS by virtue of atypical or subthreshold presentations (e.g., AN without amenorrhea or without direct verbal endorsement of fear of weight gain), highlighting the importance of a transdiagnostic perspective with an appreciation of clinical severity that transcends the DSM and the diagnostic categories therein.

Second, a "core psychopathology" of eating disorders has been proposed by Fairburn and colleagues (Fairburn, 2008; Fairburn et al., 2003) both to explain mechanisms of symptom maintenance across AN, BN, and EDNOS and to inform a transdiagnostic cognitive-behavioral approach to treatment. This core pathology is thought to underlie the majority of clinically significant eating disorder presentations—regardless of whether and how they are formally codified in the DSM—and consists mainly of the cognitive features of overevaluation of shape and weight and their control, which are expressed in a range of disordered thoughts and behaviors (Fairburn, 2008; Fairburn et al., 2003). A recent randomized controlled trial (RCT) comparing two versions of the transdiagnostic, "enhanced" cognitive-behavioral therapy (CBT-E) for BN and EDNOS (body mass index > 17.5; Fairburn et al., 2009), found that patients improved in both treatments and that DSM diagnosis did not moderate treatment effects, even at 60-week follow-up, suggesting that DSM diagnosis has little predictive validity with regard to outcome and, in turn, perhaps limited clinical utility. Third, eating disorders typically have their onset in adolescence (Lewinsohn, Striegel-Moore, & Seeley, 2001; Lucas, Beard, O'Fallon, & Kurland, 1991), with initial presentations frequently appearing subthreshold or atypical relative to DSM-defined AN or BN (Workgroup for Classification of Eating Disorders in Children and Adolescents [WCEDCA], 2007, 2010). Although in a percentage of these cases the symptoms may be transient, the subsyndromal state can be associated with marked clinical severity and risk, similar to full-threshold presentations (Binford & Le Grange, 2005; Crow, Agras, Halmi, Mitchell, & Kraemer, 2002; Le Grange et al., 2006; Le Grange, Loeb, Van Orman, & Jellar, 2004; McIntosh et al., 2004; Ricca et al., 2001; Watson & Andersen, 2003; Wonderlich et al., 2005), and a portion of EDNOS cases will ultimately go on to meet full criteria for an eating disorder (Ben-Tovim et al., 2001; Herzog, Hopkins, & Burns, 1993; Le Grange et al., 2004). One possibility is that we are misdiagnosing AN and BN as EDNOS in younger populations (Le Grange & Loeb, 2007), as DSM makes very few allowances for age-specific manifestations of eating disorders (WCEDCA, 2007, 2010). For example, whereas the DSM-IV anxiety disorders criteria permit behavioral indicators of fear among children, such as crying in the presence of a feared stimulus, the criteria for eating disorders require more direct endorsement of abstract concepts such as intense fear of becoming fat, or undue influence of shape and weight on self evaluation, across the age spectrum. An obvious solution is to improve the developmental sensitivity of the existing DSM criteria for AN and BN within the current categorical diagnostic system (WCEDCA, 2007, 2010), and this was considered in the development of DSM-5 by proposing transdevelopmental revisions to the criteria that rely less on verbal expressions of psychological symptoms. Alternatively, a transdiagnostic framework for classification of eating disorders would not only arguably provide a more valid nosological assignment than EDNOS for such severe and/or potentially prodromal cases but would also elevate their perceived clinical significance. This could have positive implications for early identification and intervention and, in turn, for improved course of illness and prognosis (Deter & Herzog, 1994; Le Grange & Loeb, 2007; Ratnasuriya, Eisler, Szmukler, 1991).

This chapter describes a transdiagnostic approach to family-based treatment (FBT) for children and adolescents with eating disorders. FBT was developed at the Maudsley Hospital in England and originally tested against individual treatment among adults and adolescents with AN and BN (Eisler et al., 1997; Russell, Szmukler, Dare, & Eisler, 1987). Results from this seminal study favored the application of this approach for patients with a less-than-3-year duration of AN, and the body of studies to immediately follow therefore focused exclusively on adolescent AN (Eisler et al., 2000; Eisler, Simic, Russell, & Dare, 2007; Le Grange, Eisler, Dare, & Russell, 1992). Since the original collection of RCTs of FBT was conducted, the approach has been disseminated and tested beyond the Maudsley Hospital (Le Grange, Crosby, Rathouz, & Leventhal, 2007; Lock, Agras, Bryson, & Kraemer, 2005; Lock, Couturier, & Agras, 2006; Loeb et al., 2007; Robin et al., 1999; Schmidt et al., 2007) and is now being adapted for a more transdiagnostic spectrum. There are currently FBT manuals for the treatment of AN (Lock, Le Grange, Agras, & Dare, 2001) and BN (Le Grange & Lock, 2007), both of which have been tested in studies that included subthreshold and atypical (i.e., EDNOS) cases (Le Grange et al., 2007; Lock et al., 2005; Lock, Le Grange, Forsberg, & Hewell, 2006; Loeb et al., 2007); for the prevention of AN in symptomatic children and adolescents at high risk for developing the full disorder (Loeb, Craigen, Munk Goldstein, Lock, & Le Grange, 2011); and even for the treatment of overweight and obesity in adolescence (Loeb et al., 2006), which can be associated with disordered eating but are not categorized as psychiatric disorders. It is also being tested once again with young adult populations (Le Grange & Chen, 2007). This chapter describes the fundamentals of FBT, a transdiagnostic theoretical model of FBT and the literature supporting its clinical application, adaptations across developmental stages and the diagnostic spectrum of eating disorders, and the strengths and challenges of this approach.

FBT for Eating Disorders:
Clinical Description of the Foundation Approach

FBT is a brief (between 10 and 20 sessions) outpatient approach for the treatment of youth with eating disorders. Its specific interventions derive indirectly from a variety of schools of psychotherapy, including behavioral, family systems, and structural family therapy. Although it reflects an amalgam of approaches in practice, FBT is explicitly atheoretical with regard to etiology of illness, and the family is treated not to uncover an underlying familial pathology expressing itself in the child's eating disorder but rather to enlist the parents as a resource in the practical resolution of the problem. In fact, FBT incorporates an overt agenda of blame reduction toward both the parents and the patient and directly corrects criticism of the child. To date in the literature on FBT, mechanisms maintaining the eating disorder are at most implied by virtue of the strategies inherent in the intervention, but the mechanisms have not been delineated. In this chapter, we explicate these theoretical mechanisms of symptom maintenance in adolescent eating disorders that FBT targets and, in turn, put forth hypothesized mechanisms of action of FBT for the transdiagnostic eating disorder population.

FBT consists of three phases, typically delivered with the entire family, including siblings, present at each session. The parents' roles shift across the treatment phases, while siblings maintain a supportive role for the patient throughout the course of FBT. In the first phase, parents take charge of their child's eating disorder symptoms much as an inpatient staff might, making decisions about appropriate eating and related behaviors at a stage when the adolescent is too affected by the eating disorder pathology to engage in adequate self-care. In fact, the adolescent is explicitly depicted as a distinct entity from the eating disorder, but with the healthy self temporarily eclipsed by a pernicious disorder. In Phase I, parents directly compensate for the effects of the illness by managing and supervising all aspects of their child's eating. In Phase II, as the eating disorder begins to remit, control over eating is gradually transferred back to the child as she or he emerges into her or his appropriate developmental stage and corresponding level of autonomy. Phase III attends to broader issues of adolescent development and family functioning. Inherent in FBT is a belief that the acute symptoms of the eating disorder must be resolved and basic functioning restored before the adolescent will experience any relief from the cognitive symptoms of the eating disorder, such as extreme shape and weight concerns. In FBT, food, regular eating, and cessation of eating disorder behaviors are the potent medicine, with parents delivering the treatment in an authoritative manner that blends firmness, kindness, and resolve. Parents never apply force in FBT but rather create a zero-tolerance environment for the eating disorder.

FBT is most frequently applied in a conjoint format, that is, with all family members who live at home expected to attend treatment sessions. Moreover, it is a focused treatment and requires the therapist to "stay with" the symptoms of self-starvation or binge eating and purging until these behaviors begin to dissipate or have been resolved. This focus leaves the therapist with relatively little time early in treatment to attend to the adolescent in the same way that is possible in more traditional individual psychotherapeutic approaches. FBT has also been studied in a separated format (Eisler et al., 2000; Le Grange et al., 1992) that allows for equal time being spent with the adolescent and with her or his parents but sequentially instead of together. Despite this "extra" time being available for the adolescent, these studies have shown treatment outcome to be similar across the two treatment formats. However, separated FBT appears to be more effective for families with high levels of expressed emotion, particularly criticism (Eisler et al., 2000; Le Grange et al., 1992).

FBT has been adapted for pediatric obesity (FBT-PO; Loeb et al., 2006) and was tested in a two-site (Mount Sinai School of Medicine and the University of Chicago) RCT comparing conjoint FBT-PO with nutritional education counseling delivered to parents and children in a separated format by one of the authors (Loeb). Inherent in the FBT model is a mission to increase parental empowerment, competence, and efficacy in facilitating healthy behaviors and outcomes for children and unapologetically assuming appropriate parental influence. Beyond this, FBT provides a strong foundation for application to the significant problem of pediatric obesity because of its attention to parental engagement strategies, its demonstrated efficacy in correcting maladaptive eating and related behaviors, its explicit agenda of blame reduction, its disease-based model, and its emphasis on promoting normal physical and psychosocial development for the child or adolescent. In applying the FBT model to pediatric obesity, specific differences between eating disorders and obesity were carefully addressed. FBT-PO has transdevelopmental applicability in that younger children and older adolescents may benefit from an appropriate level of family involvement in weight control. Our adaptation recognizes that obesity is not a psychiatric disorder and that children and adolescents are not developmentally regressed as they are in severe eating disorders. Therefore, FBT-PO modulates the quality and intensity of parental involvement as a function of developmental stage. FBT-PO is designed to empower parents within the existing family structure and dynamics, allowing flexibility along cultural lines. It also recognizes specific challenges of socioeconomically diverse populations (e.g., built environment, reduction in school-based physical activity), the challenges of concordance of overweight across family members, and the need for parents to model attitudes and dietary and physical activity habits associated with healthy weight. Finally, FBT-PO addresses the multisystemic toxic environment in which obesogenic choices are readily available as the default selections (Wadden, Brownell, & Foster, 2002) that contribute to pediatric obesity and focuses on parent-driven, family-level change.

A Transdiagnostic Model of FBT

As noted earlier, FBT posits no mechanism by which family or individual variables may have given rise to the eating disorder, nor are maintenance factors directly explored in the existing FBT literature. However, the key interventions and principles of FBT and their effectiveness in the aggregate (no specific dismantling studies have been conducted to date) suggest the following transdiagnostic model of the approach. This model is designed to explain how the disorder can influence family-level variables, which in turn might limit the resolution of the disorder. FBT targets these family variables and mechanisms explicitly by directly labeling, conceptualizing, and prescribing interventions to address each. FBT also affects individual variables and mechanisms, but only implicitly. For example, as introduced shortly, FBT is hypothesized to correct eating-disorder-specific maladaptive reinforcement patterns (e.g., fear conditioning) via new associative learning during exposure that occurs naturalistically in the context of FBT (Hildebrandt, Bacow, Markella, & Loeb, 2012). However, FBT is not framed as exposure treatment, and exposure exercises per se are not planned or developed in a hierarchy in this intervention. The transdiagnostic model of family-based therapy for youth with eating disorders is depicted in Figure 16.1.

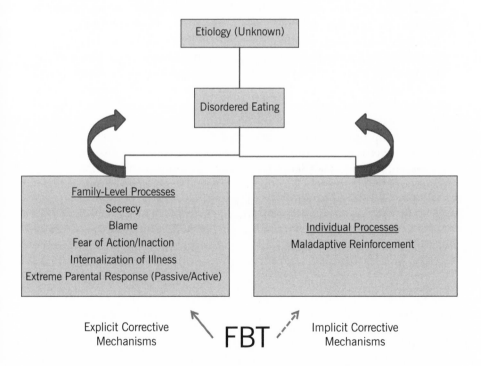

FIGURE 16.1. Transdiagnostic model of family-based therapy for youth with eating disorders.

Family-Level and Individual-Level Processes of Eating Disorders: A Transdiagnostic Perspective in the Context of FBT

At the family level, we propose that the eating disorder elicits secrecy, fear, blame, and a belief that the adolescent has control over her or his symptoms (internalization of the illness). These mechanisms operate both intrapersonally, reflecting internal experiences within each family member, as well as interpersonally, between parents, siblings, and the affected child or adolescent. These variables are not hypothesized to reflect premorbid relational patterns within the family that may have either contributed to a general familial vulnerability to psychopathology or to a specific risk for eating disorders; rather, they are processes that the eating disorder initiates and that collectively inhibit symptom resolution. Secrecy, fear, blame, and internalization of illness function transdiagnostically, across formally recognized categories of eating disorders and within clinically significant but more vaguely codified eating disorder presentations. The effectiveness of FBT may be due in part to the intervention extinguishing each of these mechanisms.

Secrecy involves either the direct concealment of or the failure to explicitly recognize or acknowledge eating disorder symptoms. For example, patients who purge might either go to extreme measures to hide their symptoms (e.g., surreptitiously purging in the shower) or display a public quality to their secretive behaviors (e.g., abruptly leaving the table in the middle of dinner to "use" the bathroom while her family sits silently suspecting her true motives and behaviors). In this respect, the eating disorder can become the "elephant in the room," with the adolescent protecting the symptoms through secrecy and the parents and siblings unsure how to effectively confront the adolescent. Parents may also hide their adolescent's eating disorder from the outside world, fearing stigma, judgment, and blame, thereby limiting their social support and coping strategies. Fear manifests in multiple additional ways. The siblings often fear for their ill sister or brother's health and at times that they too will contract an eating disorder. The ill adolescent fears symptom arrest, while the healthy part of the adolescent (an explicit conceptualization in FBT is that during active stages of an eating disorder, the former occludes the latter) fears symptom progression and a failure on the part of parents and professionals to adequately intervene. This theory is consistent with frequent anecdotal clinical presentations in which the most actively resistant patients during Phase I of FBT will later express appreciation toward parents and therapist alike for persisting in their efforts; even in the midst of Phase I, in which resistance to treatment efforts is expected, some patients will "tell" on parents to the therapist for failing to supervise a meal adequately. A somewhat parallel internal conflict between action and inaction exists within the parents, who fear exacerbating the condition with active involvement—a fear sometimes reinforced by clinical recommendations to stay out of the child's eating matters lest their efforts be perceived as intrusive and inadvertently worsen their child's putative maladaptive attempts at separation and control as expressed through the eating disorder. At the same time, they fear that inaction will lead to their child's further deterioration. This conflict leads to an extreme but ineffective response on the parents' part, either active or passive in nature. For example, parents may try to actively convince their child that symptom cessation is in the child's best interest by attempting to mobilize her or his affect (e.g., "Can't you see how thin you are? Please eat!" or "You'll ruin your health if you keep vomiting!"). Conversely, parents may feel too paralyzed to intervene at all, terrified that confronting their child or taking charge will have a deleterious effect on both the parent–child relationship and an already fragile clinical state. Such extreme responses are invariably misguided and ineffective and will likely potentiate intrafamilial blame for the illness (parents toward themselves, patient toward her- or himself, parent toward patient, patient toward parent). They may also reinforce the erroneous belief that the child has direct control over her or his symptoms (internalization of illness), heightening criticism. Notably, as reviewed shortly, familial expressed emotion, particularly criticism, is associated with a poorer response to FBT (Le Grange et al., 1992; Szmukler, Eisler, Russell, & Dare, 1985).

At the individual (patient) level, eating disorder symptoms are generally maintained and exacerbated through maladaptive reinforcement, although the function of symptom maintenance may differ for each individual. These mechanisms are not conceptualized to operate via interpersonal or relational family processes but are believed to occur intrapersonally. Self-starvation in low-weight eating disorders, for example, may become chronic through fear conditioning, that is, fear of eating (Hildebrandt et al., 2012). In eating disorder presentation with binge-eating and purging patterns, negative reinforcement plays a prominent role (e.g., vomiting reduces immediate fear of weight gain). Transdiagnostically, extreme dietary restriction is negatively reinforcing in that it reduces shape and weight concerns (overevaluation of shape and weight and their control are also considered the core pathology in the transdiagnostic model of CBT for eating disorders; Fairburn, 2008; Fairburn et al., 2003) in the short term, and weight loss is directly positively reinforcing. FBT is not designed around an assumption that these individual mechanisms are operative, nor does FBT prescribe specific interventions within a conditioning framework, the environmental changes FBT imposes promote extinction of some of these behaviors via new associative learning. In fact, it has been argued that FBT functions as a form of parent-facilitated exposure to feared stimuli (Hildebrandt et al., 2012). With notable distinctions from explicit behavioral interventions of this nature (e.g., lack of a corresponding psychoeducational frame, absence of exposure hierarchies, allowance of distraction to mitigate discomfort), FBT, in particular Phase I of the treatment, provides a naturalistic context for exposure and escape extinction. For instance, the second session of FBT involves a family meal in which the parents are asked to bring a picnic, including food that challenges the core disordered eating symptoms of their ill adolescent. Parents are then asked, in vivo, to facilitate their child's consumption of at least a minimum quantity of the difficult food(s). Depending on the specific pathology, this food can represent just barely eating (e.g., a bite of an apple in low-weight eating disorders), eating a food that triggers binge eating or purging (e.g., chocolate), or eating a broadly avoided food (e.g., carbohydrates) or a full meal in the case of normal weight but highly restrictive eating disorder presentations. Parents, empowered by this experience, continue these efforts in the home environment, tackling various aspects of their adolescent's fundamental eating pathology by presenting food and insisting firmly and empathically, without force, criticism, or threat of punishment—on its consumption without active symptom engagement or escape. Although many of these principles and strategies apply to other eating-disorder treatment milieus, such as in inpatient settings, FBT has the significant advantage of being conducted in the patient's natural environment, with maximum potential for potency, durability, and generalizability of exposure effects (Hildebrandt et al., 2012).

Fear of weight gain, a cognitive eating disorder symptom, is addressed in several ways (Hildebrandt et al., 2012). First, there is exposure to the weight itself, and, in cases of low-weight eating disorders, to the increasing number on the scale over the course of treatment. The therapist weighs the patient at the beginning of each session during time alone with the adolescent, and the weight is openly discussed and charted once the family convenes. This confronts avoidance behaviors concerning weight and scales that extend from fear of weight gain; at the same time, checking rituals, such as frequent weighing and trying on small-sized clothes, are curtailed by parents at home. Moreover, in FBT, no precise numeric weight is set for patients in need of nutritional rehabilitation; rather, FBT looks for functional markers of weight restoration, such as resumption or onset of menses and a reduction in pathological shape and weight concerns. With no declared ceiling weight, patients are also exposed to the anxiety pertaining to the unknown that is embedded in their fear of weight gain. Finally, by creating a zero-tolerance environment with regard to self-starvation and weight loss, FBT allows the patient to maintain a normal weight long enough that expectancies regarding feared consequences of weight gain can be modified via new associative learning (Foa & Kozak, 1986; Hildebrandt et al., 2012).

In summary, FBT directly targets each of the family-level mechanisms that may collectively be creating an environment in which the eating disorder is left unchecked, worsening through individual mechanisms. FBT reverses secrecy by promoting discussion of symptom status, progress, and strategies as a family. The eating disorder is externalized, and the therapist draws a Venn diagram to depict the current overlap between the child and the eating disorder and the ultimate goal to separate them. It empowers parents to channel their efforts in the most effective manner possible, reducing their fear and facilitating recovery actively and without criticism, blame, or negotiation with the illness. Although FBT provides a mission statement for parents to reverse their child's illness and, with these concepts, a frame in which they can be successful, a key tenet of FBT is that "parents know best." In this respect, many (but not all) of the details of treatment are left for the parents to determine in an effort to restore their confidence as caregivers and to recognize the idiosyncratic needs of different patients and families. FBT encourages parents to follow their instinct to intervene and reminds parents of all they have accomplished in their parenting capacity to date. At the same time, the FBT therapist functions as the expert on eating disorders and provides consultation and parameters to prevent missteps or failure on the part of the parents. Unaffected siblings and the patient's premorbid healthy status are noted as evidence of the eating disorder being a result not of poor parenting but of vulnerability factors still poorly understood by the scientific field. Importantly, by creating a family environment that curtails symptom expression, FBT implicitly functions as a form of exposure therapy, targeting individual-level mechanisms such as fear conditioning in the generalized context of the affected individual's home (Hildebrandt et al., 2012). We propose that although FBT remains atheoretical with regard to etiology of eating disorders, its strategies and their collective effectiveness imply several mechanisms that maintain the illness, with family-level processes explicitly addressed in treatment and family-based strategies enlisted to target suggested individual-level processes.

Evidence in Support of FBT as a Transdiagnostic Intervention for Adolescents with Eating Disorders

There are only eight published RCTs of eating disorders in children and adolescents—six studies with adolescents with AN-spectrum disorders (Eisler et al., 2000; Gowers et al., 2007; Le Grange et al., 1992; Lock et al., 2005, 2010; Robin et al., 1999; Russell et al., 1987), and two with adolescents with BN presentations (Le Grange et al., 2007; Schmidt et al., 2007). Of these studies, only one (Gowers et al., 2007) did not employ family therapy as a treatment arm in these comparisons. Collectively, these studies offer strong support for FBT not only for acute weight restoration but also for long-term maintenance of gains in AN (Eisler et al., 1997; 2007;

Lock, Couturier, & Agras, 2006). Specifically, FBT appears to yield superior outcomes relative to individual forms of psychotherapy in earlier, smaller trials (Robin et al., 1999; Russell et al., 1987), as well as more recent and better powered research (Lock et al., 2010). Lock and colleagues (2010) demonstrated that FBT-AN was superior to individual ego-oriented psychotherapy (also called adolescent-focused therapy) in terms of full remission rates at 6- and 12-month follow-up. Fewer studies of FBT for BN have been conducted, and these studies show a more mixed picture. Schmidt and colleagues (2007) found no differences in abstinence rates for binge eating and purging between FBT and cognitive-behavioral therapy–guided self-help, while Le Grange and colleagues (2007) found that FBT showed greater abstinence rates at the end of treatment and follow-up compared with individual supportive therapy. Notably, in light of the developmental concerns with regard to diagnostic criteria outlined previously (Peebles, Wilson, & Lock, 2006; WCEDCA, 2007, 2010), treatment studies of adolescents with AN or BN have typically accommodated subthreshold and atypical presentations, essentially capturing a more transdiagnostic population of youth with eating disorders. For instance, participants who did not meet the amenorrhea diagnostic criterion for AN were included in at least two recent RCTs (Lock et al., 2005, 2010). Similarly, the inclusion criteria for both RCTs with binge-eating and purging adolescents allowed for participants who did not meet full DSM criteria for BN (Le Grange et al., 2007; Schmidt et al., 2007). There is no evidence that FBT performs differently for those adolescents who meet full DSM criteria for AN versus those who fall into the EDNOS category (Lock et al., 2005, 2010). For BN, the picture is somewhat different, with patients with the least severe psychological and behavioral manifestations of the disorder faring better in FBT than in the individual comparison treatment and no difference in outcome between treatments for those with the most severe eating disorder pathology (Le Grange, Crosby, & Lock, 2008). Collectively, such research suggests the transdiagnostic efficacy of FBT across eating disorder conditions (Loeb, Lock, Le Grange, & Greif, 2012).

FBT across Developmental Stages and the Diagnostic Spectrum of Eating Disorders

FBT was specifically developed as an intervention for adolescents as opposed to other treatments that have been adapted for the treatment of adolescents. Several reasons can be put forward to explain the development of FBT specifically for adolescents with eating disorders, but the main driving force that gave rise to this therapy is probably twofold. First, the Maudsley team of clinical researchers in London (e.g., Dare, 1983) argued that hospitalization of one's child for any reason is almost always experienced as traumatic and therefore should be avoided if possible. Second, such hospitalizations often cause the parents to feel disempowered, that is, that they have "failed" in taking care of their child. This places parents at a considerable disadvantage when they are presented with the crisis of the eating disorder and the need to take care of their offspring once she or he is discharged from inpatient care. FBT aims to prevent hospitalization if it is medically appropriate and instead seeks to bolster parental skills to take charge of their adolescent's weight restoration and/ or to curtail binge eating and purging. From a developmental perspective these strategies may come across as out of place given that patients seen in FBT are mostly teens. However, these interventions are temporary, and the ultimate goal is to encourage adolescents' independence and to support them on their developmental trajectory unencumbered by the eating disorder.

Most adolescents are embedded in their families and, in many respects, are dependent on their parents, a situation that provides the parents with considerable leverage over their adolescent. Consequently, it would seem appropriate to expect parents to utilize this advantageous position, in conjunction with their caretaking skills and affection for their child, to "arrest" the eating disorder from their child. As stated earlier, this intervention is time-limited, as FBT is ultimately most respectful of the adolescent and her or his nascent independence. A key tenet of FBT is to separate the illness from the adolescent (externalization) and is perhaps the most tangible way in which respect for the adolescent is demonstrated. In addition, this process of externalization also helps parents to view the eating disorder as something that has overtaken their teen and in turn allows them (the parents) to be effective in their interventions.

FBT is consistent in the application of its core strategies and therapeutic interventions across the developmental spectrum of childhood through adolescence. This consistency often surprises parents and clinicians alike, who assume that prescriptions such as parental control over eating should be modulated to reflect chronological age. Although developmental stage must be respected with regard to the patient's general life and broad psychosocial domains, the eating disorder is a leveling force that renders the child or adolescent regressed with regard to ability to appropriately self-regulate food intake. Thus parental control should be (1) focused only on the eating disorder symptoms, (2) temporary until sufficient weight is restored for the cognitive symptoms of the eating disorder to improve and motivation for wellness to set in, and (3) only as extreme as the eating disorder is ego-syntonic, with low-weight eating disorder presentations generally requiring more initial parental control and normal-weight binge eating and purging clinical profiles allowing for more collaboration between parents and child in navigating symptom management. As discussed previously, the one FBT-application exception to this algorithm is for pediatric obesity, a nonpsychiatric disorder. Unlike eating disorders, obesity does not affect insight and judgment, although it may be associated with or exacerbated by disordered eating patterns. For this medical condition, degree and intensity of parental control should precisely match developmental stage, attenuating as the child ages, even in early phases of treatment.

The distinctions between FBT for AN, BN, EDNOS, and pediatric obesity, for which there are separate manuals (Le Grange & Lock, 2007; Lock et al., 2001; Loeb et al., 2006, 2011), can be resolved within a trans-diagnostic framework by combining weight status (low vs. normal to high) and specific behavioral symptoms (restriction vs. restriction plus binge eating and/or purging vs. other forms of excessive eating), yielding the following algorithm:

• Low-weight patients will benefit from principles and practices in the AN treatment that are more categorically defined, especially in terms of the allocation and timing of autonomy and control over eating.

   o Low-weight patients with bulimic symptoms will benefit more from the behavioral techniques drawn from the BN protocol, which target binge eating and purging behaviors.

• For normal- to higher-weight adolescents, for whom symptoms may be experienced as more ego-dystonic, the more collaborative parent–child approach described in the BN manual is appropriate.

• For EDNOS, especially for those children and adolescents in whom a more serious eating disorder may be in the process of unfolding, severity, chronicity, and breadth of the eating disorder symptoms must also be considered. Such symptom-driven guidelines may be more useful than age- or developmentally based ones, as clinical observations suggest that a low-weight eating disorder renders a regressed state with regard to self-care that is fairly equivalent across childhood, adolescence, and even adulthood. For individuals above a minimally normal weight threshold, and especially for overweight patients without an eating disorder, maturational stages will serve as a better guide for the intensity and quality of parental involvement in Phase I of FBT.

Strengths and Challenges of FBT

Therapeutic Alliance and Treatment Acceptability

Some studies have examined therapeutic alliance and acceptability of FBT for adolescents with AN (Krautter & Lock, 2004; Le Grange & Gelman, 1998; Pereira, Lock, & Oggins, 2006) and BN (Zaitsoff, Celio-Doyle,

Hoste, & Le Grange, 2008). FBT is a highly demanding therapy in that one of its primary goals is to empower parents to play a significant role in addressing their adolescent's eating disorder. For instance, early on in treatment, the adolescent is not allowed to make independent decisions about eating and weight-related behaviors. This is especially true for AN, and most adolescents become quite resistant to their parents' efforts. It is therefore particularly salient whether this treatment is acceptable for both adolescents and parents. An early qualitative description of FBT in a modest sample of adolescents with AN demonstrated that this form of therapy was ultimately acceptable for adolescents and their families (Le Grange & Gelman, 1998). Additional empirical support for this notion was provided in a larger study of patient satisfaction with FBT for AN in which both quantitative and qualitative evaluations were employed (Krautter & Lock, 2004). In this study, treatment effectiveness and therapeutic alliance were both rated quite high; however, almost a third of participants expressed a desire for individual therapy in addition to the FBT they received. In the most sophisticated study of therapeutic alliance in FBT conducted to date (Pereira et al., 2006), independent assessors scored early and late therapeutic alliances for patients and parents using recorded sessions from an RCT for adolescent AN. Therapeutic alliance throughout treatment was strong for both adolescents and their parents. An early alliance with adolescents predicted early treatment response in terms of weight gain, a strong early alliance with parents prevented dropout, and a strong late parental alliance predicted their child's total weight gain over the course of treatment. To date, only one study has examined the therapeutic alliance and treatment acceptability across FBT and an individual supportive psychotherapy (Zaitsoff et al., 2008). Ratings were positive in both treatments and generally did not differ. Within FBT-BN, more severe eating disorder symptomatology pretreatment was related to lower alliance ratings mid-treatment. However, reductions in binge and purge behaviors over the course of treatment were not related to alliance or acceptability for participants in FBT-BN.

Dissemination and Implementation

Early efforts to disseminate FBT have been documented (Couturier, Isserlan, & Lock, 2010; Loeb et al., 2006). Several factors support the dissemination of FBT. First, detailed clinician manuals are available for AN (Lock et al., 2001), BN (Le Grange & Lock, 2007), EDNOS (Loeb et al., 2011), and obesity (Loeb et al., 2006), and regular workshops are being conducted to train clinicians in FBT (*www.train2treat4ed.com*). Second, FBT is theoretically agnostic in terms of etiology of illness, and, from an implementation perspective, this agnosticism enables therapists from a variety of backgrounds to practice FBT relatively free from any specific theoretical prescriptions. Third, FBT has a substantial behavioral and educational focus, especially for the first part of therapy. Consequently, interventions are relatively straightforward to describe in these treatment manuals, and the process of implementing and mastering these therapeutic techniques can therefore be rehearsed and scrutinized during the training of aspiring therapists.

Potential Barriers to the Implementation of FBT

Therapist Variables

FBT is a behaviorally focused treatment and first addresses eating disorder symptoms before attending to psychosocial concerns. Therefore, FBT focuses on the here-and-now, and insight is not a prerequisite for change. Some therapists may find the initial emphasis on symptomatic behavior appealing because they are able to compartmentalize or postpone any "distractions" and retain their focus on the eating disorder. It also removes the almost insurmountable challenge for the therapist to uncover the "underlying issues" that explain the eating pathology. Yet other therapists may find it irresistible not to attend to the countless psychological "events" that occur during the course of any one psychotherapeutic encounter. Therapists who feel unduly tempted to attend to such events may find FBT a challenge as they sacrifice the initial focus on weight restoration, which is a hallmark of FBT for AN. Another issue for consideration is the FBT therapist's "joining" the family in a non-authoritarian stance. This complex task requires stamina or therapeutic endurance, expert knowledge of eating disorders and basic human nutrition, and taking on the role as team leader and liaison, among others, and ultimately calls for the therapist to take on an authoritative position. Although it is important in the successful implementation of this therapy, this role can be experienced by some therapists as arduous.

Patient and Family Variables

Although FBT can be experienced by many therapists as demanding, it is fair to say that it is even more grueling for parents. A considerable time and effort commitment on the part of the parents is expected. For instance, the first part of treatment requires parents to be available for constant supervision of their adolescent at times when she or he will not be attending school and every meal is eaten at home. During this part of treatment, mealtimes are almost uniformly experienced as stressful by both the parents and their family. Compounding this potential barrier to successful treatment, parents who are critical of their child's eating-disordered behavior (as measured by expressed emotion) could be at risk to drop out of treatment prematurely (Szmukler et al., 1985). Should such critical parents remain in treatment, there is increased probability that the symptomatic behavior will not abate and treatment outcome will be compromised (Le Grange et al., 1992). In such instances it has been shown that a separated format of FBT (meeting with the adolescent and the parents but not together) may be more advantageous (Eisler et al., 2000).

Single parents of adolescents with AN who present with high levels of obsessive and/or compulsive traits are particularly at risk for being taxed beyond their capacity and might require more treatment than in cases in which two parents are present (Lock et al., 2005). On the other hand, single parents of patients with BN do not appear to be at a disadvantage (Doyle, McLean, Washington, Hoste, & Le Grange, 2009).

Conclusions

FBT is a promising outpatient treatment for AN, BN, and their EDNOS variants. The transdiagnostic model of FBT posits that although the etiology of an eating disorder is unknown, the pathology affects the family and home environment in ways that inadvertently allow for symptom maintenance and progression. FBT directly targets and resolves family-level variables, including secrecy, blame, internalization of illness, and extreme active or passive parental responses to the eating disorder. Future research will test these mechanisms, which are currently theoretical.

ACKNOWLEDGMENTS

Work on this chapter was supported in part by grants from the National Institutes of Health (No. R01MH079979, Daniel Le Grange, Principal Investigator; No. K23MH074506, Katharine L. Loeb, Principal Investigator). We thank Terri Bacow for her comments on the manuscript. Daniel Le Grange receives royalties from The Guilford Press for the sale of the published treatment manuals mentioned in this report. Daniel Le Grange and Katharine L. Loeb receive honoraria from the Training Institute for Child and Adolescent Eating Disorders, LLC.

REFERENCES

American Psychiatric Association. (1980). *Diagnostic and statistical manual of mental disorders* (3rd ed.). Washington, DC: Author.

American Psychiatric Association. (1987). *Diagnostic and statistical manual of mental disorders* (3rd ed., rev.). Washington, DC: Author.

American Psychiatric Association. (2000). *Diagnostic and statistical manual of mental disorders* (4th ed., text rev.). Washington, DC: Author.

American Psychiatric Association. (2013). *Diagnostic and statistical manual of mental disorders* (5th ed.). Arlington, VA: Author.

Ben-Tovim, D. I., Walker, K., Gilchrist, P., Freeman, R., Kalucy, R., & Esterman, A. (2001). Outcome in patients with eating disorders: A five-year study. *Lancet, 357,* 1254–1257.

Binford, R. B., & Le Grange, D. (2005). Adolescents with bulimia nervosa and eating disorder not otherwise specified—purging only. *International Journal of Eating Disorders, 38,* 157–161.

Crow, S. (2007). Eating disorder not otherwise specified: Next steps. *International Journal of Eating Disorders, 40,* S104–S106.

Crow, S. J., Agras, W. S., Halmi, K., Mitchell, J. E., & Kraemer, H. C. (2002). Full syndromal versus subthreshold anorexia nervosa, bulimia nervosa, and binge eating disorder: A multicenter study. *International Journal of Eating Disorders, 32,* 309–318.

Couturier, J., Isserlan, L., & Lock, J. (2010). Family-based treatment for adolescents with anorexia nervosa: A dissemination study. *International Journal of Eating Disorders, 43,* 199–209.

Dare, C. (1983). *Family therapy for families containing an anorectic youngster.* Columbus, OH: Ross Laboratories.

Deter, H. C., & Herzog, W. (1994). Anorexia nervosa in a long-term perspective: Results of the Heidelberg–Mannheim study. *Psychosomatic Medicine, 56,* 20–22.

Doyle, A. C., McLean, C., Washington, B. N., Hoste, R. R., & Le Grange, D. (2009). Are single-parent families different from two-parent families in the treatment of adolescent bulimia nervosa using family-based treatment? *International Journal of Eating Disorders, 42,* 153–157.

Eddy, K. T., Dorer, D. J., Franko, D. L., Tahilani, K., Thompson-Brenner, H., & Herzog, D. B. (2008). Diagnostic crossover in anorexia nervosa and bulimia nervosa: Implication for DSM-V. *American Journal of Psychiatry, 165,* 245–250.

Eisler, I., Dare, C., Hodes, M., Russell, G., Dodge, E., & Le Grange, D. (2000). Family therapy for adolescent anorexia nervosa: The results of a controlled comparison of two family interventions. *Journal of Child Psychology and Psychiatry and Allied Disciplines, 41,* 727–736.

Eisler, I., Dare, C., Russell, G. F. M., Szmukler, G., Le Grange, D., & Dodge, E. (1997). Family and individual therapy in anorexia nervosa: A five-year follow-up. *Archives of General Psychiatry, 54,* 1025–1030.

Eisler, I., Simic, M., Russell, G. F. M., & Dare, C. (2007). A randomized controlled treatment trial of two forms of family therapy in adolescent anorexia nervosa: A five-year follow-up. *Journal of Child Psychology and Psychiatry, 48,* 552–560.

Fairburn, C. G. (2008). *Cognitive behavior therapy and eating disorders.* New York: Guilford Press.

Fairburn, C. G., & Cooper, Z. (2007). Thinking afresh about the classification of eating disorders. *International Journal of Eating Disorders, 40,* S107–S110.

Fairburn, C. G., Cooper, Z., Bohn, K., O'Connor, M. E., Doll, H. A., & Palmer, R. L. (2007). The severity and status of eating disorder NOS: Implications for DSM-V. *Behavior Research and Therapy, 45,* 1705–1715.

Fairburn, C. G., Cooper, Z., Doll, H. A., O'Connor, M. E., Bohn, K., Hawker, D. M., et al. (2009). Transdiagnostic cognitive-behavior therapy for patients with eating disorders: A two-site trial with a 60-week follow up. *American Journal of Psychiatry, 166,* 311–319.

Fairburn, C. G., Cooper, Z., & Shafran, R. (2003). Cognitive behavior therapy for eating disorders: A "transdiagnostic" theory and treatment. *Behaviour Research and Therapy, 41,* 509–528.

Fichter, M. M., & Quadflieg, N. (2007). Long-term stability of eating disorder diagnoses. *International Journal of Eating Disorders, 40,* S61–S66.

Fichter, M. M., Quadflieg, N., & Hedlund, S. (2006). Twelve-year course and outcome predictors of anorexia nervosa. *International Journal of Eating Disorders, 39,* 87–100.

Foa, E. B., & Kozak, M. J. (1986). Emotional processing of fear: Exposure to corrective information. *Psychological Bulletin, 99,* 20–35.

Gowers, S. G., Clark, A., Roberts, C., Griffiths, A., Edwards, V., Bryan, C., et al. (2007). Clinical effectiveness of treatments for anorexia nervosa in adolescents: Randomised controlled trial. *British Journal of Psychiatry, 191,* 427–435.

Herzog, D. B., Hopkins, J. D., & Burns, C. D. (1993). A follow-up study of 33 subdiagnostic eating disordered women. *International Journal of Eating Disorders, 14,* 261–267.

Hildebrandt, T., Bacow, T., Markella, M., & Loeb, K. L. (2012). Anxiety in anorexia nervosa and its management using family-based treatment. *European Eating Disorders Review, 20,* e1–e16.

Krautter, T., &, Lock, J. (2004). Is manualized family-based treatment for adolescent anorexia nervosa acceptable to patients?: Patient satisfaction at end of treatment. *Journal of Family Therapy, 26,* 65–81.

Le Grange, D., Binford, R., Peterson, C., Crow, S., Crosby, R., Klein, M., et al. (2006). DSM-IV threshold versus sub-threshold bulimia nervosa. *International Journal of Eating Disorders, 39,* 462–467.

Le Grange, D., & Chen, E. (2007). *Family-based treatment for young adults with anorexia nervosa.* Unpublished manual, University of Chicago.

Le Grange, D., Crosby, R. D., & Lock, J. (2008). Predictors and moderators of outcome in family-based treatment for adolescent bulimia nervosa. *Journal of the American Academy of Child and Adolescent Psychiatry, 47,* 464–470.

Le Grange, D., Crosby, R. D., Rathouz, P. J., & Leventhal, B. L. (2007). A randomized controlled comparison of family-based treatment and supportive psychotherapy for adolescent bulimia nervosa. *Archives of General Psychiatry, 64,* 1049–1056.

Le Grange, D., Eisler, I., Dare, C., & Hodes, M. (1992). Family criticism and self-starvation: A study of expressed emotion. *Journal of Family Therapy, 14,* 177–192.

Le Grange, D., Eisler, I., Dare, C., & Russell, G. F. M. (1992). Evaluation of family treatments in adolescent anorexia nervosa: A pilot study. *International Journal of Eating Disorders, 12,* 347–357.

Le Grange, D., & Gelman, T. (1998). The patient's perspective of treatment in eating disorders: A preliminary study. *South African Journal of Psychology, 28,* 182–186.

Le Grange, D., & Lock, J. (2007). *Treating bulimia in adolescence: A family-based approach.* New York: Guilford Press.

Le Grange, D., & Loeb, K. L. (2007). Early identification and treatment of eating disorders: Prodrome to syndrome. *Early Intervention in Psychiatry, 1,* 27–39.

Le Grange, D., Loeb, K. L., Van Orman, S., & Jellar, C. C. (2004). Bulimia nervosa in adolescents: A disorder in evolution? *Archives of Pediatrics and Adolescent Medicine, 158,* 478–482.

Lewinsohn, P. M., Striegel-Moore, R. H., & Seeley, J. R. (2001). Epidemiology and natural course of eating disorders in young women from adolescence to young adulthood. *Journal of the American Academy of Child and Adolescent Psychiatry, 39,* 1284–1292.

Lock, J., Agras, W. S., Bryson, S., & Kraemer, H. C. (2005). A comparison of short- and long-term family therapy for adolescent anorexia nervosa. *Journal of the American Academy of Child and Adolescent Psychiatry, 44,* 632–639.

Lock, J., Couturier, J., & Agras, W. S. (2006). Comparison of long term outcomes in adolescents with anorexia nervosa treated with family therapy. *Journal of the American Academy of Child and Adolescent Psychiatry, 46,* 666–672.

Lock, J., Le Grange, D., Agras, W. S., & Dare, C. (2001). *Treatment manual for anorexia nervosa: A family-based approach.* New York: Guilford Press.

Lock, J., Le Grange, D., Agras, S., Moye, A., Bryson, S., & Jo, B. (2010). Randomized clinical trial comparing family-based treatment to adolescent-focused individual therapy for adolescents with anorexia nervosa. *Archives of General Psychiatry, 67,* 1025–1032.

Lock, J., Le Grange, D., Forsberg, S., & Hewell, K. (2006). Is family therapy useful for treating children with anorexia nervosa?: Results of a case series. *Journal of the American Academy of Child and Adolescent Psychiatry, 45,* 1323–1328.

Loeb, K. L., Celio Doyle, A., Le Grange, D., Bremer, J., Hildebrandt, T., & Hirsch, A. (2006). *Family-based treatment for child and adolescent overweight: A transdevelopmental approach.* Unpublished manual, Mount Sinai School of Medicine.

Loeb, K. L., Craigen, K. E., Munk Goldstein, M., Lock, J., & Le Grange, D. (2011). Early treatment of eating disorders. In D. Le Grange & J. Lock (Eds.), *Handbook of assessment and treatment for children and adolescents with eating disorders* (pp. 337–361). New York: Guilford Press.

Loeb, K. L., Lock, J., Le Grange, D., & Greif, R. (2012). Transdiagnostic theory and application of family-based treatment for youth with eating disorders. *Cognitive and Behavioral Practice, 19,* 17–30.

Loeb, K. L., Walsh, B. T., Lock, J., Le Grange, D., Jones, J., Marcus, S., et al. (2007). Open trial of family-based treatment for full and partial anorexia nervosa in adolescence: Evidence of successful dissemination. *Journal of the American Academy of Child and Adolescent Psychiatry, 46,* 792–800.

Lucas, A. R., Beard, C. M., O'Fallon, W. M., & Kurland, L. T. (1991). 50-year trends in the incidence of anorexia nervosa in Rochester, Minn.: A population-based study. *American Journal of Psychiatry, 148,* 917–929.

McIntosh, V. V., Jordan, J., Carter, F. A., McKenzie, J. M., Luty, S. E., Bulik, C. M., et al. (2004). Strict versus lenient weight criterion in anorexia nervosa. *European Eating Disorders Review, 12,* 51–60.

Milos, G., Spindler, A., Schnyder, U., & Fairburn, C. G. (2005). Instability of eating disorder diagnoses: Prospective study. *British Journal of Psychiatry, 187,* 573–578.

Peebles, R., Wilson, J. L., & Lock, J. D. (2006). How do children with eating disorders differ from adolescents with eating disorders at initial evaluation? *Journal of Adolescent Health, 39,* 800–805.

Pereira, T., Lock, J., & Oggins, J. (2006). The role of therapeutic alliance in family therapy for adolescent anorexia nervosa. *International Journal of Eating Disorders, 39*, 677–684.

Ratnasuriya, R. H., Eisler, I., Szmukler, G. I., & Russell, G. F. (1991). Anorexia nervosa: Outcome and prognostic factors after 20 years. *British Journal of Psychiatry, 158*, 495–502.

Ricca, V., Mannucci, E., Mezzani, B., Di Bernardo, M., Zucchi, T., Paionni, A., et al. (2001). Psychopathological and clinical features of outpatients with an eating disorder not otherwise specified. *Eating and Weight Disorders, 6*, 157–165.

Robin, A. L., Siegel, P. T., Moye, A. W., Gilroy, M., Dennis, A. B., & Sikand, A. (1999). A controlled comparison of family versus individual therapy for adolescents with anorexia nervosa. *Journal of the American Academy of Child and Adolescent Psychiatry, 38*, 1482–1489.

Russell, G. F. M., Szmukler, G. I., Dare, C., & Eisler, I. (1987). An evaluation of family therapy in anorexia nervosa and bulimia nervosa. *Archives of General Psychiatry, 44*, 1047–1056.

Schmidt, U., Lee, S., Beecham, J., Perkins, S., Treasure, J., Yi, I., et al. (2007). A randomized controlled trial of family therapy and cognitive behavior therapy guided self-care for adolescents with bulimia nervosa and related disorders. *American Journal of Psychiatry, 164*, 591–598.

Stice, E., Killen, J. D., Hayward, C., & Taylor, C. B. (1998). Support for the continuity hypothesis of bulimic pathology. *Journal of Consulting and Clinical Psychology, 66*, 784–790.

Szmukler, G. I., Eisler, I., Russell, G. F. M., & Dare, C. (1985). Anorexia nervosa, parental "expressed emotion" and dropping out of treatment. *British Journal of Psychiatry, 147*, 265–271.

Tozzi, F., Thornton, L. M., Klump, K. L., Fichter, M. M., Halmi, K. A., Kaplan, A. S., et al. (2005). Symptom fluctuation in eating disorders: Correlates of diagnostic crossover. *American Journal of Psychiatry, 162*, 732–740.

Wadden, T. A., Brownell, K. D., & Foster, G. D. (2002). Obesity: Responding to the global epidemic. *Journal of Consulting and Clinical Psychology, 70*, 510–525.

Waller, G. (2008). A "trans-transdiagnostic" model of the eating disorders: A new way to open the egg? *European Eating Disorders Review, 16*, 165–172.

Watson, T. L., & Andersen, A. E. (2003). A critical examination of the amenorrhea and weight criteria for diagnosing anorexia nervosa. *Acta Psychiatric Scandinavia Supplement, 108*, 175–182.

Wentz, E., Gillberg, C., Gillberg, I., & Rastam, M. (2001). Ten-year follow-up of adolescent anorexia nervosa: Psychiatric disorders and overall functioning scales. *Journal of Child Psychology and Psychiatry, 42*, 613–622.

Wilfley, D. E., Bishop, M. E., Wilson, G. T., & Agras, W. S. (2007). Classification of eating disorders: Toward DSM-V. *International Journal of Eating Disorders, 40*, S123–S129.

Wonderlich, S., Crosby, R., Joiner, T., Peterson, C. B., Bardone-Cone, A., Klein, A., et al. (2005). Personality subtyping and bulimia nervosa: Psychopathological and genetic correlates. *Psychosomatic Medicine, 35*, 649–657.

Wonderlich, S. A., Crosby, R. D., Mitchell, J. E., & Engel, S. G. (2007). Testing the validity of eating disorder diagnoses. *International Journal of Eating Disorders,* *40,* S40–S45.

Wonderlich, S. A., Joiner, T. E., Keel, P. K., Williamson, D. A., & Crosby, R. D. (2007). Eating disorder diagnoses: Empirical approaches to classification. *American Psychologist, 62,* 167–180.

Workgroup for Classification of Eating Disorders in Children and Adolescents. (2007). Classification of child and adolescent eating disturbances. *International Journal of Eating Disorders, 40,* S117–S122.

Workgroup for Classification of Eating Disorders in Children and Adolescents. (2010). Classification of eating disturbance in children and adolescents: Proposed changes to the DSM-V. *European Eating Disorders Review, 18,* 79–89.

Zaitsoff, S., Celio-Doyle, A., Hoste, R., & Le Grange, D. (2008). How do adolescents with bulimia nervosa rate the acceptability and therapeutic relationship in family-based treatment? *International Journal of Eating Disorders, 41,* 390–398.

CHAPTER 17

Unified Protocol for Youth with Chronic Pain in Pediatric Medical Settings

Laura A. Payne, Jennie C. I. Tsao, and Lonnie K. Zeltzer

Health problems in children and adolescents can have a significant impact on social, family, and academic functioning. Short-term effects of significant medical problems include missed school, withdrawal from social and physical activities, and family stress and tension. However, long-term effects of health problems in youth may be even more deleterious. In addition to placing them at risk for future health problems, significant medical conditions can also lead to chronic illness, premature death, and emotional disorders (Power, DuPaul, Shapiro, & Parrish, 1998). In fact, the high rate of comorbid emotional disorders, particularly anxiety and depression, has proved to be an obstacle to the effective treatment of chronic pain (Eccleston et al., 2012; Keefe et al., 2001). Because chronic pain is a common pediatric medical condition and involves the interaction of biological, social, and psychological factors (Gatchel, Peng, Peters, Fuchs, & Turk, 2007), it is well suited to psychosocial intervention. This chapter focuses largely on the psychosocial transdiagnostic conceptualization of pediatric chronic nonmalignant pain with comorbid anxiety and depression.

Definition of Transdiagnostic Theory in Relation to Medical Conditions

A transdiagnostic approach may represent a more efficient, and possibly more efficacious, way to ameliorate overlapping emotional disorder symptomatology (comorbidity), in addition to facilitating effective dissemination of empirically supported treatments to practicing clinicians

(Allen, Ehrenreich, & Barlow, 2005). We believe that chronic pain disorders naturally fit within this transdiagnostic paradigm, given that many patients present with multiple chronic pain complaints (Perquin et al., 2000). Evidence supporting a pain and emotional transdiagnostic approach is also found in the high rates of psychological comorbidity in chronic pain populations, common neurobiological underpinnings, evidence of emotion dysregulation associated with chronic pain, and the efficacy of cognitive-behavioral strategies for managing chronic pain. The treatment presented here is an adaptation of the Unified Protocol for the Treatment of Emotional Disorders in Adolescents (UP-A; Ehrenreich-May et al., 2008; Ehrenreich, Goldstein, Wright, & Barlow, 2009) for use with adolescents (ages 12–17) with a chronic pain disorder and self-reported symptoms of anxiety and/or depression. Our adaptation of the protocol differs substantially from the UP-A by emphasizing emotional reactions to discomfort *and pain*—an area that is only minimally addressed in the UP-A in the context of interoceptive exposure and panic attacks.

The Unified Protocol for the Treatment of Emotions in Youth with Pain (UP-YP; Allen, Tsao, Zeltzer, Ehrenreich-May, & Barlow, 2010) is a transdiagnostic treatment using cognitive-behavioral principles to address both pain-related and emotional dysfunction. This unified approach differs from the transdiagnostic approaches described in the current literature (e.g., Masia Warner, Reigada, Fisher, Saborsky, & Benkov, 2009; Reigada, Fisher, Cutler, & Masia Warner, 2008) in a number of important ways. First, from a theoretical perspective, the UP-YP goes beyond the application of general cognitive-behavioral strategies to pain and anxiety and instead focuses on identifying and modifying maladaptive emotion regulation (ER) and response strategies associated with the experience of pain. Although the techniques may be similar to traditional cognitive-behavioral therapy (CBT), the function is different. In the UP-YP, the therapist aims to implement more adaptive ER skills using a variety of situations and contexts, and this theoretical shift allows the UP-YP to be applied to any emotional experience, regardless of whether it stems from pain or is related to anxiety, depression, anger, or other emotions. Second, as this theoretical perspective implies, therapists will not be limited to working with only certain types of pain disorders or emotional comorbidity (including depressive disorders). Even though the particular situations and contexts may vary depending on symptom presentation, the function of the treatment strategies is similar, that is, to assist patients in learning adaptive ways to manage their emotional distress.

Description of the Clinical Population

Chronic pain, including functional disorders such as complex regional pain Syndrome Type 1 (CRPS-1), chronic daily headaches, fibromyalgia, myofascial pain disorders, and recurrent abdominal pain, is a significant medical problem among youth. Chronic pain has been defined as recurrent or continuous pain lasting more than 3 months (Perquin et al., 2000). Epidemiological work indicates that more than 45% of children ages 10–18 report chronic pain, most commonly headaches, abdominal pain, limb pain, and back pain (Perquin et al., 2000; Roth-Isigkeit, Thyen, Raspe, Stoven, & Schmucker, 2004). There are significant economic costs associated with medical problems such as chronic pain. For example, use of health-care services is higher in adolescents with chronic pain, resulting in significant financial burdens to families and government programs. One study of 70 adolescents with juvenile rheumatoid arthritis found that the mean annualized direct cost per child was $7,905, with extra school costs estimated at $1,449 and family costs at $1,524 per year (Allaire, DeNardo, Szer, Meenan, & Schaller, 1992). More recently, annual costs for each child with chronic pain in the United Kingdom are estimated at £8000 (approximately $12,170 in U.S. currency), resulting in a yearly nationwide cost of £3840 million (Sleed, Eccleston, Beecham, Knapp, & Jordan, 2005).

Youth with chronic pain can also exhibit patterns of "doctor seeking" and overutilization of medications, as well as high levels of psychosocial distress and dysfunction (Palermo, Krell, Janosy, & Zeltzer, 2008; Zeltzer & Krell, 2007). A significant concern for children and adolescents with chronic pain is the high rate of comorbid anxiety and depression in this patient population (Campo et al., 2004; Campo, Comer, Jansen-McWilliams, Gardner, & Kelleher, 2002; Dorn et al., 2003; Ghanizadeh et al., 2007; Lipsitz et al., 2005; Ramchandani, Fazel, Stein, Wiles, & Hotopf, 2007). Generally, results across these studies indicate a greater risk of comorbid anxiety and/or unipolar mood disorders, as well as increased levels of anxiety and depression symptoms in individuals with chronic pain. These data highlight the significant overlap between physical and psychological disorders.

UP-YP Treatment Approach

The UP-YP is a flexible, modular-based individual treatment protocol. A full course of treatment can consist of between eight and twenty-one 50-minute sessions, all occurring within a 6-month time frame. It is recommended that, at least initially, sessions occur on a weekly basis. However, as termination approaches, sessions may be spaced out to every 2 weeks. Therapists using the UP-YP are expected to have some level of familiarity with traditional CBT protocols; however, initial research has shown that even junior-level therapists are able to successfully use the original Unified Protocol for the Transdiagnostic Treatment of Emotional Disorders (UP; Barlow et al., 2010) (Ellard, Fairholme, Boisseau, Farchione, & Barlow, 2010) and the UP-A (Ehrenreich et al., 2009).

The UP-YP modules are as follows (described in more detail subsequently): (1) psychoeducation about emotions and pain, (2) awareness of emotions and pain, (3) flexibility in thinking, (4) modifying emotion-driven behaviors through exposures, and (5) treatment review and relapse prevention. In addition, several optional modules are available for therapists, which include: (1) building and keeping motivation, (2) keeping safe (for adolescents with suicidal ideation or intent), and (3) parenting the emotional adolescent with pain. Regarding delivery of the UP-YP, it is important to note that some of the basic procedures described in the protocol are not necessarily different from the procedures a therapist might employ using a traditional CBT protocol. In fact, it is the theoretical underpinnings and conceptualization that makes the UP-YP unique and different from traditional CBT. Whereas CBT aims to improve emotional reactions through modification of maladaptive cognitions and elimination of conditioned associations with environmental cues, the UP-YP aims to modify both pain and emotions based on emotion theory using an ER framework—that is, creating emotional change through reduced emotional avoidance and modification of action tendencies. Therefore, although the techniques may appear similar for clients with similar diagnoses or symptoms, the potential value of the UP-YP is in teaching therapists the necessary targets of emotional change so that strategies can be applied flexibly and individually across clients with various presenting complaints.

UP-YP Modules

Module 1: Psychoeducation about Emotions and Pain

The first module of the UP-YP consists primarily of psychoeducation about emotions and pain responses. Treatment begins with a review of the functional/adaptive nature of emotions and pain, describing how both are signals that can give important information about the environment. Clients are instructed in and asked to monitor the *three-component model of pain* by reviewing thoughts, physical sensations, and behaviors associated with pain responses. Then the cycle of pain is discussed in relation to the concept of negative reinforcement. For example, with a 14-year-old boy with chronic daily headache, the relationship between physical sensations (head pain), thoughts (e.g., "If I go out with my friends, my head pain will get worse and it will never get better"), and behaviors (staying home in a dark room) were explicitly discussed, emphasizing how this cycle contributes to more frequent and intense levels of head pain. In addition, this particular boy's *emotional* response to head pain (i.e., anxiety) was discussed as an additional factor that contributes to the cycle of pain. Clients are also asked to monitor pain levels, moods, and anxiety over the course of each week. Because the UP-YP is heavily focused on emotions and (eventual) modification of subsequent responses, these practices begin to develop the skill of emotional awareness, which is essential for implementing future aspects of the protocol.

Module 2: Awareness of Emotions and Pain

The second module of the UP-YP focuses specifically on awareness of emotions through the use of practices designed to elicit different emotions. The first awareness skill involves using diaphragmatic breathing as an opportunity for the client to become more aware of what he or she is feeling, both physically and emotionally. Consistent with an emotional acceptance-based approach and in contrast to traditional CBT, the UP-YP does not emphasize breathing as a way to "relax," as this may have the unintended effect of creating increased levels of anxiety/stress because of the implied goal of suppressing any "nonrelaxing" experiences. In this sense, breathing is only used as a tool to increase awareness. The client is also asked to engage in some brief exposures designed to trigger at least mild pain symptoms. During these exposures, the goal is not to create or exacerbate this pain per se; rather, clients are encouraged to practice being aware of *emotional responses* to the pain. In this sense, the UP-YP targets the emotional dysregulation (affective component) related to pain rather than the sensory experience of pain. A 15-year-old girl with chronic low back pain and generalized anxiety disorder (GAD) practiced slowly bending over until she began to feel the sensation of pain in her back, noticing those sensations and her emotional reactions for a minute and then returning to a standing posture. As she continued to practice this exercise, she became more aware that even subtle sensations in her back triggered an anxious response, and thus she was better able to understand the connection between her physical sensations of pain and her anxiety.

During this module, the UP-YP also emphasizes the role of *emotional avoidance* and its relationship to pain responses. Emotional avoidance strategies include any action that attempts to minimize, control, or dampen an emotion. The conceptualization of emotional avoidance and its contribution to pain is a unique and specific goal of the transdiagnostic approach inherent in the UP-YP. Whereas traditional CBT protocols, or protocols addressing pain and anxiety, may identify specific behavioral targets of change (e.g., exposures), the UP-YP focuses on identifying and modifying potentially any situation in which the individual is attempting to control, avoid, or escape from emotions. For adolescents with chronic pain and anxiety/depression, emotional avoidance strategies can comprise a wide range of behaviors. A client with chronic head pain may wear sunglasses to prevent excessive light that could exacerbate head pain and anxiety, whereas a client with recurrent abdominal pain may avoid certain foods in an attempt to regulate stomach discomfort and anxiety. Another adolescent with fibromyalgia and depression may avoid physical contact with her parents, as hugging them triggers both body pain and increased feelings of loneliness. Most important during this module, the therapist must begin to pay close attention to the ways in which each client attempts to manage his or her pain and emotional responses, as these are often a clue to the emotional avoidance strategies used.

Module 3: Flexibility in Thinking

Module 3 addresses the cognitive component of pain and emotional experiences. First, "thoughts" are described as "interpretations," and clients are asked to consider how interpretations are subject to personal experience and emotional reactions. This notion is illustrated through the presentation of an ambiguous picture. Each client is asked to determine what the picture means. Then each interpretation is discussed as a function of what information the client focused on to generate that interpretation, as well as the emotional state that the client is experiencing at the time. Subsequently, alternative interpretations are generated in session, and the importance of flexibility in thinking is highlighted. Next, the specific skills for responding to automatic interpretations are reviewed, including identification of "thinking traps" (i.e., negative or unhelpful ways of thinking that are easy to get "stuck" in, such as "jumping to conclusions" or "thinking the worst") and "detective questioning" (i.e., using evidence from past experience to consider whether automatic interpretations are accurate). These skills help clients consider the broader context of interpretations, particularly the influence of emotional states on attention to information to generate interpretations. In chronic pain, cycles of negative interpretations lead to maladaptive behaviors, such as social withdrawal and isolation. Challenging interpretations about the consequences or impact of pain can help modify this negative cycle.

The skills of this module are illustrated in the example of a girl with recurrent abdominal pain, whole-body pain, and depression. This client was able to identify a core thought related to her experience of pain (i.e., "I'll never be allowed to leave my parents' house if I have chronic pain"), as well as a core depressive thought (i.e., "No one understands me"). Both these thoughts were identified as thinking traps ("jumping to conclusions" and "thinking the worst," respectively). Detective questioning skills were used to help her consider that her interpretations were at least partly a function of her mood and to help her generate alternative interpretations of her physical and emotional pain experiences.

Module 4: Modifying Emotion-Driven Behaviors through Exposures

The fourth module of the UP-YP involves specifically designing and executing situational exposures that trigger uncomfortable emotions so that behaviors that occur during the experience of emotion (i.e., "emotion-driven behaviors," usually escape during the experience of fear or discomfort) can be modified and emotional avoidance and safety behaviors reduced or eliminated. In this module, triggers can vary from interoceptive (e.g., pain) to situational (e.g., in vivo), so that the therapist has greater flexibility to design effective emotion exposures. This module typically begins with in-session interoceptive exercises using a symptom induction test, in which clients are asked to engage in three exercises: spinning while standing, hyperventilating, and breathing through a thin straw. These exercises are designed to induce a mild to moderate degree of physical discomfort, and the exercise that triggers the most discomfort is assigned for practice out of session. Through repeated practice, the connection between the physical discomfort and the client's emotional reaction begins to weaken, as he or she learns that physical discomfort is to some degree under his or her control and does not necessarily lead to catastrophic consequences. Although these exercises are typically used with clients who have panic disorder, interoceptive cues can be a strong trigger for a variety of emotional disorders (including depression), as well as chronic pain, given the strong relationship of anxiety sensitivity to pain responses (Tsao et al., 2004).

Other out-of-session practices can focus on designing any situation that will elicit the emotion or physical sensation that is dysregulated and avoided. It is not necessary to focus on one particular situation or emotion (e.g., assigning only social situational exposures for a child who has social anxiety); rather, the flexibility of the UP-YP allows the therapist to assign exposures that can be very broadly focused to target the emotional dysregulation inherent in chronic pain. Through these exposures, avoidance is reduced or eliminated.

Some examples of emotion exposures in adolescents with chronic pain and anxiety/depression have included reading poetry out loud (both in session and later in class) for social anxiety, writing poetry and short paragraphs about sadness and isolation for depression, and touching bathroom walls for anxiety about contamination. Examples of exposures specific to emotions related to pain include going on a school field trip without a parent for anxiety related to head pain, attending band practice while in mild physical discomfort for depression related to whole-body pain, and drinking a large amount of water for anxiety related to recurrent abdominal pain.

Module 5: Treatment Review and Relapse Prevention

The final module (Module 5) typically consists of one session to review progress and anticipate future difficulties. At this session, progress over the course of treatment is highlighted, and skills learned during each module are reviewed. Clients are asked to consider future obstacles and how to implement skills learned to deal with these obstacles.

Optional Modules

Three optional modules are also included in the UP-YP. The first is *Building and Keeping Motivation*, which encourages therapists to use motivational enhancement techniques (e.g., expressing empathy, developing discrepancy, rolling with resistance, supporting self-efficacy) to motivate and engage the client in the treatment strategies (for a review of motivational interviewing strategies, see Miller & Rollnick, 2012). The strategies provided in this module may be especially important at the beginning of the therapy but may also be beneficial as the therapy progresses into more challenging sessions, when disengagement from the therapy is common (Ehrenreich-May et al., 2008). The second optional module, *Keeping Safe/ Dealing with Difficult Times*, is designed for adolescents who struggle with depression and suicidal ideation. This module can last up to three flexible sessions, in which the therapist deviates from the module in an effort to address events that indicate a substantial worsening of functioning and may interfere with the delivery of the protocol. Some of the strategies in this module include developing a safety plan (in the case of suicidal ideation) and building positive experiences and events into an activity schedule. The third optional module, *Parenting the Emotional Adolescent with Pain*, can include up to three sessions in which the therapist meets with the parent(s) to review the treatment rationale, to discuss how to respond to distressed adolescents, and to discuss common conflicts between adolescents and parents. Parent sessions may be scheduled separately from the individual sessions with the client.

The optional modules are particularly important for youth with pain. Often hopelessness and despair about the future associated with a chronic health condition (such as pain) can pervade a child's or adolescent's thoughts and may trigger thoughts of self-harm. Parenting skills are also critical, as parents may have unwittingly been reinforcing the pain experience in their child through negative reinforcement or encouraging coping with avoidance.

Support for Mechanisms Underlying Chronic Pain and Emotions

The biopsychosocial model of pain purports that chronic pain represents a complex interaction of biological, psychological, and social factors (Gatchel et al., 2007). Pain itself is a multidimensional construct incorporating both sensory (e.g., intensity, duration) and affective (emotional) aspects. Recognition of the affective dimension of pain has focused attention on the ways in which mood states influence the pain experience. For example, higher levels of anticipatory anxiety about an upcoming pain task have been shown to predict increased pain responses to that pain task in children and adolescents (Tsao et al., 2004). Research over the past several decades has begun to provide support for the concept of common mechanisms underlying both pain and emotions.

Neurobiological Mechanisms

Although the mechanisms by which emotions influence pain (and vice versa) are unclear, it is possible that pain and emotions share similar neurobiological pathways. A recent study explored the neural correlates of pain anticipation in a sample of participants with and without major depressive disorder (MDD) (Strigo, Simmons, Matthews, Craig, & Paulus, 2008). Results suggested that anticipation of the pain task led to increased activity in brain areas associated with emotional reactivity only for participants with MDD. Furthermore, in participants with MDD only, greater activation in the right amygdala during anticipation of pain was associated with greater levels of perceived helplessness. The authors suggest that the presence of MDD may lead to an impaired ability to modulate painful experiences due to activation of these emotional centers of the brain (Strigo et al., 2008). Others have highlighted the role of the endogenous opioid system in the modulation of both pain and stress (anxiety; Ribeiro, Kennedy, Smith, Stohler, & Zubieta, 2005).

Emotion Regulation

Given the prominent role of mood in modulating the pain experience, it follows that difficulties in regulating emotions may have an adverse impact on pain. ER refers to attempts to change subjective experiential, cognitive, behavioral, or physiological emotional responses in oneself or others. Although some approaches are adaptive, growing evidence suggests that *excessive* and rigid attempts to control, suppress, or hide emotional experiences results in increased levels, intensity, and duration of the very emotion the individual is attempting to regulate (Barrett, Rapee, Dadds, & Ryan, 1996; Gross, 2002; Keefe et al., 2001; Zeman, Cassano, Perry-Parrish, & Stegall, 2006).

Although evidence now supports the concept of emotion dysregulation as both a contributing and a maintaining factor for emotional disorders, more recently this concept has been extended to physical health and pain. Initial findings highlight a potentially important role of ER in pain responses, with evidence pointing especially to problems with emotion identification and expression (Lumley, Beyer, & Radcliffe, 2008; Mattila et al., 2008; Tuzer et al., 2010). Similarly, the tendency to inhibit or suppress feelings appears to have deleterious consequences with regard to pain. In laboratory studies, students instructed to suppress thoughts of pain demonstrated poorer recovery following a cold-pressor pain task as compared with students who were asked to monitor pain responses. In addition, recall of pain intensity was significantly higher in the suppression group (Cioffi & Holloway, 1993). In a separate investigation, when individuals were asked to suppress thoughts about pain prior to a pain task, they reported significantly more intrusive thoughts about the pain and greater pain severity as compared with those who were not asked to suppress (Sullivan, Rouse, Bishop, & Johnston, 1997). In chronic pain patients (women with fibromyalgia), intensity of affect was related to more severe pain only for those individuals who also had difficulty identifying and expressing feelings (van Middendorp et al., 2008). These findings suggest that interventions aimed at improving ER and psychological flexibility (i.e., flexibility in behavioral responding to various emotional states) may assist in the amelioration of chronic pain.

Support for Transdiagnostic Treatment Approaches to Chronic Pain in Children

Psychologically based therapies are commonly used to assist individuals with chronic pain to improve function and reduce disability (Jensen, Nielson, & Kerns, 2003). In a recent review, Eccleston and colleagues (2012) found that psychological therapies (such as CBT, biofeedback, hypnosis, and relaxation) were effective for treating pain in children with headache, abdominal pain, and musculoskeletal pain. Similar results were obtained in a meta-analysis of psychological therapies for children with pain (Palermo, Eccleston, Lewandowski, Williams, & Morley, 2010). Even though CBT has been shown to be efficacious for a number of specific pain conditions, evidence suggests that youth often present with multiple pain complaints (Perquin et al., 2000), which may require a more comprehensive treatment approach.

In response to this need, a number of transdiagnostic treatment approaches have been developed for adolescents with chronic pain. A modification of acceptance and commitment therapy (ACT; Hayes, Strosahl, & Wilson, 1999)—a cognitive-behavioral approach that uses exposures in combination with acceptance—has been applied to adolescents with chronic pain. ACT strategies focus on helping the client determine his or her personal *values* and encouraging participation in valued activities while accepting what the client cannot change in the situation (e.g., levels of pain in that moment, negative thoughts and feelings). The components and strategies are conceptualized as universal processes in individuals with pain and therefore are not specific to any particular pain or emotional condition. Initial pilot testing of this protocol in adolescents with chronic pain revealed that adolescents treated with ACT showed significant improvements in functional ability, school attendance, catastrophizing, and pain (i.e., intensity and interference) following treatment, and these gains were maintained at 3- and 6-month follow-up assessments (Wicksell, Melin, & Olsson, 2007). More recently, a randomized controlled trial of this protocol demonstrated success as compared with a multidisciplinary treatment approach that included amitriptyline (Wicksell, Melin, Lekander, & Olsson, 2009).

Another promising approach that addresses the high rate of comorbidity of anxiety seen in chronic pain conditions is the treatment for anxiety and physical symptoms (TAPS), specifically for adolescents with chronic pain and comorbid separation, social, or generalized anxiety disorders (Reigada et al., 2008). The TAPS program was developed to jointly address anxiety and uncomfortable physical symptoms (i.e., pain) through identifying situations in which both anxiety and pain are experienced and may interact to exacerbate one another. The protocol, based on the Coping Cat workbook (Kendall, 1992), uses a standard cognitive-behavioral approach, including psychoeducation, relaxation, cognitive restructuring, and exposures. The Coping Cat approach is modified in several specific ways to make it more applicable to anxiety and pain-related sensations, including emphasizing the connection between anxiety and somatic sensations, specific instruction in diaphragmatic breathing for the purpose of reducing physical discomfort, broadening the focus of cognitive restructuring strategies to include thoughts related to somatic symptoms, planning and executing exposures that target pain, and increasing parent involvement. In a pilot, single-arm study, seven children (ages 8–15) with abdominal pain and anxiety received 12 weekly sessions of individual TAPS treatment, with all participants classified as treatment responders (reductions in diagnostic severity, anxiety, and pain; Masia Warner et al., 2009). Although additional data are needed to confirm these findings in a larger, more diverse sample, these results at least initially suggest that a transdiagnostic approach targeting physical symptoms and anxiety is a feasible and efficacious method of addressing chronic pain in children.

Empirical Support for the UP-YP

The UP-YP has not yet been extensively tested in an open or randomized controlled trial. However, an initial pilot study using a multiple baseline across-subjects design demonstrated improvements in functional disability, anxiety and depression, and positive and negative affect (Allen, Tsao, & Zeltzer, 2009). In addition, two cases of adolescents who received treatment using the UP-YP have been described in detail in a recent manuscript

(Allen, Tsao, Seidman, Ehrenreich-May, & Zeltzer, 2012) In brief, over the course of treatment, a 14-year-old boy with chronic daily headache, high functioning autism spectrum disorder (ASD), and social anxiety demonstrated improvement in levels of functional disability and self-reported symptoms of anxiety and depression; emotional awareness and expression increased, and somatization decreased. Continued improvements occurred over the course of the 3-month follow-up period. Interestingly, this adolescent's pain levels changed little over treatment but did show some improvement over follow-up. Another 17-year-old girl with whole-body pain, abdominal pain, and depression demonstrated little improvement in functional disability, pain, depression, and somatization over the course of treatment. However, she showed improvement on all measures across follow-up, suggesting that she may have been able to implement some of the skills she learned after treatment ended. Her parents also reported a notable change in her overall mood and irritability at follow-up.

These data provide some initial support for the UP-YP as a comprehensive, transdiagnostic treatment protocol that can address both pain-related and emotional dysfunction in adolescents. There may be several potential mechanisms by which the UP-YP is able to address a broad range of symptoms. It is possible that the strategies used target common, underlying processes contributing to both pain and emotional dysfunction. Another possibility is that teaching a core set of skills allows a client to apply those skills to each disorder individually. However, regardless of the mechanism, these cases suggest that broadening the scope of applicability of ER skills and cognitive-behavioral treatment strategies may be both feasible and helpful for individuals with complex medical and psychological conditions.

Developmental Considerations

The current version of the protocol is for use with adolescents ages 12–17, and the lower age limit of 12 was set keeping in mind the complexities of the protocol and the emotional and cognitive development of children. At its core, the UP-YP is directed at improving emotional identification and regulation skills, both in the context of emotions and pain. The flexibility of the protocol, both with regard to the specific strategies (e.g., emotion exposures) designed by the therapist and the number of sessions in each module, allows for some individual variation depending on emotional skill level. However, in our experience, it is important for the child to already have some emotion identification and regulation abilities in order to fully participate in the sessions. Emotion identification, understanding, and regulation are closely tied to cognitive development (Saarni, 1999), and as such this protocol may not be appropriate for participants younger than age 12 or who have severe deficits in emotional understanding. Previous research suggests that children with anxiety disorders have greater difficulty regulating (Suveg & Zeman, 2004) and understanding emotions (Southam-Gerow & Kendall, 2000). Given that this protocol is directed toward adolescents who experience pain and anxiety and/or depression, a careful analysis of emotional development would be an important step for the therapist to take prior to delivering this or a similar CBT protocol (Kingery et al., 2006).

Similarly, cognitive developmental level is an important consideration for implementing the thinking skills module of the protocol. Even though the development of problem-solving and metacognitive skills is much more pronounced in adolescence, the therapist may need to modify this module to some degree to accommodate adolescents with developmentally appropriate cognitive limitations (Kingery et al., 2006). For example, with adolescents in the lower age range, the therapist may have to first discuss the concept of "thoughts" and "interpretations" as mental activities that help a person understand a situation. A younger adolescent may find it more challenging to identify "core" thoughts, and the therapist may instead focus on interpretations specific to individual situations. Similarly, older adolescents may struggle with challenging some of their fears by considering alternative interpretations, particularly in social contexts. Because social interactions and relationships are a critical component of adolescence, asking the client to consider alternatives to negative thoughts about how others view him or her may be a challenge. The therapist must consider these factors when using detective questioning skills and help the adolescent consider alternatives to strongly held beliefs about social relationships.

With regard to designing and executing emotion exposures, this component of the UP-YP allows the therapist a great degree of flexibility to accommodate children with various levels of cognitive and emotional development. The therapist can select exposures that are developmentally appropriate and directly related to the client's daily experience, such as helping improve school attendance, developing peer relationships, or increasing activity level.

Future Directions

An ER-based treatment approach represents a new and potentially more comprehensive treatment approach to improving pain and disability in children with medical problems. The treatment described here, the UP-YP, incorporates specific ER skills that aim to reduce the *affective* component of pain, as well as co-occurring anxiety and depression symptoms, through psychoeducation, emotional awareness and prevention of emotional avoidance, flexibility in thinking, and engaging in emotion exposures. Initial data from a pilot study (Allen et al., 2009) and case examples (Allen et al., 2012) suggest that the UP-YP may jointly target pain and anxiety and depression in adolescents with chronic pain conditions.

There may be several potential mechanisms by which the UP-YP is able to address a broad range of emotional and physical symptoms. Most importantly, initial evidence suggests that inclusion of ER skills and cognitive-behavioral treatment strategies may be important in psychological treatments for individuals with both medical and psychological conditions. Future research should further explore the relationship of ER to pain responses, as well as the applicability of the UP-YP to children and adolescents with diverse pain and emotional disorders, as well as other chronic health conditions seen in pediatric medical settings.

ACKNOWLEDGMENTS

This research was supported by Grant No. F32MH084424, awarded by the National Institute of Mental Health (Laura B. Allen, Principal Investigator), and Grant No 2R01DE012754, awarded by the National Institute of Dental and Craniofacial Research (Lonnie K. Zeltzer, Principal Investigator).

REFERENCES

Allaire, S. H., DeNardo, B. S., Szer, I. S., Meenan, R. F., & Schaller, J. G. (1992). The economic impacts of juvenile rheumatoid arthritis. *Journal of Rheumatology, 19,* 952–955.

Allen, L. B., Ehrenreich, J. T., & Barlow, D. H. (2005). A unified treatment for emotional disorders: Applications with adults and adolescents. *Japanese Journal of Behavior Therapy, 31,* 3–31.

Allen, L. B., Tsao, J. C. I., Seidman, L. C., Ehrenreich-May, J. T., & Zeltzer, L. K. (2012). A unified, transdiagnostic treatment for adolescents with chronic pain and comorbid anxiety and depression. *Cognitive and Behavioral Practice, 19,* 56–67.

Allen, L. B., Tsao, J. C. I., & Zeltzer, L. K. (2009, March). *Development and applications of a unified cognitive-behavioral therapy (CBT) for adolescents with chronic pain and comorbid anxiety/depression.* Workshop conducted at the 8th International Symposium on Pediatric Pain, Acapulco, Mexico.

Allen, L. B., Tsao, J. C. I., Zeltzer, L. K., Ehrenreich-May, J. T., & Barlow, D. H. (2010). *Unified protocol for treatment of emotions in youth with pain (UP-YP).* Los Angeles: University of California, Los Angeles, Pediatric Pain Program.

Barlow, D. H., Farchione, T. J., Ellard, K. K., Fairholme, C. P., Boisseau, C. L., Allen, L. B., et al. (2010). *The unified protocol for the transdiagnostic treatment of emotional disorders: Therapist guide.* New York: Oxford University Press.

Barrett, P. M., Rapee, R. M., Dadds, M. R., & Ryan, S. M. (1996). Family enhancement of cognitive style in anxious and aggressive children. *Journal of Abnormal Child Psychology, 24*, 187–203.

Campo, J. V., Bridge, J., Ehmann, M., Altman, S., Lucas, A., Birmaher, B., et al. (2004). Recurrent abdominal pain, anxiety, and depression in primary care. *Pediatrics, 113*, 817–824.

Campo, J. V., Comer, D. M., Jansen-McWilliams, L., Gardner, W., & Kelleher, K. J. (2002). *Journal of Pediatrics, 141*, 76–83.

Cioffi, D., & Holloway, J. (1993). Delayed costs of suppressed pain. *Journal of Personality and Social Psychology, 64*, 274–282.

Dorn, L. D., Campo, J. C., Thato, S., Dahl, R. E., Lewin, D., Chandra, R., et al. (2003). Psychological comorbidity and stress reactivity in children and adolescents with recurrent abdominal pain and anxiety disorders. *Journal of the American Academy of Child and Adolescent Psychiatry, 42*, 66–75.

Eccleston, C., Palermo, T. M., Williams, A. C., Lewandowski, A., Morley, S., Fischer, E., et al. (2012). Psychological therapies for the management of chronic and recurrent pain in children and adolescents. *Cochrane Database of Systematic Reviews*, Issue 2 (Article No. CD003968), DOI: 10.1002/14651858. CD003968.pub3.

Ehrenreich, J. T., Goldstein, C. M., Wright, L. R., & Barlow, D. H. (2009). Development of a unified protocol for the treatment of emotional disorders in youth. *Child and Family Behavior Therapy, 31*, 20–37.

Ehrenreich-May, J. T., Buzzella, B. A., Trosper, S. E., Bennett, S. M., Wright, L. R., & Barlow, D. H. (2008). *Unified protocol for the treatment of emotional disorders in youth (UP-Y)*. Boston: Boston University.

Ellard, K. K., Fairholme, C. P., Boisseau, C. L., Farchione, T. J., & Barlow, D. H. (2010). Unified protocol for the transdiagnostic treatment of emotional disorders: Protocol development and initial outcome data. *Cognitive and Behavioral Practice, 17*, 88–101.

Gatchel, R. J., Peng, Y. B., Peters, M. L., Fuchs, P. N., & Turk, D. C. (2007). The biopsychosocial approach to chronic pain: Scientific advances and future directions. *Psychological Bulletin, 133*, 581–624.

Ghanizadeh, A., Moaiedy, F., Imanieh, M. H., Askani, H., Haghighat, M., Dehbozorgi, G., et al. (2008). Psychiatric disorders and family functioning in children and adolescents with functional abdominal syndrome. *Journal of Gastroenterology and Hepatology, 23*, 1132–1136.

Gross, J. J. (2002). Emotion regulation: Affective, cognitive, and social consequences. *Psychophysiology, 39*, 281–291.

Hayes, S. C., Strosahl, K. D., & Wilson, K. G. (1999). *Acceptance and commitment therapy: An experiential approach to behavior change*. New York: Guilford Press.

Jensen, M. P., Nielson, W. R., & Kerns, R. D. (2003). Toward the development of a motivational model of pain self-management. *Journal of Pain, 4*, 477–492.

Keefe, F. J., Lumley, M., Anderson, T., Lynch, T., Studts, J. L., & Carson, K. L. (2001). Pain and emotion: New research directions. *Journal of Clinical Psychology, 57*, 587–607.

Kendall, P. C. (1992). *Coping Cat workbook*. Ardmore, PA: Workbook Publishing.

Kingery, J. N., Roblek, T. L., Suveg, C., Grover, R. L., Sherrill, J. T., & Bergman,

R. L. (2006). They're not just "little adults": Developmental considerations for implementing cognitive-behavioral therapy with anxious youth. *Journal of Cognitive Psychotherapy, 20,* 263–273.

Lipsitz, J. D., Masia, C., Apfel, H., Marans, Z., Gur, M., Dent, H., et al. (2005). Noncardiac chest pain and psychopathology in children and adolescents. *Psychosomatic Research, 59,* 185–188.

Lumley, M. A., Beyer, J., & Radcliffe, A. (2008). Alexithymia and physical health problems: A critique of potential pathways and a research agenda. In A. Vingerhoets, I. Nyklicek, & J. Denollet (Eds.), *Emotion regulation: Conceptual and clinical issues* (pp. 43–68). New York: Springer.

Masia Warner, C., Reigada, L. C., Fisher, P. H., Saborsky, A. L., & Benkov, K. (2009). CBT for anxiety and somatic complaints in pediatric medical settings: An open pilot study. *Journal of Clinical Psychology in Medical Settings, 16,* 169–177.

Mattila, A. K., Kronholm, E., Jula, A., Salminen, J. K., Koivisto, A. M., Mielonen, E. L., et al. (2008). Alexithymia and somatization in general population. *Psychosomatic Medicine, 70,* 716–722.

Miller, W. R., & Rollnick, S. (2012). *Motivational interviewing: Helping people change* (3rd ed.). New York: Guilford Press.

Palermo, T. M., Eccleston, C., Lewandowski, A. S., Williams, A. C., & Morley, S. (2010). Randomized controlled trials of psychological therapies for management of chronic pain in children and adolescents: An updated meta-analytic review. *Pain, 148,* 387–397.

Palermo, T. M., Krell, H., Janosy, N., & Zeltzer, L. K. (2008). Pain and somatoform disorders. In M. Wolraich, D. Drotar, P. Dworkin, & E. Perrin (Eds.), *Developmental and behavioral pediatrics: Evidence and practice* (pp. 711–741). Philadelphia: Mosby.

Perquin, C. W., Hazebroek-Kampschreur, A. A., Hunfeld, J. A., Bohnen, A. M., van Suijlekom-Smit, L. W., Passchier, J., et al. (2000). Pain in children and adolescents: A common experience. *Pain, 87,* 51–58.

Power, T. J., DuPaul, G. J., Shapiro, E. S., & Parrish, J. M. (1998). Role of the school-based professional in health-related services. In L. Phelps (Ed.), *Health-related disorders in children and adolescents* (pp. 15–26). Washington, DC: American Psychological Association.

Ramchandani, P. G., Fazel, M., Stein, A., Wiles, N., & Hotopf, M. (2007). The impact of recurrent abdominal pain: Predictors of outcome in a large population cohort. *Acta Paediatrica, 96,* 697–701.

Reigada, L. C., Fisher, P. H., Cutler, C., & Masia Warner, C. (2008). An innovative treatment approach for children with anxiety disorders and medically unexplained somatic complaints. *Cognitive and Behavioral Practice, 15,* 140–147.

Ribeiro, S. C., Kennedy, S. E., Smith, Y. R., Stohler, C. S., & Zubieta, J. K. (2005). Interface of physical and emotional stress regulation through the endogenous opioid system and mu-opioid receptors. *Progress in Neuro-psychopharmacology and Biological Psychiatry, 29,* 1264–1280.

Roth-Isigkeit, A., Thyen, U., Raspe, H. H., Stoven, H., & Schmucker, P. (2004). Reports of pain among German children and adolescents: An epidemiological study. *Acta Paediatrica, 93,* 258–263.

Saarni, C. (1999). *The development of emotional competence.* New York: Guilford Press.

Sleed, M., Eccleston, C., Beecham, J., Knapp, M., & Jordan, A. (2005). The economic impact of chronic pain in adolescence: Methodological considerations and a preliminary costs-of-illness study. *Pain, 119,* 183–190.

Southam-Gerow, M. A., & Kendall, P. C. (2000). A preliminary study of the emotion understanding of youths referred for treatment of anxiety disorders. *Journal of Clinical Child Psychology, 29,* 319–327.

Strigo, I. A., Simmons, A. N., Matthews, S. C., Craig, A. D., & Paulus, M. P. (2008). Major depressive disorder is associated with altered functional brain response during anticipation and processing of heat pain. *Archives of General Psychiatry, 65,* 1275–1284.

Sullivan, M. J. L., Rouse, D., Bishop, S., & Johnston, S. (1997). Thought suppression, catastrophizing, and pain. *Cognitive Therapy and Research, 21,* 555–568.

Suveg, C., & Zeman, J. (2004). Emotion regulation in children with anxiety disorders. *Journal of Clinical Child and Adolescent Psychology, 33,* 750–759.

Tsao, J. C., Myers, C. D., Craske, M. G., Bursch, B., Kim, S. C., & Zeltzer, L. K. (2004). Role of anticipatory anxiety and anxiety sensitivity in children's and adolescents' laboratory pain responses. *Journal of Pediatric Psychology, 29,* 379–388.

Tuzer, V., Dogan Bulut, S., Bastug, B., Kayalar, G., Göka, E., & Bestepe, E. (2010). Causal attributions and alexithymia in female patients with fibromyalgia or chronic low back pain. *Nordic Journal of Psychiatry, 65,* 1–7.

van Middendorp, H., Lumley, M. A., Jacobs, J. W., van Doornen, L. J., Bijlsma, J. W., & Geenen, R. (2008). Emotions and emotional approach and avoidance strategies in fibromyalgia. *Journal of Psychomatic Research, 64,* 159–167.

Wicksell, R. K., Melin, L., Lekander, M., & Olsson, G. (2009). Evaluating the effectiveness of exposure and acceptance strategies to improve functioning and quality of life in longstanding pediatric pain: A randomized controlled trial. *Pain, 141,* 248–257.

Wicksell, R. K., Melin, L., & Olsson, G. L. (2007). Exposure and acceptance in the rehabilitation of adolescents with idiopathic chronic pain: A pilot study. *European Journal of Pain, 11,* 267–274.

Zeltzer, L. K., & Krell, H. (2007). Pain management in children. In R. E. Behrman, R. M. Kliegman, H. B. Jenson, & B. F. Stanton (Eds.), *Nelson textbook of pediatrics* (18th ed., pp. 475–484). Philadelphia: Saunders.

Zeman, J., Cassano, M., Perry-Parrish, C., & Stegall, S. (2006). Emotion regulation in children and adolescents. *Journal of Developmental and Behavioral Pediatrics, 27,* 155–168.

PART V

Conclusions and Future Directions

CHAPTER 18

Transdiagnostic Treatments

Issues and Commentary

Thomas H. Ollendick, Maria G Fraire, and Susan H. Spence

The transdiagnostic approach focuses on underlying psychopathological processes that are hypothesized to characterize two or more psychiatric disorders. In turn, transdiagnostic treatments are designed to target these underlying processes and, in doing so, address multiple disorders concurrently. The purpose of this chapter is to comment on some important issues when considering a transdiagnostic approach and to suggest future directions for research and practice. For example, what does "transdiagnostic" really mean, and what are the boundaries surrounding its use? When should one take a transdiagnostic approach, and for whom is this approach most beneficial? What is the evidentiary base for this approach at this time?

The transdiagnostic approach is based on research and theory that emphasizes the commonalities among disorders rather than differences. As indicated by Fairburn, Cooper, and Shafran (2003), Barlow, Allen, and Choate (2004), and Harvey, Watkins, Mansell, and Shafran (2004), there is considerable support for the notion that cognitive, emotional, and behavioral processes are shared across multiple disorders and contribute to the development and maintenance of these disorders. For example, Harvey and colleagues (2004) identified 12 such processes within the domains of attention, memory, reasoning, thought, and behavior. Indeed, many of these processes, including recurrent negative thinking, avoidance behaviors, and biases in interpretation, are addressed in many cognitive-behavioral therapies (CBT) for many diverse disorders. The high rates of comorbidity between psychiatric disorders such as anxiety and depression and between the eating disorders, depression, and substance use, among others, are offered as further support of such shared psychological and biological processes (Barlow et al., 2004). Moreover, some research has shown that successfully treating any one of the co-occurring disorders typically leads to the reduction of other comorbid disorders (for adults, see Norton & Philipp, 2008; for children, see Ollendick, Öst, Reuterskiöld, & Costa, 2010). Given these observations and findings, the transdiagnostic approach has been offered as a more parsimonious account for understanding psychopathology; furthermore, it has been suggested that an integrated treatment protocol that addresses multiple processes and disorders at the same time allows for greater dissemination of evidence-based treatments and their "uptake" in applied clinical settings. Building on this, integrated treatment protocols have been, and continue to be, developed to target these commonalities. In essence, the transdiagnostic framework offers a way to target multiple comorbid disorders with one "integrated" approach without relying on disorder-specific interventions. This approach has been viewed not only as a way to disseminate evidence-based treatments for more widespread use by reducing the number of manualized treatments that a clinician would need to master but also as a way to reduce the amount of time a client spends in therapy, thereby reducing both financial and time cost (see Ehrenreich-May & Chu, Chapter 1, and Chu, 2012, for further discussion of this issue).

A review of the transdiagnostic literature reflects a focus on a host of underlying processes, including biological and genetic factors, emotion regulation processes, attentional biases, negative affect, avoidance behaviors, coping styles, and family and interpersonal processes (see Harvey, Chapter 2; Compas, Watson, Reising, & Dunbar, Chapter 3; Arditte & Joormann, Chapter 4; Chu, Skriner, & Staples, Chapter 5; La Greca & Lai, Chapter 6; and Smith & Dishion, Chapter 7, as well as Harvey et al., 2004; McManus, Shafran, & Cooper, 2010). Often, evidence to support transdiagnostic processes comes from research that originated outside the transdiagnostic framework. For example, Mansell, Harvey, Watkins, and Shafran (2009) drew from the attentional processing literature in general to highlight how these processes underlie a variety of disorders in adults, as do Racer and Dishion (2012; see also Arditte & Joormann, Chapter 4) with children and adolescents. However, less empirical work has been undertaken specifically within the transdiagnostic context. This not only suggests great potential for future research but also reminds us that there is still a great deal to be understood about the transdiagnostic process itself, its specificity within any set of disorders, and the treatments emanating from this approach.

Current Status of Transdiagnostic Approaches with Emotional Disorders

Given that the extension of transdiagnostic work is still in its early stages for most psychiatric disorders in children and adolescents (as is evident in the various chapters in this volume), here we concentrate on the emotional or internalizing disorders for which there is more research. In doing so, we first turn to the adult literature to frame our comments about the current status of transdiagnostic work with children and adolescents. Based on advances in basic research on the psychopathological processes associated with various adult disorders, Barlow and his colleagues developed the Unified Protocol (UP) for the Transdiagnostic Treatment of Emotional Disorders (Barlow, Ellard, et al., 2011; Barlow, Farchione, et al., 2011). This CBT program, designed to treat all anxiety and unipolar mood disorders, incorporates existing strategies used in previously established evidence-based interventions for the treatment of anxiety and mood disorders: restructuring maladaptive cognitive appraisal, changing maladaptive action tendencies associated with emotions, preventing emotional avoidance, and utilizing emotion exposure procedures. To date, this treatment has been evaluated in two open trials and one randomized control trial (RCT) by this group. In the open trials with 18 and 15 patients, respectively, the treatment appeared promising with patients with principal anxiety disorders (Ellard, Fairholme, Boisseau, Farchione, & Barlow, 2010). In these open trials, approximately 60% of the patients achieved high end-state functioning with respect to their anxiety disorders, their symptoms of depression were reduced, and, importantly, negative affect (the underlying process dimension shared in common with anxiety and depression) was reduced as well. These encouraging results led to a recently completed RCT comparing the UP treatment to a wait-list control condition (WLC) in 37 outpatients who met criteria for an anxiety disorder (Farchione et al., 2012). In the 37 patients, diverse principal anxiety disorders were represented: seven with generalized anxiety disorder (GAD), eight with obsessive–compulsive disorder (OCD), eight with social anxiety disorder (SOC), eight with panic disorder with agoraphobia (PDAG), two with anxiety disorder not otherwise specified (NOS), one with posttraumatic stress disorder (PTSD), and three with coprincipal anxiety disorders (two anxiety diagnoses of equal severity). Several had co-occurring anxiety disorders in addition to their principal diagnoses, and 9 of the 37 met criteria for a mood disorder. Using a 2:1 allocation ratio, 26 patients were assigned to the UP condition and 11 to WLC. The UP treatment consisted of eighteen 60-minute individual sessions. In terms of outcomes at posttreatment, significantly more patients in the UP treatment achieved subclinical status on their principal diagnosis than did those in the WLC (50% compared with 0%); in addition, more of the UP patients no longer met criteria for any of their comorbid diagnoses compared with those in the WLC at posttreatment (50% versus 17%), although this difference did not reach statistical significance. Other analyses of self-reported anxiety, depression, negative and positive affect, work and social adjustment, and clinician ratings of anxiety and depression also favored the UP condition. Of special significance to the transdiagnostic process, 6 of the 9 patients with a mood disorder achieved subclinical status at posttreatment, and these effects were maintained at a 6-month follow-up. Similar encouraging results were found in a recent RCT comparing a WLC with Internet-delivered transdiagnostic treatment for adults presenting with anxiety and/or depression (Titov et al., 2011).

These initial open trials and recent RCTs provide reason for optimism about the transdiagnostic approach. However, caution is recommended because the bulk of the evidence was obtained from uncontrolled open trials, the number of participants in the studies has been limited, rigorous treatment fidelity and adherence measures have not been obtained, and, perhaps most important for the transdiagnostic approach, changes in transdiagnostic processes such as positive and negative affect have not been shown to mediate changes in anxiety and depression. Furthermore, none of these studies have examined the utility and efficacy of this approach with individuals with a principal diagnosis of a mood disorder. In fact, most of the patients in these trials have not even had a comorbid mood disorder, raising the question as to whether evidence for a "transdiagnostic" approach is available. Finally, it remains to be determined whether the impact of the transdiagnostic intervention exceeds that resulting from nonspecific, attention placebo factors. Studies indicate that the majority of symptom reduction in traditional CBT for depression and anxiety occurs in the first 3–4 weeks of treatment, suggesting that much of the impact of CBT may be attributable to nonspecific therapy factors rather than specific cognitive or behavioral mediation processes (Ilardi & Craighead, 1994). It is not clear at this time whether changes in the underlying processes that are common to anxiety and depression and that characterize transdiagnostic therapy can be differentiated from nonspecific therapy processes such as increased expectancies for positive change, perceptions of social support, and feelings of being valued and respected. These are questions for future research to establish the unique contributions of a transdiagnostic approach.

Questions also remain as to when a transdiagnostic treatment would be the best treatment option. Should a transdiagnostic approach work for all comorbid disorders, or are there specific combinations for which it is more effective? Although there is limited research to suggest that all anxiety-related disorders, including OCD and PTSD, share underlying processes and can be targeted in a transdiagnostic approach (Norton & Philipp, 2008), it is not at all clear how the differing symptoms of these disorders might be targeted efficiently and effectively. Although they do not examine transdiagnostic processes and treatments specifically, two studies in the adult area highlight this issue. Craske et al. (2007) reported on an RCT in which 65 patients with panic disorder were allocated to either a dual target intervention focusing on panic disorder and their most severe comorbid disorder (usually other anxiety disorders, but also mood and somatization disorders) or to an intervention focusing only on their panic disorder. Interestingly, those whose intervention focused only on panic disorder had better outcomes both at posttreatment and at 1-year follow-up, not only in terms of their panic disorder but also on the severity of their comorbid disorders. These results indicate that remaining focused on the single evidence-based treatment for panic disorder resulted in better outcomes for both the principal and comorbid diagnoses than did attempting to combine evidence-based treatments for the two disorders. Tantalizingly, Craske and her colleagues subtitled their paper "More of the same, or less of more?" In a similar RCT, Randall, Thomas, and Thevos (2001) randomized 93 patients with social anxiety disorder and alcoholism to receive either cognitive treatment for alcoholism and social anxiety or treatment for alcoholism alone. Patients receiving the combined treatment had worse outcomes for their primary diagnosis of alcoholism than those treated for alcoholism alone; moreover, they showed no benefit in terms of their comorbid social anxiety. As noted by McManus and colleagues (2010), these studies suggest, contrary to what might have been expected, that simply combining evidence-based interventions in patients with comorbid disorders may actually dilute the efficacy of the treatments for the primary disorders and not lead to improvements in the comorbid disorders. Expanding the range of therapy techniques to be acquired may make it difficult for patients to fully learn and consolidate the skills and knowledge of either of the treatment approaches. Using the catchphrase of Craske and colleagues, in some instances, more of the same might be better. However, in fairness to the transdiagnostic approach, it should be noted that this integrated approach should be differentiated from those that combine treatments that aim to change different underlying processes of more than one condition, as was the case in the Craske and colleagues (2007) and Randall and colleagues (2001) studies. Rather, the transdiagnostic approach requires identification of and change in the common, underlying processes of multiple disorders. Such was not done in the studies by Craske and colleagues and Randall and colleagues.

Additionally, less empirical research has focused on truly delineating and assessing the underlying processes that occur across disorders. To date there does not appear to be a great deal of research speaking to which transdiagnostic processes should be targeted for change, how those transdiagnostic processes should be measured, or, for that matter, how or if changes in these presumed underlying processes mediate treatment outcomes. It appears that often diagnostic symptoms are used to determine the commonality across disorders and that treatment outcomes are based on reduction of those symptoms and subsequent changes in diagnostic status, not the candidate underlying processes. In the adult literature, McEvoy, Nathan, and Norton (2009) reviewed outcome studies that had investigated the efficacy of transdiagnostic treatments and found that a majority of the studies used only symptom-based measures, providing little empirical evidence that the underlying processes were being effectively addressed in the unified treatments. It seems to us that it is especially important that research into transdiagnostic therapies investigate the purported common underlying processes to determine whether they are present, whether they are being targeted in treatment, whether there is significant change in the processes as a result of treatment, and whether those changes mediate outcomes.

We also note that transdiagnostic theory provides less of an explanation as to why clinical presentations are so very different between disorders if they do indeed share a set of common processes. Harvey and colleagues (2004) suggest that symptom presentation depends on the "concerns" of the individual at the point in time that these differing behaviors occur and when they seek treatment. This analysis potentially focuses on the shared underlying processes; however, less attention is afforded the unique processes related to differing disorders. Others have argued that, although there are differences, the commonalities are more prominent and that, as such, targeting the commonalities may be more beneficial than remaining disorder-specific (McEvoy et al., 2009). Much research remains to be conducted on when it would be more appropriate to apply a disorder-specific treatment or a transdiagnostic treatment. At what point is the decision made that targeting the underlying processes between anxiety and depression, for example, is better than focusing solely on the anxiety or the depression? Common underlying processes may explain only part of symptom development with a given presenting problem, and transdiagnostic treatment may not address the processes and factors involved in the etiology and maintenance of some of the more unique features of disorders. Thus further research is needed to determine whether transdiagnostic treatments are as effective as disorder-specific approaches. Similarly, it would be valuable to determine whether a staged approach might be more effective, in which treatment begins with a transdiagnostic approach and branches off to disorder- (or symptom-) specific therapy elements for those cognitive and behavioral features that have not responded to the transdiagnostic component.

Indeed, very little research has focused on a direct comparison between disorder-specific treatments and transdiagnostic treatments. To our knowledge, no such treatment studies have yet been conducted. However, Farchione and colleagues (2012) indicate that such a trial is about to begin with adults, and Spence and her colleagues have such a trial under way with youth who present with social anxiety disorder (Spence,

Donovan, March, & Kenardy, 2012). In the Spence and colleagues (2012) Internet-based trial, the relative efficacy of a transdiagnostic online CBT approach is being compared with an online CBT approach that specifically targets social anxiety disorder and with a WLC. In the past few years, Spence and her group have systematically developed and evaluated an Internet-based CBT program for the treatment of diverse anxiety disorders (e.g., GAD, social anxiety disorder, separation anxiety disorder) in children and adolescents that has proven to be highly successful (March, Spence, & Donovan, 2009; Spence et al., 2011). The fully online CBT program incorporates minimal e-mail–based therapist contact but produces effects that rival those of therapist-delivered interventions, with approximately 68% of youth in the Internet condition free of disorder at follow-up and with those gains maintained or enhanced at follow-up intervals. In the RCT under way, a specific online program targeting social anxiety is being compared with this effective transdiagnostic approach to determine whether such enhanced gains might be realized. As noted, fully one-third of individuals receiving the transdiagnostic online intervention do not respond to the treatment—rates very similar to those found in clinician-delivered interventions (see Seligman & Ollendick, 2011, for a review). The targeted intervention includes two components that are specific to social anxiety disorder but that might be less relevant to other childhood anxiety disorders: social skills and assertiveness training on the one hand and interpretation biases and self-focused attention on the other. These features, though frequently evident in social anxiety disorder, are frequently not included, or at least not highlighted, in extant evidence-based CBT programs for childhood anxiety disorders. The diagnosis-specific intervention highlights specific causal and maintaining factors for social anxiety in youth, addresses thinking errors and interpretation biases specific to social anxiety, uses highly specific exposure hierarchies, and teaches social skills and assertiveness. As noted, the trial is under way, but Spence and her colleagues hypothesize greater treatment gains with the disorder-specific intervention.

Some support for such specificity can be found in other research with socially anxious youth. For example, Beidel, Turner, and Morris (2000) developed a behavioral treatment program to specifically target social anxiety in children. This program, social effectiveness therapy for children (SET-C), aims to enhance social skills and reduce social anxiety. After SET-C treatment, 67% of the children no longer met criteria for social anxiety, and these gains were maintained at both short-term and long-term (5-year) follow-up (Beidel, Turner, & Young, 2006). SET-C also demonstrated efficacy in comparison to fluoxetine and a pill placebo (Beidel et al., 2007). Moreover, improved social skills, assertiveness, and overall social competency were witnessed only in the SET-C condition. These findings are used as an example to highlight how disorder-specific treatments can be highly beneficial. An example of a treatment that provides a broader, transdiagnostic approach to the treatment of child anxiety is Kendall's (1994) Coping Cat program. In this program, children with social anxiety disorders are frequently treated alongside children with GAD and separation anxiety disorder. The "generic" treatment is applied across disorders, inasmuch as these disorders share an underlying anxiety construct (Bell-Dolan & Brazeal, 1993), as well as underlying negative affectivity (Seligman & Ollendick, 1998). Kendall and his colleagues (Kendall, 1994; Kendall et al., 1997; Kendall, Hudson, Gosch, Flannery-Schroeder, & Suveg, 2008) reported that of the children who participated in their Coping Cat treatment program for anxious youth, about 53–61% no longer met criteria for their principal anxiety disorders posttreatment. As noted, this program was designed to treat anxiety more broadly (i.e., across anxiety disorders) and in that sense transdiagnostically.

In a recent analysis of the outcomes of socially anxious youth in these more generic, transdiagnostic programs, Scharfstein and Beidel (in press) noted three major trends and concerns: (1) only about 15% of the youth in these treatment studies had social anxiety disorder, and hence these disorders are underrepresented in these larger studies; (2) these generic treatment programs rarely include training in social skills, assertiveness, and social competency more broadly defined; and (3) in those studies that examined diagnostic recovery, youth with social anxiety disorder fared worse than their counterparts without social anxiety. For example, Crawley, Beidas, Benjamin, Martin, and Kendall (2008) reported that 40.1% of the youth with social anxiety no longer met diagnostic criteria in their trials compared with 67.2% of those youth with separation anxiety disorder and 71.2% of those with GAD. Shortt, Barrett, and Fox (2001) reported similar outcomes with their generic FRIENDS program in Australia, as did Hudson and colleagues (2009) with their generic Cool Kids program, also in Australia. In this latter study, only 25% of youth with social anxiety disorder were free of their diagnoses at posttreatment, compared with 51% of those with GAD or separation anxiety disorder. Notably, these differential findings were obtained even after controlling for mood disorders. Collectively, these findings suggest that diagnosis-specific treatment programs for socially anxious youth may be more effective than generic, transdiagnostic (across anxiety disorders) programs, although a direct test of these findings is yet to be conducted. To our knowledge, Spence and colleagues' (2012) online trial is the first to make this direct comparison.

What Is the Current Status of Recent Transdiagnostic Approaches with Children with Emotional Disorders?

As noted earlier, a considerable amount of work on generic transdiagnostic approaches across the anxiety disorders in youth has already occurred. In general these studies show that these evidence-based CBT interventions for youth with diverse anxiety disorders are effective; yet approximately one-third to one-half of the youth do not respond positively to these anxiety-focused treatment programs (see Seligman & Ollendick, 2011, for a review). Efforts to explore the moderators of treatment outcome in these studies have been undertaken, and, although the evidence is sparse, a few studies reveal that the co-occurrence of anxiety and depression may be associated with treatment failure. For example, Berman, Weems, Silverman, and Kurtines (2000) showed that diagnoses of a comorbid mood disorder, as well as self-reported depressive symptomatology, were associated with lower levels of treatment success both in group and individual CBT programs for anxiety-disordered youth. So, too, did Crawley and colleauges (2008) in a reanalysis of outcomes associated with Kendall's (1994) Coping Cat program. These authors concluded that comorbid affective disorders likely contributed to differential treatment outcomes, especially for those youth who had a principal diagnosis of social anxiety disorder. However, it should be noted that these effects associated with mood disorders were shown in only 2 of the now more than 25 studies examining these generic transdiagnostic treatments. Unfortunately, many of these studies failed to report on those patients with depressive comorbidities, and, even when they did, the number of such youth was relatively small (e.g., less than 5% of the 166 youth in Crawley et al., 2008, were diagnosed with a secondary mood disorder). Furthermore, a high clinical level of comorbid depression is frequently an exclusion criterion in clinical trials of the treatment of anxiety disorders in youth, which limits the capacity to examine the impact of comorbid depression in these trials. Thus the conclusions based on co-occurrence of depressive disorders must be viewed as preliminary at best.

Recently, in an effort to address both anxiety and depression symptoms in the same integrated treatment, Ehrenreich and her colleagues have extended Barlow and colleagues' UP to adolescents and children (Ehrenreich, Goldstein, Wright, & Barlow, 2009). Parent sessions were added, and the language and therapeutic exercises were modified to make the protocol more developmentally appropriate and relevant for an adolescent and child population. In the first study, Ehrenreich and colleagues (2009) conducted a multiple-baseline design study of their modified treatment protocol with three adolescents presenting an array of anxiety and depression symptoms. All of the youth had a principal diagnosis of one of the major anxiety disorders, and one of the youth had a comorbid mood disorder. All three youth benefited from this 16-session treatment, at least as evidenced by reductions in the clinical severity level of their principal anxiety diagnoses at posttreatment; however, two of the three remained at a clinical level at that time, and the youth who had a mood disorder retained that diagnosis at posttreatment as well. At 6-month follow-up, however, all diagnoses, including the mood disorder, were subclinical, suggesting continued gains. Although it is indicated that a multiple baseline design was enlisted in this study, results for such are not presented, and essentially what we have here is a wait-list treatment design. Moreover, it is difficult to determine what produced the gains following treatment, as they were not present at posttreatment. Finally, only one of the three youth had a mood disorder, and hence the "transdiagnostic" value of this treatment demonstration remains unclear.

In the second study, additional modifications to the adolescent protocol were made, and the protocol was applied to two young children in an open trial (Ehrenreich-May & Bilek, 2012). The new protocol, dubbed "UP for Children: Emotion Detectives" (UP-C:ED), is designed to be a group treatment program for comorbid anxious and depressed youth. One child in this open trial, an 8-year-old boy, possessed diagnoses of generalized anxiety disorder and social phobia and a subclinical diagnosis of a specific phobia of the dark. The second child, a 7-year-old girl, possessed a diagnosis of separation anxiety disorder and subclinical diagnoses of GAD, social phobia, and depressive disorder not otherwise specified. Both children responded positively to the 15-session intervention, and their principal diagnoses were no longer clinically significant at posttreatment. Of course, as an open trial and with only two participants, the scientific value of this demonstration is found wanting, albeit interesting. It is also of note that neither of the children was diagnosed with a mood disorder (although the second child was subclinical), and the "transdiagnostic" value of the treatment remains unclear.

Recently, Bilek and Ehrenreich (2012) reported on findings for 22 children between 7 and 12 years of age who participated in an open trial of the UP-C:ED program (two of the 22 children were reported on in the Ehrenreich and Bilek open trial described previously). All of the children met a principal diagnosis of one of the anxiety disorders; additionally, most met criteria for at least one other comorbid anxiety disorder, and seven (32%) met criteria for a comorbid subclinical or clinical mood disorder (clinical severity rating [CSR] > 3). Four of the 22 participants (18%) terminated treatment prematurely. For those 18 children who completed treatment, 14 (78%) were free of their pretreatment clinical diagnoses; however, this rate dropped to 64% in the intent-to-treat analyses. For those with a comorbid depressive disorder, four of the five (80%) who completed treatment were free of their mood disorder at posttreatment; however, this number dropped to 57% for the intent-to-treat analyses. Moreover, those who dropped out of treatment reported greater depressive symptoms at intake. Overall, then, the treatment was effective for the majority of the youth, but at rates comparable to those seen in other anxiety-diagnosis-specific programs such as Coping Cat, FRIENDS, and Cool Kids. The results for depression are less clear and seem to suggest that the presence of elevated depressive symptoms may lead to early termination. It is also not clear what common underlying processes the intervention was designed to target and whether the intervention was effective in producing change in these variables. As noted earlier, future research into transdiagnostic therapies must address these issues.

In addition to these efforts by Ehrenreich and colleagues, Weersing and colleagues (Weersing, Gonzalez, Campo, & Lucas, 2008; Weersing, Rozenman, Maher-Bridge, & Campo, 2012) and Chu and colleagues (Chu, Colognori, Weissman, & Bannon, 2009; Chu, Merson, Zandberg, & Areizaga, 2012) have independently explored integrated treatment protocols for the treatment of children and adolescents with anxiety, depression, and somatic disorders. However, like the studies of Ehrenreich and colleagues, these studies have consisted largely of uncontrolled pilot case studies and have not tracked underlying transdiagnostic processes throughout treatment nor shown changes in these processes following treatment.

Summary and Commentary

As is evident from adult studies but most assuredly from child and adolescent studies, transdiagnostic treatment approaches are in their infancy, with primary support coming from small open clinical trials, underpowered RCTs, and designs that do not allow us to conclude that the transdiagnostic treatment is any more effective than placebo or disorder-specific therapies. In many respects, at this time these approaches must be considered "experimental" in terms of evidence-based nomenclature (see Chambless & Ollendick, 2001). To date, to our knowledge, results are not yet available comparing transdiagnostic approaches directly with diagnosis-specific and/or placebo treatments. Indeed, the limited research available suggests that they may be no more effective than diagnosis-specific treatments and, in fact, might be less effective. Moreover, in reference to treating anxiety and mood disorders transdiagnostically, studies have rarely included patients with diagnosed mood disorders, and these individuals have frequently done less well in treatment when included. Furthermore, no studies to our knowledge have included patients with principal diagnoses of mood disorders. As a result, we really do not know the extent of their reach to "emotional" disorders more broadly speaking.

Additionally, a great deal of the transdiagnostic research appears to revolve around treatment, without the foundational work of empirically validating the underlying processes that are believed to co-occur in emotional disorders. Although there is clearly a great deal of research in the various domains (e.g., cognitive biases, negative affect, attentional processes), research specifically detailing these underlying processes within a transdiagnostic conceptualization is limited. Strengthening the transdiagnostic theory will come from additional research focused on elucidating and empirically validating these underlying processes and then showing that these underlying processes not only change as a function of a transdiagnostic treatment but are causally related to the reduction of symptoms and diagnoses. To our knowledge, no studies employing this approach have demonstrated that the cognitive, emotional, and behavioral processes that are shared by various emotional disorders mediate treatment outcomes. Although we have noted that these processes have been shown to change in some studies, along with symptoms of anxiety and depression, it has not been demonstrated that these changes are related to or causal of treatment outcomes. Such studies and demonstrations will be critical to testing the basic assumptions underlying the transdiagnostic approach.

This chapter has mainly focused on the transdiagnostic approach as applied to anxiety disorders and depression and between different forms of anxiety disorders. Future studies will no doubt examine the common underlying features of other disorders in young people in which common underlying mechanisms can be demonstrated, such as depression and eating disorders, or social phobia and substance use, or conduct and attentional problems. The various chapters in this volume attest to the exciting work under way in these nascent areas. Also, we have concentrated predominantly on the treatment of anxiety and depressive disorders, but a case can be made for a transdiagnostic approach to the prevention of anxiety and depression and other disorders. Interventions that are designed to tackle the cognitive and familial risk factors associated with these and other disorders, such as problem-solving skills training, cognitive coping strategies, and parent training, offer promise as targeted transdiagnostic prevention approaches for these disorders (Dozois, Seeds, & Collins, 2009).

It is our hope that the current volume will go far to address some of these shortcomings and will pave the way for more scientific evidence both on the transdiagnostic processes that characterize emotional disorders and the integrated, transdiagnostic treatments that emanate from this approach. Until then, and in the absence of more compelling and scientifically acceptable evidence, we suggest that the promulgation and dissemination of these unified procedures may be premature and that we need to proceed with caution. Nonetheless, the transdiagnostic approach appears most promising and is most deserving of our continued attention and careful analysis.

REFERENCES

Barlow, D. H., Allen, L. B., & Choate, M. L. (2004). Toward a unified treatment for emotional disorders. *Behavior Therapy, 35*(2), 205–230.

Barlow, D. H., Ellard, K. K., Fairholme, C. P., Farchione, T. J., Boisseau, C. L., Allen, L. B., et al. (2011). *The unified protocol for transdiagnostic treatment of emotional disorders: Client workbook.* New York: Oxford University Press.

Barlow, D. H., Farchione, T. J., Fairholme, C. P., Ellard, K. K., Boisseau, C. L., Allen, L. B., et al. (2011). *The unified protocol for transdiagnostic treatment of emotional disorders: Therapist guide.* New York: Oxford University Press.

Beidel, D. C., Turner, S. M., & Morris, T. L. (2000). Behavioral treatment of childhood social phobia. *Journal of Consulting and Clinical Psychology, 68,* 1072–1080.

Beidel, D. C., Turner, S. M., Sallee, F. R., Ammerman, R. T., Crosby, L. A., & Pathak, S. (2007). SET-C versus fluoxetine in the treatment of childhood social phobia. *Journal of the American Academy of Child and Adolescent Psychiatry, 46,* 1622–1632.

Beidel, D. C., Turner, S. M., & Young, B. J. (2006). Social effectiveness therapy for children: Five years later. *Behavior Therapy, 37,* 416–425.

Bell-Dolan, D. J., & Brazeal, T. (1993). Separation anxiety disorder, overanxious disorder, and school refusal. *Child and Adolescent Psychiatric Clinics of North America, 2,* 563–580.

Berman, S. L., Weems, C. F., Silverman, W. K., & Kurtines, W. M. (2000). Predictors of outcome in exposure-based cognitive and behavioral treatments for phobic and anxiety disorders in children. *Behavior Therapy, 31,* 713–731.

Bilek, E. L., & Ehrenreich-May, J. (2012). An open trial investigation of a transdiagnostic group treatment for children with anxiety and depressive symptoms. *Behavior Therapy, 43,* 887–897.

Chambless, D. L., & Ollendick, T. H. (2001). Empirically supported psychological interventions: Controversies and evidence. *Annual Review of Psychology, 52,* 685–716.

Chu, B. C. (2012). Translating transdiagnostic approaches to children and adolescents. *Cognitive and Behavioral Practice, 19,* 1–4.

Chu, B. C., Colognori, D., Weissman, A., & Bannon, K. (2009). An initial description and pilot of group behavioral activation therapy for anxious and depressed youth. *Cognitive and Behavioral Practice, 16,* 408–419.

Chu, B. C., Merson, R. A., Zandberg, L. J., & Areizaga, M. (2012). Calibrating for comorbidity: Clinical decision-making in youth depression and anxiety. *Cognitive and Behavioral Practice, 19,* 5–16.

Craske, M. G., Farchione, T. J., Allen, L. B., Barrios, V., Stoyanova, M., & Rose, R. (2007). Cognitive-behavioral therapy for panic disorder and comorbidity: More of the same or less of more? *Behaviour Research and Therapy, 45,* 1095–1109.

Crawley, S. A., Beidas, R. S., Benjamin, C. L., Martin, E., & Kendall, P. C. (2008). Treating socially phobic youth with CBT: Differential outcomes and treatment considerations. *Behavioural and Cognitive Psychotherapy, 36,* 379–389.

Dozois, D. J. A., Seeds, P. M., & Collins, K. A. (2009). Transdiagnostic approaches to the prevention of depression and anxiety. *Journal of Cognitive Psychotherapy, 23,* 44–59.

Ehrenreich, J. T., Goldstein, C. R., Wright, L. R., & Barlow, D. H. (2009). Development of a unified protocol for the treatment of emotional disorders in youth. *Child and Family Behavior Therapy, 31,* 20–37.

Ehrenreich-May, J., & Bilek, E. L. (2012). The development of a transdiagnostic, cognitive-behavioral group intervention for childhood anxiety disorders and co-occurring depression symptoms. *Cognitive and Behavioral Practice, 19,* 41–55.

Ellard, K. K., Fairholme, C. P., Boisseau, C. L., Farchione, T. J., & Barlow, D. H. (2010). Unified protocol for the transdiagnostic treatment of emotional disorders: Protocol development and initial outcome data. *Cognitive and Behavioral Practice, 17,* 88–101.

Fairburn, C. G., Cooper, Z., & Shafran, R. (2003). Cognitive behaviour therapy for eating disorders: A "transdiagnostic" theory and treatment. *Behaviour Research and Therpy, 41,* 509–528.

Farchione, T. J., Fairholme, C. P., Ellard, K., Boisseau, C. L., Thompson-Hollands, J., Carl, J. R., et al. (2012). Unified protocol for transdiagnostic treatment of emotional disorders: A randomized controlled trial. *Behavior Therapy, 43,* 666–678.

Harvey, A., Watkins, E., Mansell, W., & Shafran, R. (2004). *Cognitive behavioural processes across psychological disorders: A transdiagnostic approach to research and treatment.* New York: Oxford University Press.

Hudson, J. L., Rapee, R. M., Deveney, C., Schniering, C. A., Lyneham, H. J., & Bovopoulos, N. (2009). Cognitive-behavioral treatment versus an active control for children and adolescents with anxiety disorders: A randomized trial. *Journal of the American Academy of Child and Adolescent Psychiatry, 48,* 533–544.

Ilardi, S. S., & Craighead, W. E. (1994). The role of nonspecific factors in cognitive-behavior therapy for depression. *Clinical Psychology: Science and Practice, 1,* 138–156.

Kendall, P. C. (1994). Treating anxiety disorders in children: Results of a randomized clinical trial. *Journal of Consulting and Clinical Psychology, 62,* 100–110.

Kendall, P. C., Flannery-Schroeder, E., Panichelli-Mindel, S. M., Southam-Gerow, M., Henin, A., & Warman, M. (1997). Therapy for youths with anxiety disorders: A second randomized clinical trial. *Journal of Consulting and Clinical Psychology, 65,* 366–380.

Kendall, P. C., Hudson, J. L., Gosch, E., Flannery-Schroeder, E., & Suveg, C. (2008). Cognitive–behavioral therapy for anxiety disordered youth: A randomized clinical trial evaluating child and family modalities. *Journal of Consulting and Clinical Psychology, 76,* 282–297.

Mansell, W., Harvey, A., Watkins, E., & Shafran, R. (2009). Conceptual foundations of the transdiagnostic approach to CBT. *Journal of Cognitive Psychotherapy, 23,* 6–19.

March, S., Spence, S. H., & Donovan, C. L. (2009). The efficacy of an Internet-based cognitive-behavioral therapy intervention for child anxiety disorders. *Journal of Pediatric Psychology, 34,* 474–487.

McEvoy, P. M., Nathan, P., & Norton, P. J. (2009). Efficacy of transdiagnostic treatments: A review of published outcome studies and future research directions. *Journal of Cognitive Psychotherapy, 23,* 20–33.

McManus, F., Shafran, R., & Cooper, Z. (2010). What does a "transdiagnostic" approach have to offer the treatment of anxiety disorders? *British Journal of Clinical Psychology, 49,* 491–505.

Norton, P. J., & Philipp, L. M. (2008). Transdiagnostic approaches to the treatment of anxiety disorders: A quantitative review. *Psychotherapy: Theory, Research, Practice, Training, 45,* 214–226.

Ollendick, T. H., Öst, L.-G., Reuterskiöld, L., & Costa, N. (2010). Comorbidity in youth with specific phobias: Impact of comorbidity on treatment outcome and the impact of treatment on comorbid disorders. *Behaviour Research and Therapy, 48,* 827–831.

Racer, K. H., & Dishion, T. J. (2012). Disordered attention: Implications for understanding and treating internalizing and externalizing disorders in childhood. *Cognitive and Behavioral Practice, 19,* 31–40.

Randall, C. L., Thomas, S., & Thevos, A. K. (2001). Concurrent alcoholism and social anxiety disorder: A first step toward developing effective treatments. *Alcoholism: Clinical and Experimental Research, 25,* 210–220.

Scharfstein, L. A., & Beidel, D. C. (in press). Behavioral and cognitive-behavioral treatment for children with social phobia. *Journal of Experimental Psychopathology.*

Seligman, L. D., & Ollendick, T. H. (1998). Comorbidity of anxiety and depression in children and adolescents: An integrative review. *Clinical Child and Family Psychology Review, 1,* 125–144.

Seligman, L. D., & Ollendick, T. H. (2011). Cognitive-behavioral therapy for anxiety disorders in youth. *Child and Adolescent Psychiatric Clinics of North America, 20,* 217–238.

Shortt, A. L., Barrett, P. M., & Fox, T. L. (2001). Evaluating the FRIENDS Program: A cognitive-behavioral group treatment for anxious children and their parents. *Journal of Clinical Child Psychology, 30,* 525–535.

Spence, S. H., Donovan, C. L., March, S., Gamble, A., Anderson, R. E., Prosser, S., et al. (2011). A randomized controlled trial of online versus clinic-based CBT for adolescent anxiety. *Journal of Consulting and Clinical Psychology, 79,* 629–642.

Spence, S. H., Donovan, C. L., March, S., & Kenardy, J. (2012). *Evaluation of transdiagnostic versus disorder-specific, Internet-based cognitive behaviour therapy for social phobia in young people* (Grant No. 12611000901909). Canberra, Australia: National Health and Medical Research Council.

Titov, N., Dear, B. F., Schwencke, G., Andrews, G., Johnston, L., Craske, M. G., et al. (2011). Transdiagnostic Internet treatment for anxiety and depression: A randomised controlled trial. *Behaviour Research and Therapy, 49,* 441–452.

Weersing, V. R., Gonzalez, A., Campo, J. V., & Lucas, A. N. (2008). Brief behavioral therapy for pediatric anxiety and depression: Piloting an integrated treatment approach. *Cognitive and Behavioral Practice, 15,* 126–139.

Weersing, V. R., Rozenman, M. S., Maher-Bridge, M., & Campo, J. V. (2012). Anxiety, depression, and somatic distress: Developing a transdiagnostic internalizing toolbox for pediatric practice. *Cognitive and Behavioral Practice, 19,* 68–82.

CHAPTER 19

Transdiagnostic Research and Treatment in Youth

Revolution or Evolution?

Brian C. Chu and Jill Ehrenreich-May

Even a cursory review of the preceding chapters in this book impresses on the reader the magnitude of research and treatment development that has occurred in an extremely brief amount of time. The first mention of the term *transdiagnostic therapy* was published in 2003 by Fairburn and colleagues in their description of common maintaining processes across eating disorders. At the same time, Barlow and colleagues (2004) were detailing their case for a "unified protocol" across a wide spectrum of disorders. Simultaneously, Harvey and colleagues (2004) were laying out a detailed exposition of basic science that supported the presence of common cognitive and behavioral mechanisms that explained the onset and maintenance of adult psychological disorders. And, finally, the first explicit description of a transdiagnostic intervention in youth population occurred in Ehrenreich, Buzzella, and Barlow's (2007) extension of the unified protocol across the lifespan. It cannot be overstated that the explicit, intentional study of transdiagnostic mechanisms and unified treatments is in its very nascent stages and has far to go. And yet impressive progress has been made.

Revisiting Definitions

At this point, it is worth revisiting the definitions that guide this developing field. After reviewing the preceding chapters in this volume and considering the multiple approaches to this literature, it makes every sense to refine our basic terms. The diverse array of approaches represented within this volume calls for a broad, flexible set of definitions. At its heart, transdiagnostic research encompasses any research that explicitly looks to understand the common processes that link or differentiate multiple disorders. Such mechanism research can aim to explain the differences among two or more problem sets, but problem sets have been used to include diagnoses, disorder classes (anxiety vs. mood disorders), or behavioral–emotional–interpersonal clusters (e.g., internalizing vs. externalizing symptoms). Transdiagnostic treatments aim to treat multiple disorders or problem sets using a common set of techniques or interventions. However, it is important to note that the defining feature of transdiagnostic interventions is that they target an *identified set of core underlying processes*. This distinguishes them from therapeutic eclecticism, in which therapists select interventions from a wide array of therapeutic strategies, predominantly for pragmatic reasons in an ad hoc fashion. This "kitchen sink" approach helps the therapist feel that he or she is taking a comprehensive approach (i.e., "no stone is left unturned"), but it risks dilution of key interventions. Transdiagnostic interventions prescribe a core set of interventions that target common processes. Transdiagnostic theories help bridge the findings from basic science with treatment application. Theories provide guidance for which specific strategies are chosen for a given intervention based on the presumed underlying mechanisms.

Benefits of a Transdiagnostic Approach

Implicit to these definitions is the expectation that studying multiple processes across multiple disorders adds some explanatory power beyond what could be achieved simply by studying those same processes within a single disorder. We are beginning to see the fruits of this labor in the empirical research represented in this volume. The actual transdiagnostic processes under study represent a broad array of cognitive, behavioral, emotional, social, and systems factors. From a review of the chapters herein, we can point to good evidence that there are indeed a number of good candidates that meet initial criteria as transdiagnostic processes, including stress and coping (Compas, Watson, Reising, & Dunbar, Chapter 3), attention and interpretation biases (Arditte and Joormann, Chapter 4), avoidant behaviors (Chu, Skriner, & Staples, Chapter 5), and peer and family interactions (La Greca & Lai, Chapter 6; Smith & Dishion, Chapter 7). This basic research may not have been conducted within an explicit transdiagnostic framework, but we suspect that approaching research in this way (as multiple processes across multiple disorders) will likely reveal more truths and interrelations rather than fewer.

Transdiagnostic treatment implies that addressing core processes conveys a number of benefits. Transdiagnostic treatments can be more efficient by treating multiple problem sets by targeting a core set of processes. By targeting core processes, rather than symptoms and problem lists, interventions might also produce more robust and generalizable outcomes. We have seen an emerging foundation for this contention across an array of treatment populations, including anxiety and depression (Ehrenreich-May, Queen, Bilek, Remmes, & Marciel, Chapter 12), eating disorders (Le Grange & Loeb, Chapter 16), substance use disorders (Suarez, Ellis, & Saxe, Chapter 15), health and pain (Allen Payne, Tsao, & Zeltzer, Chapter 17), anger and aggression (Lochman, Powell, Boxmeyer, Ford, & Minney, Chapter 13), and delinquent behaviors (Schoenwald, Chapter 14). The universal processes targeted represent a diverse range of mechanisms, including cognitive, behavioral, distress tolerance, family dynamics, and multiple levels of community systems. And ultimately, when it comes to training novice therapists and disseminating interventions (once empirically supported), it might be easier to train several core techniques than to train many separate empirically supported single-disorder treatments. These theories remain to be tested, and yet there is promise.

Revolution or Evolution?

In the end, should we consider the advances offered in transdiagnostic research an evolution or a revolution in clinical science? In Barlow and colleagues' (2004) case for a unified understanding of emotional disorders, they described the return to the science of a "negative affect syndrome" as the "revolution of the last 40 years" in how it brought broader and deeper understanding to psychopathology (p. 224). Of course, the authors were referring to the broader context of clinical science applying rigorous empirical practices to what had been a predominantly theory-driven discipline. Nevertheless, it raises the question: To what degree do transdiagnostic methods and aims jettison the field forward in a transformative way?

The views and evidence recited in this volume have us viewing transdiagnostic work in a refined way, at least when it comes to youth-based populations. In youth-based domains, transdiagnostic research and treatment appear to be a natural extension of the "best practices," developmentally sensitive research that child and adolescent researchers have been advocating for a long time. Although many researchers on adult disorders may consider it "revolutionary" to study multiple disorders at once, cross-diagnostic research has been commonplace in studies of youth disorders for years. This is in no small part due to the realities of youth-based work, in which co-occurrence of disorders is the norm rather than the exception. Youth researchers are also forced to acknowledge and accommodate rapid developmental changes and diverse expressions of common problems. In this sense, transdiagnostic research represents more of a natural *evolution* of the methodology used in developmental psychopathology and developmentally sensitive clinical research for decades. Nevertheless, transdiagnostic research offers a unique and valuable extension to these prior approaches.

Transdiagnostic Theories as an Extension of Developmental Psychopathology

Nolen-Hoeksema and Watkins (2011) explicate this position by drawing a direct connection between transdiagnostic aims and traditional developmental concepts, including continuous and discontinuous development, multi- and equifinality, and convergent and divergent trajectories. Their model provides a heuristic by which to explore transdiagnostic mechanisms, including assessment of multiple mechanisms, risk factors, and disorders over time. In this model, transdiagnostic research offers a unique advantage over single-disorder research in explaining divergent trajectories, or why individuals with the same initial risk factors manifest different problem sets. Their focus is on explaining the mechanisms that link distal (environmental context, congenital biological abnormalities) and proximal (emotional, behavioral, or cognitive tendencies) risk factors and on identifying moderators (environmental, interpersonal, individual conditions) that predict expression of various disorders. The simultaneous study of multiple disorders within this developmental paradigm permits an explicit study of multiple mechanisms and moderating conditions that would not be possible in a single-disorder approach.

Likewise, in Chapter 3, Compas and colleagues present three models in which transdiagnostic research can proceed: multiple processes explaining a single disorder, a single process explaining multiple disorders, and multiple processes explaining multiple disorders. Compas and colleagues encourage this third model as the most complete approach to yielding comparative evidence for a single or multiple mechanism in relation to the disorders under study.

Both the Nolen-Hoeksema and Watkins (2011) and Compas and colleagues models aim to explicate the initial development and maintenance of disorders over time. Chu and colleagues (Chapter 5), offer a model that narrows the focus to a more immediate time frame surrounding a specific trigger and behavioral response. Given a similar trigger, they explored how a single process (avoidance) could potentially differentiate disorders according to how it influences behavioral responses at different time points in relation to the initial trigger. With a focus on a more immediate time frame, it was hypothesized that this model could provide a more direct link to treatment applications.

Taking all these studies together, we propose that transdiagnostic research provides a unifying frame that joins the empirical study of basic science, developmental psychopathology, and treatment research (Figure 19.1). It acknowledges that the study of multiple disorders within the same research agenda can illuminate novel relationships within and across each domain of inquiry. It provides the glue that justifies studying multiple problem sets at once within a single research agenda. In studying multiple disorders at once, it promises to accelerate the generation, dissemination, and translation of findings across multiple lines of inquiry. The potential for these benefits will come, in large part, from borrowing the methodologies encouraged in developmental psychopathology. These include multidimensional foci (e.g., diagnosis, symptom, basic mechanisms), openness to continuous and discrete entities, multimethod and multireporter assessment, and the explicit investigation of convergent and divergent trajectories over varying periods of time.

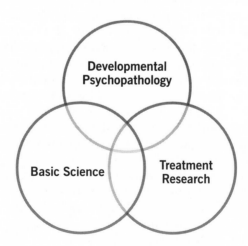

FIGURE 19.1. Transdiagnostic research provides a "unifying framework" to study developmental psychopathology, basic science, and treatment research.

Challenges to the Transdiagnostic Approach

From basic research conducted in a developmental framework, we can build efficacious, robust treatments that acknowledge both discrete disorders and continuous processes. The research described herein attests to this. However, transdiagnostic research is not without its challengers. Ollendick, Fraire, and Spence (Chapter 18) have laid out a number of points worth considering as transdiagnostic research moves forward. We highlight and respond to several of the key issues.

- *Challenge 1: "Why veer from what works?"* In this line of argument, critics contest that the field has already established a library of well-tested evidence-based treatment protocols. And even after substantial investment and rigorous testing, overall success rates typically hover around 60% (see Silverman & Hinshaw, 2008). Critics note that early trials of transdiagnostic interventions also produce about 60% efficacy rates. If the two approaches deliver relatively equivalent treatment effects, why commit resources and effort into developing a new brand of therapies? Critics remind us further that transdiagnostic treatments should theoretically improve on traditional success rates given their contention that greater robustness in outcomes should follow the targeting of common processes. In response, we think it fair to acknowledge that transdiagnostic interventions are still in the nascent stages of development and that it might be unfairly premature to compare overall success rates with established behavioral treatments. Traditional treatments have refined their techniques and methods over decades, and so transdiagnostic treatments will likely require time to identify their ideal blend of strategies and interventions.

Furthermore, it is not entirely clear that overall success rates are the most important criterion by which to judge transdiagnostic approaches. It is natural to want more, better, faster. However, an equally valuable contribution would be for transdiagnostic treatments to help a *different* set of people than traditional evidence-based therapies. Even if overall success rates peak at 60% for transdiagnostic treatments, there will be distinctive value if a different set of 60% of people are helped (e.g., those with complex comorbidities). This hypothesis needs to be tested, but it would be premature to stifle any area of investigation because of skepticism about what it has not yet produced at the outset of inquiry.

- *Challenge 2: "Transdiagnostic treatments could dilute potent evidence-based interventions by encouraging eclecticism."* Ollendick and colleagues (Chapter 18) summarize a set of literature that appears to support the superiority of a single-disorder focus over multiple-disorder treatments. For example, Craske and colleagues (2007) completed a study subtitled

"More of the same, or less of more?" in which a more focused cognitive-behavioral protocol reduced severity in both primary and secondary diagnoses. Sixty-five adults with panic disorder all received the same exposure-based group treatment, but then half were randomly assigned to receive semiweekly individual sessions that continued to review the same material covered in the group. The other half received flexible individual therapy in which therapists could focus on the clients' second-most severe problem. Both conditions led to improvements across primary and secondary problems, but the focused protocol contributed to better outcomes, at least at posttreatment. Randall, Thomas, and Thevos (2001) demonstrated that a treatment focused exclusively on alcoholism proved superior to a combined treatment that focused on alcoholism and social anxiety. In the child literature, a series of secondary analyses from clinical trials suggest that youth with social anxiety fare worse after receiving various multiproblem interventions compared with youth with other disorders (e.g., generalized anxiety disorder, separation anxiety disorder; Crawley, Beidas, Benjamin, Martin, & Kendall, 2008; Hudson et al., 2009; Shortt, Barrett, & Fox, 2001).

We would point out that none of the treatment interventions used in these prior studies were intentionally transdiagnostic. Instead, the protocols were eclectic in nature, which we have already cautioned against. For example, the Craske and colleagues (2007) study compared an intensive treatment focused on panic disorder alone with a treatment in which individual therapists could choose to use diverse cognitive-behavioral skills to address the secondary problem. As Ollendick and colleagues point out in Chapter 18, this eclectic approach threatens to divert the therapist's attention away from the primary target and dilute the efficacy of treatments for the primary disorder. However, this interpretation neglects our definition of transdiagnostic interventions, which endorses use of a core set of skills that focus on universal underlying processes. It is the focus on the core processes that makes it a transdiagnostic treatment, and this is where the promise for greater efficacy and generalizability exist. The two adult studies tested additive models of therapy in which a secondary set of therapy skills was added onto a core set of skills. Depending on the selection of the second set of skills, this additive model can either help or dilute a focused attempt. Transdiagnostic interventions use a focused set of interventions that, by design, address multiple problems. In this way, transdiagnostic treatments can provide "more of the same" while still addressing multiple problems.

In the youth anxiety studies cited before, all of the findings were secondary moderator analyses that indicated that social anxiety fared less well than other disorders in a common treatment. Youth with social anxiety were not randomly assigned to receive either a transdiagnostic treatment or a treatment focused solely on social anxiety. It may be the case that social anxiety is simply more difficult to treat than other anxiety disorders, no matter the treatment. Spence, Donovan, March, and Kenardy (2011) are currently initiating such a test, and we agree that this type of trial is very valuable, both for demonstrating overall efficacy rates of transdiagnostic interventions and for examining more interesting explanatory pathways of clinical improvement (i.e., how interventions work differentially for different people).

We feel compelled to note that several modular-based therapies are gaining traction as a way to address multiple problems within a single treatment protocol (e.g., Chorpita & Weisz, 2009; Weisz et al., 2012). We find several of these modular approaches appealing and promising for some of the same reasons that excite us about transdiagnostic therapy. Modular approaches identify common treatment elements across diverse intervention packages and create a single treatment protocol using the most potent treatment procedures. The protocol usually supplies a decision-making flowchart that helps the therapist choose which procedures to use in different clinical contexts. Modular treatments promise an efficiency similar to what transdiagnostic interventions offer by distilling treatment into its most potent components. However, modular treatments tend to focus on commonalities among treatment *procedures* across disorder classes (e.g., problem solving, cognitive restructuring), and less on universal maintaining *processes*. It is important to remember that "modular treatment" is simply a description of a delivery system, not a theory of change. Transdiagnostic interventions (focused on universal processes) can make use of a modular format just as eclectic treatment interventions can be modular. Nevertheless, modular and transdiagnostic interventions represent novel directions in psychology. It will be interesting and important to compare these treatment approaches as they develop.

- *Challenge 3: "What's new?"* In a final challenge, critics of transdiagnostic treatments wonder whether this represents a truly novel approach or reflects more of an extension of current evidence-based clinical research. As we have acknowledged, we have come to view transdiagnostic research and treatment as a natural extension of developmental psychopathology, basic science, and evidence-based treatment research. The treatment section of this book reflects a diverse set of established treatments that were designed to address multiple problems simultaneously. These did not develop out of an explicit transdiagnostic focus but to address the natural realities of studying youth populations, in which comorbidity is the rule rather than the exception. We happily did not have to work hard to find many examples of evidence-based therapies that fit the broad criteria of "transdiagnostic." Several of the exemplar treatments presented were not designed within a transdiagnostic framework (e.g., Kendall et al., Chapter 8; Lochman et al., Chapter 13), whereas others were (e.g., Ehrenreich-May et al., Chapter 12; Allen Payne et al., Chapter 17). It was interesting to witness some authors reconceptualize their work into a novel transdiagnostic framework and arrive at new insights.

We believe that the main contribution offered by a transdiagnostic framework is an expanded focus on explanatory pathways of treatment. Identifying mediators and mechanisms of treatment has been an important goal of clinical research for decades, but it has been difficult for it to gain traction (Kazdin & Nock, 2003). Various mediators are tested across studies in different settings, with varying treatment populations, and employ diverse methodologies and assessment tools. This tends to yield inconsistent findings that are difficult to interpret. In part, this results from a lack of prospective planning to collect and analyze mediators in relation to outcome. We believe that a transdiagnostic framework provides a unifying structure within which to study multiple change mediators across multiple disorders within a single treatment or across multiple treatments. Much like the models proposed by Compas and colleagues (Chapter 3), Chu and colleagues (Chapter 5), and Nolen-Hoeksema and Watkins (2011), a transdiagnostic framework encourages the study of *pathways* of change, taking into account divergent trajectories and developmental methodology. In this way, a transdiagnostic framework sets a new research agenda that emphasizes developmental and explanatory mechanisms, both in basic science and intervention research and development.

Conclusions

Ollendick and colleagues (Chapter 18) present a challenge: "It seems to us that it is especially important that research into transdiagnostic therapies investigate the purported common underlying processes to determine whether they are present, whether they are being targeted in treatment, whether there is significant change in the processes as a result of treatment, and whether those changes mediate outcomes" (p. 410). We agree that this is the challenge that confronts transdiagnostic research and treatment. The onus is ultimately on those who wish to distinguish the transdiagnostic research agenda from others. This volume highlights the conceptual, research, and intervention groundwork that has been laid, and the foundation is firm. Now, an unlimited future awaits with many challenges, but also with many exciting possibilities.

Transdiagnosis in the Land of DSM-5 and RDoC

In the course of completing this volume, two initiatives in the world of mental health have come to fruition that could have substantial impact on the landscape of transdiagnostic research and practice. First, the American Psychiatric Association (APA) has just recently released its fifth edition of the *Diagnostic and Statistical Manual of Mental Disorders* (DSM-5; APA, 2013a), which defines the diagnostic categories by which we organize multidisorder work. As discussed in Chapter 1, a number of the revisions presented in DSM-5 are very compatible with a transdiagnostic approach (Kupfer, Kuhl, & Regier, 2013). First, authors of the DSM incorporated a more naturalistic developmental approach to defining its disorders. They eliminated the separate chapter on "disorders first diagnosed in childhood" and, instead, incorporated developmental descriptions in each disorder's chapter. This approach is consistent with the developmental approach that a transdiagnostic agenda encourages. Second, it developed a dimensional system to support its classification of discrete diagnoses. DSM authors described dimensional indices of severity for symptoms both within (e.g., panic attacks in panic disorder) and across (e.g., suicidal ideation) disorders. This approach supports a transdiagnostic approach in that it recognizes the value of studying discrete disorder categories but also acknowledges the presence of important universal symptoms and processes.

One might also look at the creation of the new child and adolescent diagnosis, disruptive mood dysregulation disorder (DMDD), as an acknowledgment of transdiagnostic processes. DMDD was designed to address concerns about potential overdiagnosis of bipolar disorder in children and provides an alternative diagnosis to capture youth who exhibit persistent irritability and frequent episodes of extreme behavioral dyscontrol (APA, 2013b). Although DMDD is positioned as a distinct diagnosis, the behavioral syndrome described therein could easily describe the nonepisodic irritability and explosiveness that appears across multiple youth disorders, including unipolar depression, anxiety disorders, and attention-deficit/hyperactivity disorder (ADHD). Some have proposed using a modifier, such as "ADHD with explosive behavior," as a way to label this cluster of behaviors that occurs across disorders (Carlson, 2012). Although DSM-5 does not describe DMDD as a transdiagnostic condition, its presence suggests its authors embraced the study of symptom clusters across diagnostic boundaries.

The second initiative that has potential to have serious implications for transdiagnostic research and treatment is the National Institute for Mental Health's (NIMH) Research Domain Criteria (RDoC) project (NIMH, 2011). The goal of RDoC is to bring mental health research in line with other areas of medicine that base diagnostic systems on underlying biology and not just clinical presentations of symptoms (Insel, 2013). The strength of the DSM has always been in its ability to enhance reliability of diagnosis by ensuring researchers and clinicians use the same terms in the same ways. The DSM's weakness has been in its lack of validity because of the lack of objective "laboratory" measures to inform diagnosis. Through RDoC, NIMH plans to prioritize research studies that lay the groundwork for a psychiatric classification system based on biomarkers, including genetics, imaging, physiology, and cognitive science.

Two trends should be evident in this plan. First, NIMH is expressing a preference for transdiagnostic research. The agency is reorienting research away from strict DSM categories. It is instead supporting research that looks across current categories to identify the underlying biological or cognitive processes that explain symptomatic manifestations of disorders. This is a positive for transdiagnostic research. It should also be evident that NIMH is clearly prioritizing biological, genetic, and neural processes over behavioral and interpersonal processes as explanatory mechanisms (Belluck & Carey, 2013). In current documentation of RDoC priorities, individual behavior, interpersonal interactions, family and community systems, and broad emotional processes are conspicuously deemphasized in the list of encouraged research targets (NIMH, 2011). It is clear that transdiagnostic frameworks have a future in psychological research (as far as federal funding priorities go), but psychological researchers must be prepared to make strong cases for studying behavioral and social processes in the classification and treatment of mental health problems.

REFERENCES

American Psychiatric Association. (2013a). *Diagnostic and statistical manual of mental disorders* (5th ed.). Arlington, VA: Author.

American Psychiatric Association. (2013b). Highlights of changes from DSM-IV-TR to DSM-5. Retrieved from *www.dsm5.org/documents/changes%20from%20 dsm-iv-tr%20to%20dsm-5.pdf*.

Barlow, D. H., Allen, L. B., & Choate, M. L. (2004). Toward a unified treatment for emotional disorders. *Behavior Therapy, 35*, 205–230.

Belluck, P., & Carey, B. (2013, May 6). Psychiatry's guide is out of touch with science, experts say. *New York Times.* Retrieved from *www.nytimes.com/2013/05/07/ health/psychiatrys-new-guide-falls-short-experts-say.html?pagewanted=all*.

Carlson, G. (2012, November 19). *A new diagnosis for explosive behavior: The pros and cons of what's called disruptive mood dysregulation disorder.* New York: Child Mind Institute. Retrieved from *www.childmind.org/en/posts/articles/2012-11-19-pros-cons-disruptive-mood-dysregulation-disorder*.

Chorpita, B. F., & Weisz, J. R. (2009). *MATCH-ADTC: Modular approach to therapy for children with anxiety, depression, trauma, or conduct problems.* Satellite Beach, FL: PracticeWise.

Craske, M. G., Farchione, T. J., Allen, L. B., Barrios, V., Stoyanova, M., & Rose, R. (2007). Cognitive behavioral therapy for panic disorder and comorbidity: More of the same or less of more? *Behaviour Research and Therapy, 45*, 1095–1109.

Crawley, S. A., Beidas, R. S., Benjamin, C. L., Martin, E., & Kendall, P. C. (2008). Treating socially phobic youth with CBT: Differential outcomes and treatment considerations. *Behavioural and Cognitive Psychotherapy, 36,* 379–389.

Ehrenreich, J. T., Buzzella, B. A., & Barlow, D. H. (2007). General principles for the treatment of emotional disorders across the lifespan. In S. Hofmann & J. Weinberger (Eds.), *The art and science of psychotherapy* (pp. 191–209). New York: Routledge/Taylor & Francis Group.

Fairburn, C. G., Cooper, Z., & Shafran, R. (2003). Cognitive behaviour therapy for eating disorders: A "transdiagnostic" theory and treatment. *Behaviour Research and Therapy, 41,* 509–528.

Harvey, A., Watkins, E., Mansell, W., & Shafran, R. (2004). *Cognitive behavioural processes across psychological disorders: A transdiagnostic approach to research and treatment.* New York: Oxford University Press.

Hudson, J. L., Rapee, R. M., Deveney, C., Schniering, C. A., Lyneham, H. J., & Bovopoulos, N. (2009). Cognitive-behavioral treatment versus an active control for children and adolescents with anxiety disorders: A randomized trial. *Journal of the American Academy of Child and Adolescent Psychiatry, 48,* 533–544.

Insel, T. (2013, April 29). Transforming diagnosis. National Institute of Mental Health Director's Blog. Retrieved from *www.nimh.nih.gov/about/director/2013/transforming-diagnosis.shtml.*

Kazdin, A. E., & Nock, M. K. (2003). Delineating mechanisms of change in child and adolescent therapy: Methodological issues and research recommendations. *Journal of Child Psychology and Psychiatry, 44,* 1116–1129.

Kupfer, D. J., Kuhl, E. A., & Regier, D. A. (2013). DSM-5—The future arrived. *Journal of the American Medical Association, 309,* 1691–1692.

National Institute for Mental Health. (2011, June). NIMH Research Domain Criteria (RDoC). Retrieved from *www.nimh.nih.gov/research-priorities/rdoc/nimh-research-domain-criteria-rdoc.shtml.*

Nolen-Hoeksema, S., & Watkins, E. R. (2011). A heuristic for developing transdiagnostic models of psychopathology: Explaining multifinality and divergent trajectories. *Perspectives on Psychological Science, 6,* 589–609.

Randall, C. L., Thomas, S., & Thevos, A. K. (2001). Concurrent alcoholism and social anxiety disorder: A first step toward developing effective treatments. *Alcoholism: Clinical and Experimental Research, 25,* 210–220.

Shortt, A. L., Barrett, P. M., & Fox, T. L. (2001). Evaluating the FRIENDS Program: A cognitive-behavioral group treatment for anxious children and their parents. *Journal of Clinical Child Psychology, 30,* 525–535.

Silverman, W. K., & Hinshaw, S. P. (2008). The second special issue on evidence-based psychosocial treatment for children and adolescents: A 10-year update. *Journal of Clinical Child and Adolescent Psychology, 37,* 1–7.

Spence, S. H., Donovan, C. L., March, S., & Kenardy, J. (2011). *Evaluation of transdiagnostic versus disorder-specific, Internet-based cognitive behaviour therapy for social phobia in young people* (Grant No. 12611000901909). Canberra, Australia: National Health and Medical Research Council.

Weisz, J. R., Chorpita, B. F., Palinkas, L. A., Schoenwald, S. K., Miranda, J., Bearman, S. K., et al. (2012). Testing standard and modular designs for psychotherapy treating depression, anxiety, and conduct problems in youth: A randomized effectiveness trial. *Archives of General Psychiatry, 69,* 274–282.

Index

Page numbers followed by *f* indicate figure, *t* indicate table